VASCULAR DISEASE AND INJURY

CONTEMPORARY CARDIOLOGY

CHRISTOPHER P. CANNON

SERIES EDITOR

VASCULAR DISEASE AND INJURY

PRECLINICAL RESEARCH

Edited by

DANIEL I. SIMON, MD
CAMPBELL ROGERS, MD

Brigham and Women's Hospital
Boston, MA

Foreword by

VICTOR J. DZAU, MD

Brigham and Women's Hospital
Boston, MA

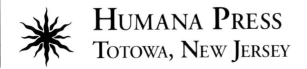

HUMANA PRESS
TOTOWA, NEW JERSEY

© 2001 Humana Press Inc.
999 Riverview Drive, Suite 208
Totowa, New Jersey 07512

For additional copies, pricing for bulk purchases, and/or information about other Humana titles, contact Humana at the above address or at any of the following numbers: Tel.: 973-256-1699; Fax: 973-256-8341; E-mail: humana@humanapr.com or visit our Website: http://humanapress.com

Due diligence has been taken by the publishers, editors, and authors of this book to assure the accuracy of the information published and to describe generally accepted practices. The contributors herein have carefully checked to ensure that the drug selections and dosages set forth in this text are accurate and in accord with the standards accepted at the time of publication. Notwithstanding, as new research, changes in government regulations, and knowledge from clinical experience relating to drug therapy and drug reactions constantly occurs, the reader is advised to check the product information provided by the manufacturer of each drug for any change in dosages or for additional warnings and contraindications. This is of utmost importance when the recommended drug herein is a new or infrequently used drug. It is the responsibility of the treating physician to determine dosages and treatment strategies for individual patients. Further it is the responsibility of the health care provider to ascertain the Food and Drug Administration status of each drug or device used in their clinical practice. The publisher, editors, and authors are not responsible for errors or omissions or for any consequences from the application of the information presented in this book and make no warranty, express or implied, with respect to the contents in this publication.

This publication is printed on acid-free paper. ⊗
ANSI Z39.48-1984 (American National Standards Institute) Permanence of Paper for Printed Library Materials.

Cover design by Patricia F. Cleary.

Photocopy Authorization Policy:
Authorization to photocopy items for internal or personal use, or the internal or personal use of specific clients, is granted by Humana Press Inc., provided that the base fee of US $10.00 per copy, plus US $00.25 per page, is paid directly to the Copyright Clearance Center at 222 Rosewood Drive, Danvers, MA 01923. For those organizations that have been granted a photocopy license from the CCC, a separate system of payment has been arranged and is acceptable to Humana Press Inc. The fee code for users of the Transactional Reporting Service is: [0-89603-753-3/01 $10.00 + $00.25].

Printed in the United States of America. 10 9 8 7 6 5 4 3 2

Library of Congress Cataloging-in-Publication Data

Vascular disease and injury: preclinical research/edited by Daniel I. Simon, Campbell Rogers.
         p.;cm.—(Contemporary cardiology)
      Includes bibliographical references and index.
      ISBN 0-89603-753-3 (alk. paper)
         1. Blood-vessels—Diseases—Animal models. I. Simon, Daniel I. II. Rogers, Campbell.
      III. Contemporary cardiology (Totowa, N.J. : unnnumbered)
         [DNLM: 1.   Vascular   Diseases.   2.   Blood   Vessels—injuries.   3.   Blood
      Vessels—transplantation. 4. Disease Models, Animal. WG 500 V331265 2000]
      RC691.4. V35 2000
      616.1'3—dc21
                                                                              00-039603

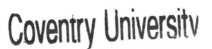

FOREWORD

We have entered an era of biomedicine marked by an explosion of new data and information and an impressively rapid translation of basic science discoveries to clinical applications. Nowhere is this more apparent than in the field of cardiovascular medicine, where in recent years significant advances have been made in our understanding of the etiology, pathophysiology, diagnosis, and therapy of coronary heart disease, atherosclerosis, hypertension, and congestive heart failure, among other diseases. New molecules, genes, and signaling pathways are being discovered at an unprecedented rate, and new drugs, devices, and surgical innovations are being developed that transform medical practice.

The most common cause of cardiovascular disorders is vascular disease. Central to the pathobiology of vascular disease is injury to the blood vessel. Data derived from experimental studies and human investigations have suggested that the major forms of vascular disease, i.e., atherosclerosis, restenosis, graft stenosis, and transplant vasculopathy, are the result of the body's response to various forms of biochemical, mechanical, infectious, and immunological injuries. The elucidation of the biological processes of response to injury (such as endothelial dysfunction, oxidation stress, inflammation, proliferation, and apoptosis) and the mediators of these processes (including nitric oxide, reactive oxygen species, cytokines, chemokines, and growth factors) have not only improved our understanding of vascular diseases, but have resulted in novel therapies. Discoveries in this area have been highly dependent on in vitro investigation, experimental animal models, and other preclinical studies. Accordingly, there is much demand for a book that brings together the voluminous preclinical information on this diverse subject: for a single source that can provide access to all the important data on vascular injury, compare and contrast the different models and conditions, provide insights into common themes and mechanisms unifying these diseases, and also identify differential processes that are specific to the various conditions. Such analysis will be of great use to students and researchers interested in vascular disease and therapy.

The rapid advances in vascular research have also created a significant challenge for researchers, especially those new to the field. Despite recent achievements in information technology, obtaining access to data that are properly linked, annotated, and interpreted is still a major difficulty. Furthermore, with the proliferation of ideas, resources, and technologies, the task of locating and then selecting sources for equipment, reagents, and animals has often become quite complicated.

For all these reasons, *Vascular Disease and Injury: Preclinical Research* is important and timely. The book is a tour de force, assembling leading experts to review the essential topics of vascular diseases under a single cover. Importantly, the book provides a "how-to" guide, paying attention to the practicality of the content by including equipment lists and sources for animals, diet, and reagents. In my opinion, this book is the most comprehensive available on this subject and will undoubtedly become a classic in the field. Simon and Rogers, through their meticulous attention and innovative efforts in developing this book, have set high standards for the definition of translational research.

Victor J. Dzau, MD
Hersey Professor of the Theory and Practice of Medicine,
Harvard Medical School
Chairman, Department of Medicine,
Brigham and Women's Hospital
Boston, MA

PREFACE

Issues related to arterial vascular injury are central to the cardiovascular practitioner and research scientist alike. Whether acute (i.e., mechanically induced) or chronic (i.e., hypertension, atherosclerosis, and immune-mediated), vascular injury and the responses it elicits are leading causes of disease today, producing such acute ischemic syndromes as transient ischemic attacks, stroke, unstable angina pectoris, and acute myocardial infarction, as well as restenosis following percutaneous angioplasty or revascularization surgeries. The development of effective cardiovascular therapeutics to treat or prevent atherosclerosis and restenosis relies on preclinical research—both cell biological studies and observations and findings from animal models.

We have found that no one resource is available for a comprehensive presentation of animal models related to vascular disease. We hope that *Vascular Disease and Injury: Preclinical Research* will provide such a medium by presenting topics related to vascular injury in an organized and comprehensive fashion. Our approach is to present issues related to vascular disease and injury in five major areas: acute mechanical injury and vascular repair, models of arterial thrombosis, chronic atherosclerotic models, vascular disease in transplanted vessels, and vascular disease in models of systemic and pulmonary arterial hypertension. We have aimed to provide a "how-to" guide and have, therefore, worked to ensure that each chapter is highly practical by including equipment lists, current sources for animals, diet and reagents, schematic diagrams and, when pertinent, photomicrographs of sample histology.

In Part I of the book, Acute Mechanical Injury and Vascular Repair, Drs. Welt and Rogers review the widely used rabbit iliac artery models of balloon- and stent-induced angioplasty. Dr. Schwartz follows with a comprehensive presentation of the classic porcine overstretch stent model, emphasizing the relationship he has characterized between the degree of vascular injury and resultant neointimal thickening that follows. Dr. Carter extends this model into an atherosclerotic milieu. Drs. Nedelman and Rogers then apply central elements of these lower animal models to nonhuman primate experimental angioplasty and stenting, a burgeoning field suited to evaluation of human-targeted biologics. Since venous conduits are used extensively with high failure rates in coronary and peripheral bypass procedures, Dr. Dzau's group provides a chapter on pathologic responses in experimental models of arterial-venous grafting. Murine systems allow cardiovascular researchers to take advantage of key transgenic and knockout strains. Therefore, we have provided extensive material on recently described models of acute and chronic vascular injury in mice. Dr. Lindner, who pioneered the use of mice in this field, discusses wire denudation and ligation models of neointimal thickening. Drs. Chen, Rogers, and Simon then describe a recently published model of arterial dilation and endothelial denudation that is accompanied by inflammatory cell recruitment and neointimal thickening. Drs. Eitzman and Westrick present a very interesting vascular photochemical model that has components of thrombosis, as well as neointimal thickening. Finally, Dr. Coller's group discusses their approach using a femoral wire injury model, a modification of the carotid wire denudation resulting in increased neointimal thickening.

In Part II, two chapters will focus on Models of Arterial Thrombosis. In the first, Drs. Fay, Parker, and Zhu use perivascular ferric chloride to induce arterial injury and thrombosis in the mouse carotid. These investigators have exploited this model to investigate the importance of plasminogen activator inhibitor-1 in modulating endogenous fibrinolysis. Finally, Dr. Folts provides a comprehensive overview of his animal preparation for studying in vivo platelet activity and platelet interactions with damaged arterial walls. This model has been instrumental in the clinical development of therapeutics for acute ischemic syndromes and percutaneous coronary interventions.

Part III focuses on Chronic Atherosclerotic Models. Drs. Palinski, Napoli, and Reaven provide an in-depth overview of mouse models of atherosclerosis, in particular the apolipoprotein E (ApoE) and low density lipoprotein (LDL) receptor knockouts. Drs. Aikawa and Libby then present their work regarding progression and regression of atherosclerosis using the classic hypercholesterolemic rabbit model. Finally, Drs. Nicolosi and Kritchevsky present the use of higher animals, including nonhuman primates, for preclinical research in atherosclerosis.

Part IV of the book concentrates on Vascular Disease in Transplanted Vessels. Drs. Shi and Hoover discuss the use of a murine carotid loop model of transplant disease that has been helpful in elucidating the important role of proteases, such as plasminogen, in transplant-related vascular disease. Dr. Mitchell then follows with an overview of heterotopic heart transplantation in the mouse. His group has used this model to study the role of cytokines and immune co-stimulatory molecules in parenchymal rejection and accelerated graft arteriosclerosis. The concluding chapter in this section by Drs. Chen and Adams presents exciting material regarding hyperacute vascular rejection in pig-to-primate xenotransplantation.

The next set of chapters in Part V concentrates on Vascular Disease in Models of Arterial Hypertension. Dr. Baumbach examines methods for investigating cerebrovascular disease in experimental systemic hypertension. Two chapters are devoted to pulmonary hypertension. In the first, Dr. Rabinovitch provides an in-depth discussion of monocrotaline-induced pulmonary hypertension. She focuses on the cellular and molecular biology of pulmonary vasculopathy, integrating dynamic interactions between smooth muscle cells, extracellular matrix, and the endothelium. This leads into the chapter by Drs. Meyrick and Tchekneva on chronic pulmonary hypertension in the hypoxic rat and in the sheep following continuous air embolization.

The final section, Part VI, provides an essential foundation in Animal Care and Tissue Processing and analysis. Dr. Marini discusses veterinary issues and anesthesia options, addressing all species covered elsewhere in the book, from mice to nonhuman primates. Key points regarding survival surgery, choice of anesthetic, and analgesia are included. Histopathologic methods are then discussed by Drs. Seifert, Rogers, and Edelman. This chapter provides the "basics" for tissue harvesting and fixation, and histology methods for routine immunology and electron microscopy.

The topics we have chosen to include in *Vascular Disease and Injury: Preclinical Research* are not meant to be all inclusive and, undoubtedly, a few areas have not been covered. We have simply tried to show the range and breadth of animal models that have been useful in translational cardiovascular research. It is important to end this discussion on a cautionary note. The track record of animal models of vascular repair after injury, as predictors of human responses, is poor. Myriad agents have been proven effective in one or another model, only to fail clinical scrutiny. This fact means that for each experimental approach, by any of the models described in this book, the purpose of research must be to further mechanistic understanding, not to recapitulate human disease in an experimental animal.

In closing, we must acknowledge the tremendous efforts of our administrative assistant, Paula McColgan, the series editor, Dr. Christopher Cannon, and the staff of Humana Press. We are indebted to Drs. Eugene Braunwald, Victor J. Dzau, Thomas W. Smith, and Peter Libby for encouraging and supporting our clinician-scientist careers. Dr. Rogers would like to thank most deeply his mentors in the study of vascular injury and repair, Drs. Morris Karnovsky and Elazer Edelman, and to dedicate this book to his wife Nathalie and three children, Camille, Genevieve, and Charles. Dr. Simon would like to honor his mentor in life and medicine, Dr. Norman M. Simon, and to dedicate this book to his wife Dr. Marcy Schwartz and three children Benjamin, Maxwell, and Aaron.

Daniel I. Simon, MD
Campbell Rogers, MD

CONTENTS

CONTRIBUTORS

DAVID H. ADAMS, MD • *Department of Surgery, Brigham and Women's Hospital, Harvard Medical School, Boston, MA*

MASANORI AIKAWA, MD, PhD • *Cardiovascular Division, Brigham and Women's Hospital, Boston, MA*

GARY L. BAUMBACH, MD • *Department of Pathology, University of Iowa College of Medicine, Iowa City, IA*

ANDREW J. CARTER, DO • *Division of Cardiovascular Medicine, Stanford University Medical Center, Stanford, CA*

RAYMOND H. CHEN, MD, DPhil • *Brigham and Women's Hospital, Harvard Medical School, Boston, MA*

ZHIPING CHEN, MS • *Cardiovascular Division, Brigham and Women's Hospital, Boston, MA*

BARRY S. COLLER, MD • *Department of Medicine, Mount Sinai School of Medicine, New York, NY*

VICTOR J. DZAU, MD • *Department of Medicine, Brigham and Women's Hospital, Boston, MA*

ELAZER R. EDELMAN, MD, PhD, FACC • *Division of Health Sciences and Technology, Brigham and Women's Hospital/Harvard-MIT, Cambridge, MA*

AFSHIN EHSAN, MD • *Research Institute and Department of Medicine, Brigham and Women's Hospital, Boston, MA*

DANIEL T. EITZMAN, MD • *Department of Internal Medicine, University of Michigan Medical School, Ann Arbor, MI*

WILLIAM P. FAY, MD • *Department of Internal Medicine, University of Michigan Medical School, Ann Arbor, MI*

JOHN D. FOLTS, PhD, FACC • *Division of Cardiology, Coronary Thrombosis Research Laboratory, University of Wisconsin-Madison Medical School, Madison, WI*

YOSHIHIRO FUKUMOTO, MD, PhD • *Cardiovascular Division, Department of Medicine, Brigham and Women's Hospital, Boston, MA*

DAVID R. HOLMES, JR., MD • *Division of Cardiovascular Diseases and Internal Medicine, Mayo Clinic, Rochester, MN*

JENNIFER L. HOOVER, BA • *Transplantation Biology, Novartis Pharmaceuticals Corporation, Summit, NJ*

CHRISTOPHER HORVATH, DVM, MS • *Millenium Pharmaceuticals Inc., Cambridge, MA*

BIRGIT KANTOR, MD • *Division of Cardiovascular Diseases and Internal Medicine, Mayo Clinic, Rochester, MN*

DAVID KRITCHEVSKY, PhD • *Wistar Institute, Philadelphia, PA*

PETER LIBBY, MD • *Cardiovascular Division, Brigham and Women's Hospital, Boston, MA*

VOLKHARD LINDNER, MD, PhD • *Division of Molecular Medicine, Maine Medical Center Research Institute, South Portland, ME*

MICHAEL J. MANN, MD • *Research Institute and Department of Medicine, Brigham and Women's Hospital, Boston, MA*

ROBERT P. MARINI, DVM • *Division of Comparative Medicine, MIT, Cambridge, MA*

BARBARA MEYRICK, PhD • *Department of Pathology and Center for Lung Research, Vanderbilt University Medical Center, Nashville, TN*

RICHARD N. MITCHELL, MD, PhD • *Department of Pathology, Brigham and Women's Hospital, Boston, MA*

CLAUDIO NAPOLI, MD • *Department of Medicine, University of California, San Diego, CA*

MARK NEDELMAN, MS • *Primedica Corporation, Worcester, MA*

ROBERT J. NICOLOSI, PhD • *Center for Chronic Disease Control, University of Massachusetts, Lowell, MA*

WULF PALINSKI, MD • *Department of Medicine, University of California, San Diego, CA*

ANDREW C. PARKER, BS • *Department of Internal Medicine, University of Michigan Medical School, Ann Arbor, MI*

MARLENE RABINOVITCH, MD • *Division of Cardiovascular Research, The Hospital for Sick Children, Toronto, Ontario, Canada*

ELENA RABKIN, MD, PhD • *Department of Pathology, Brigham and Women's Hospital, Harvard Medical School, Boston, MA*

PETER D. REAVEN, MD • *Department of Endocrinology, Carl T. Hayden VAMC, Phoenix, AZ*

ERNANE D. REIS, MD • *Department of Surgery, Mount Sinai School of Medicine, New York, NY*

CAMPBELL ROGERS, MD, FACC • *Cardiovascular Division, Brigham and Women's Hospital/Harvard-MIT, Boston, MA*

ROBERT S. SCHWARTZ, MD • *Division of Cardiovascular Diseases and Internal Medicine, Mayo Clinic, Rochester, MN*

PHILIP S. SEIFERT, MS, HTL (ASCP) • *Health Sciences and Technology Division Biomedical Engineering Center, MIT, Cambridge, MA*

VICTOR CHENGWEI SHI, MD • *Novartis Pharmaceuticals Corporation, Transplantation Biology, Summit, NJ*

DANIEL I. SIMON, MD • *Cardiovascular Division, Brigham and Women's Hospital, Boston, MA*

SUSAN S. SMYTH, MD, PhD • *Department of Medicine, Mount Sinai School of Medicine, New York, NY*

ELENA TCHEKNEVA, MD • *Department of Pathology and Center for Lung Research, Vanderbilt University Medical Center, Nashville, TN*

FREDERICK G.P. WELT, MD • *Division of Cardiology, Brigham and Women's Hospital/Harvard-MIT, Boston, MA*

RANDAL J. WESTRICK, BS • *Department of Internal Medicine, University of Michigan Medical School, Ann Arbor, MI*

YANHONG ZHU, MD • *Department of Internal Medicine, University of Michigan Medical School, Ann Arbor, MI*

COLOR PLATES

Color plates 1–9 appear as an insert following p. 236.

PLATE 1   Fig. 2. Photomicrographs of mouse carotid arteries after
               arterial dilation and endothelial denudations.
               (*See* full caption on p. 91, Chapter 7.)

PLATE 2   Fig. 2. Photomicrograph of monkey iliac artery 28 d after
               stent implantation (Verhoeff tissue elastin stain).
               (*See* full caption on p. 59, Chapter 4.)

PLATE 3   Fig. 1. The liver of cholesterol-fed rabbits with extensive
               hypercholesterolemia shows the disruption of parenchymal
               architecture and the fatty change (Masson trichrome staining).
               (*See* full caption on p. 177, Chapter 13.)

PLATE 4   Fig. 4. Interstitial collagen content in the aortic intima
               detected by the picrosirius red polarization method.
               (*See* full caption on p. 182, Chapter 13.)

PLATE 5   Fig. 6. Atherosclerotic lesion of WHHL rabbits.
               (*See* full caption on p. 185, Chapter 13.)

PLATE 6   Fig. 1. Histologic appearance of graft arteriosclerosis (GA)
               in humans and mice.
               (*See* full caption on p. 216, Chapter 16.)

PLATE 7   Fig. 2. Schematic of heterotopic grafts.
               (*See* full caption on p. 218, Chapter 16.)

PLATE 8   Fig. 1. Hyperacute rejection: wild-type pig heart transplanted
               into baboon, 60 min after implantation.
               (*See* full caption on p. 232, Chapter 17.)

PLATE 9   Fig. 1. Endovascular stainless-steel stent-implanted pig
               coronary artery, 28 d post implantation.
               (*See* full caption on p. 332, Chapter 22.)

I ACUTE MECHANICAL INJURY AND VASCULAR REPAIR

1

Mechanical Injury in Normal and Atherosclerotic Rabbit Iliac Arteries

Frederick G.P. Welt, MD,
Elazer R. Edelman, MD, PhD,
and Campbell Rogers, MD

INTRODUCTION

In the large and expanding field of research involving the vascular biology of atherosclerosis and the response to injury following intervention, animal models play a crucial initial role in understanding the mechanisms of disease and the biologic components of the response to injury, and in evaluating the safety and efficacy of new devices. In particular, the rabbit iliac artery technique offers many scientific and practical advantages.

The person credited with establishing the rabbit as a model for atherosclerosis research is Nikolaj Nikolajewitsch Anitschkow, a Russian scientist who was the first to recognize the atherogenic potential of dietary cholesterol *(1)*. His initial experiments, published in 1913, demonstrated that atherosclerotic lesions in the rabbit are proportional to the amount of cholesterol consumed *(2)*. Many of his pathologic investigations identified major chemical and cellular components of the atherosclerotic plaque which have been subsequently confirmed by immunocytochemical and molecular biologic techniques. In the 1960s, balloon

From: *Contemporary Cardiology: Vascular Disease and Injury: Preclinical Research*
Edited by: D. I. Simon and C. Rogers © Humana Press Inc., Totowa, NJ

Table 1
Selected Antibodies Available for Immunohistochemistry in Rabbit Tissues

Cell or antigen specificity	Antigen	Host/isotype	Source
Paraffin and Methacrylate			
S-phase cells	BrdU (bromodeoxyuridine)	Mouse IgG	DAKO, Carpenteria, CA
G1–M Phase	Ki-67 (clone:MIB-1)	Mouse IgG	Zymed, Raleigh, NC
All Phases	PCNA (proliferating cell nuclear antigen)	Mouse IgG	DAKO, Carpenteria, CA
Smooth-Muscle Cells and fibroblasts	SMC α-actin	Mouse IgG	DAKO, Carpenteria, CA
Endo. and platelets and plasma	von Willebrand factor (FVIII related antigen)	Rabbit/poly Goat/poly	DAKO, Carpenteria, CA
Endo. and platelets	Human CD31 (PECAM-1)	Mouse IgG	DAKO, Carpenteria, CA
Macrophages (rabbit macrophage)	RAM-11	Mouse IgG	DAKO, Carpenteria, CA
Neutrophils and Thymocytes	RPN 3/57 (rabbit thymocytes, T-cells, neutrophils, platelets)	Mouse IgG	Serotec, San Francisco, CA
Frozen Tissue			
Endothelial and Leukocytes	Rb 1/9 (VCAM-1)	Mouse IgG	P. Libby
Endothelial and Leukocytes	Rb 2/3 (ICAM-1)	Mouse IgG	P. Libby

denudation of the endothelium was found to create a lesion of intimal proliferation *(3)*, and subsequent research indicated that balloon denudation in a cholesterol-fed rabbit enhanced lesion formation *(4)*. These lesions share morphologic and cellular characteristics with human lesions.

The rabbit iliac artery model has become a well-characterized system in the literature *(5)*. One of the significant advantages of the rabbit model is the abundance of antibodies available (*see* Table 1) against rabbit antigens, which make immunocytochemical characterization possible—including cell-specific staining, quantification of proliferation through nuclear staining, and staining for a variety of cell-surface and extracellular products. The size of rabbit iliac arteries (approx 2.0–2.5 mm in diameter) also makes them suitable for dilatation with angioplasty balloons as well as commercially available coronary stents. The relatively low cost of purchase and care of rabbits offers practical advantages when compared to the costs for other larger species such as pigs and non-human primates.

ANIMAL CARE

Several species of rabbits are commercially available. The most commonly used are the New Zealand White Rabbit (discussed in detail in this chapter) and the smaller Dutch Belted Rabbit. The hyperlipidemic Watanabe Rabbit (discussed in this chapter) is also available.

Housing and Handling

Adult rabbits weighing 3–4 kg may be housed singly in cages approx 3 ft squared in area and 14 inches in height for a rabbit weighing less than 4 kg *(6)*. The animals should have free access to water at all times, and should be fed once daily. The optimal temperature for rabbits is 61°F–72°F *(6)*. Rabbits should be examined daily for signs of injury or disease. Appetite, stool production, mobility, and level of alterness should be assessed. In transferring rabbits, one should grasp them firmly by the scruff and support their hind limbs. Rabbits have long spines in proportion to their size, which—although supported by well-developed para-spinous muscles—are prone to injury. Particular care must be taken when the animals are anesthetized, because spinal fracture leading to paralysis can occur with improper handling.

Diet

Diet plays a major role in the development of atherosclerotic lesions, and by varying dietary cholesterol content with or without concomitant balloon injury, a variety of lesions can be produced (*see* Chapter 13).

Animals fed a normal diet (Purina rabbit chow: approx 2.7% fat and 1.2 mg cholesterol per 100 mg of chow) who undergo endothelial denudation develop predominantly proliferative lesions consisting of smooth-muscle cells (SMCs) with sparse macrophages evident. The addition of a chronically indwelling stent increases neointimal growth, and causes abundant adhesion and infiltration of macrophages which tend to cluster around the stent struts *(7)*.

The natural plasma cholesterol concentration in New Zealand White rabbits—approx 50 mg/dL *(8)*—can be raised dramatically through changes in diet. Atherogenic diets (ICN Nutritional Biochemicals, Warrensville Heights, OH) consist of 2–3% peanut or coconut oil enriched with 0.5–2.0% cholesterol. Bocan et al. *(8)*. fed New Zealand White rabbits a diet composed of 3% peanut oil and 3% coconut oil enriched with 0–2.0% cholesterol for a period of 9 wk and examined the subsequent lesions in balloon-denuded iliac arteries and un-injured thoracic arteries. At total cholesterol levels greater than 700 mg/dL, total plasma cholesterol exposure was linearly related, with total thoracic aorta coverage ($r = 0.66$) and thoracic aortic cholesterol ester content ($r = 0.74$). In injured iliac arteries, total cholesterol exposure was linearly correlated with lesion cholesterol ester content ($r = 0.80$) and macrophage/lesion ratio ($r = 0.64$). In addition, at total cholesterol levels greater than 700 mg/dL, more than 75% of these lesions are fibrofoamy in nature, with macrophage/lesion ratios of 0.46–0.55. The authors have concluded that atherosclerotic lesion content, type, and grade can be determined by total cholesterol exposure and by the use of endot-helial denudation. Such persistent hypercholesterolemia can lead to signs of systemic hyperlipidosis.

The duration of time required to produce an atherosclerotic lesion through diet and arterial injury depends on the type of lesion desired. A mainly prolif-erative lesion consisting of SMCs is well-established at 14 d postinjury in rab-bits fed a normal diet *(9)*. Early fatty streaks can be produced in approx 6 wk in a rabbit fed a hypercholesterolemic diet, achieving a total cholesterol of approx 500–700 mg/dL. In an effort to achieve rapid induction of atherosclerosis with-out evidence of systemic lipidosis, Saso et al. *(10)* fed Japanese white rabbits an atherogenic diet consisting of 6% peanut oil and 0.2% cholesterol for 4 wk, and then performed balloon endothelial denudation. Animals were sacrificed at 8 wk, and serum lipid measurements at this time revealed total cholesterol levels of 338 ± 79 mg/dL. Morphometry revealed significant intimal thickening (ab-dominal aorta greater than thoracic aorta), and pathologic examination revealed the content of the lesions to be abundant SMCs, foam cells, increased collagen, and occasional areas of calcification.

Watanabe Heritable Hyperlipidemic Rabbit

An alternative to diet in producing an atherogenic lesion is the use of the Watanabe heritable hyperlipidemic (WHHL) rabbit *(11)*. As in human patients with familial hypercholesterolemia, homozygous WHHL rabbits have a defi-ciency of cell-surface LDL receptors. They exhibit hypercholesterolemia, with total cholesterol levels of 650–950 mg/dL. WHHL rabbits fed a normal choles-terol chow (<2 mg/d of cholesterol) develop age-dependent lesions of athero-sclerosis from early fatty streaks at 4–5 mo of age, to advanced lesions with necrotic cores, abundant foam cells, and fibrous caps at 15 mo. In addition, like human patients with familial hypercholesterolemia, WHHL rabbits develop xanthomatous lesions. Thus, the WHHL rabbit has been touted as a good ani-mal model of human familial hypercholesterolemia.

Postsurgical Care

Animals are placed in their cages after surgery when they are awake and able to walk. Commercially available collars (Lomir, Co., Quebec, Canada) are used for the first 3–7 d after surgery to prevent the rabbits from irritating their incisions. The animals are examined daily to evaluate the incision sites for integrity, hematoma development, and signs of infection. Infection is very rare, and we do not recommend routine use of antibiotics post surgery. Appetite, stool production, and the animal's overall level of alertness are also assessed daily.

SURGERY

A list of equipment needed for the procedure and companies from which the equipment can be purchased is included in Table 2.

Presurgical Considerations

We recommend that animals be allowed to acclimate to their new environment for 2–3 d before surgery. Animals scheduled to receive stents should be given aspirin (Sigma Chemical Co., St. Louis, MO) in their drinking water at 0.07 mg/mL to achieve an approximate dose of 5 mg/kg/d. This regimen, designed to reduce the incidence of subacute thrombosis, should be continued for the duration of the experiment unless contraindicated by the experimental design.

Intravenous substances can be delivered to the rabbit with the use of subcutaneously implanted osmotic minipumps (Alza Corporation, Palo Alto, CA). These miniature implantable pumps, made of an outer membrane of cellulose ester surrounding a plastic drug reservoir, are available in a variety of sizes with varying delivery rates. When implanted, the outer membrane absorbs fluid, displacing drug from the inner reservoir at a constant rate. Specific instructions for preparing the pumps are available from the manufacturer. In brief, one fills the reservoir with the desired drug in a compatible solvent, attaches a tube (prefilled with the substance to be infused) to the nipple of the pump, and allows the pump to equilibrate in 0.9% normal saline at 37°C overnight.

Anesthesia

A variety of anesthetic agents are available for use in the rabbit (12) (see Chapter 21). For ease of use, we recommend a combination of the α-2 agonist xylazine (5 mg/kg) and the dissociative anesthetic ketamine (35 mg/kg). This combination provides adequate anesthesia for procedures lasting approx 1 h, and has relatively few side effects, although hypotension and bradycardia can occur. While it is important to watch for respiratory depression, routine intubation is unnecessary. These anesthetics may be administered through an IM injection into the anterior thigh, with careful avoidance of vascular structures and

Table 2
Necessary Equipment List for Performance of the Rabbit Iliac
Artery Balloon/Stent Injury Model

Presurgical equipment	Company
Anesthetic:	
Ketamine	Fort Dodge Animal Health Co., Fort Dodge, IA
Xylazine	Fermenta Animal Health Co., Kansas City, MO
Nembutal	Abbot Laboratories, North Chicago, IL
Isofluorane (gas machine needed)	Mallinckrodt Veterinary Inc., Mundelein, IL
IV catheters	Terumo Medical Corp., Elkton, MD
Eye lubricant	Pharmaderm Co., Melville, KY
Shavers	Oster professional Products, McMinnville, TN
Surgical scrub supplies	The Purdue Frederick Co.Norwalk, CT
IV solutions (LR, NS, etc.)	Baxter Healthcare Corp., Deerfield, CT
Osmotic pumps if needed	Alza Corp., Palo Alto, CA
Surgery	
Sterile gown and gloves	Johnson and Johnson Corp., Arlington, TX
Sterile drape or towels	"
Bowl with sterile saline	"
Gauze	"
Blade handle with #10 or	
#11 blade	Biomedical Research Instruments, Rockville, MD
Forceps:	"
1 Rat-toothed	"
1 Curved tissue	"
1 Straight tissue	"
1 Microdissecting	"
Hemostats:	
4 Kelly (curved or straight)	Biomedical Research Instruments, Rockville, MD
Scissors:	
1 Suture	Biomedical Research Instruments, Rockville, MD
1 Metzenbaum	"
1 Microdissecting	"
1 Iris	"
1 Needle holder	"
Towel clamps	"
1 Vein lifter	"

Table 2 (Continued)

Presurgical equipment	Company
Sutures:	
3-0 Dacron on a cutting needle	Johnson and Johnson Corp., Arlington, TX
2-0 Silk	"
3.0-mm Fogarty balloon catheter	Baxter Healthcare Corp., Deerfield, CT
Angioplasty and/or stent catheters as needed	
Indeflator for angioplasty catheters	
If pump used	
3-0 Macron on a taper needle	Johnson and Johnson Corp., Arlington, TX
2-0 silk on a straight needle	"
Tubing for securing pump	
0.125-inch I.D. Tygon	Norton Performance Plastic Corp, Akron, OH
0.125-inch Sylastic	Dow Corning Corp, Midland, MI
Postsurgical	
Collars	Lomir Company, Quebec, Canada

the sciatic nerve. Adequate anesthesia is confirmed throughout the procedure by assessing response to painful stimuli and by assessing the corneal reflex. If additional anesthesia is needed, several options are available. An additional dose of ketamine and xylazine may be given at one-third the original dose. Small boluses (0.1 cc at a time) of IV nembutal, or another barbiturate, can be administered with careful monitoring for excessive respiratory depression. If available, an inhaled anesthetic (such as isofluorane at 1–4%) delivered through a mask can provide very reliable anesthesia, although careful monitoring of vital signs is necessary.

Surgical Preparation

The ear is shaved and IV access is obtained with a 20- to 24-gauge catheter in the lateral marginal ear vein. Wiping the ear with alcohol before placing the catheter will be adequate for antisepsis and will also engorge the vein. As rabbits do not close their eyes completely during surgery, we place a small amount of lubricating ointment into their eyes to avoid dessication of the cornea. The groin and lower abdomen are shaved and the area is prepped with surgical scrub,

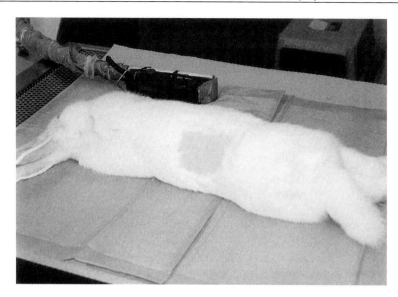

Fig. 1. Photograph of animal after shaving of the flank in anticipation of placement of a subcutaneous osmotic mini pump.

isopropyl alcohol, and betadyne. If an osmotic pump is to be used, an area on the right flank is also shaved and prepped (Fig. 1). The animal is then placed on the operating table, and the legs are secured in order to expose the surgical site.

Exposure and Anatomy of the Groin

In order to expose the femoral artery and vein, an incision approx 2 cm long is made parallel with and approx 1 cm below the inguinal ligament (*see* Fig. 2). The neurovascular bundle is visible underneath several layers of fascia. Using blunt dissection with nontoothed tissue forceps followed by careful incision with Metzenbaum scissors, the bundle is exposed. The femoral nerve lies most lateral in the bundle and appears to be white. The easily identified femoral vein lies most medial in the bundle. The femoral artery lies in the middle and posterior to the nerve and vein, and can be found by careful blunt dissection between the femoral vein and nerve. After isolating a length of the artery (approx 1 cm), two pieces of suture are placed around the artery, taking care to avoid the vein and nerve within the loop. The distal suture is used to tie off the artery, while a double loop is placed around the proximal segment. A short piece of suture is also inserted through the double loop in order to make it easier to loosen the loop as needed (Fig. 3). Leaving the proximal loop loose, a small amount of 1% lidocaine without epinephrine can be used to bathe the artery and cause dilatation. The proximal loop is then tightened, and a small incision is made with

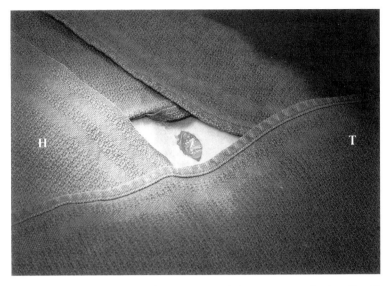

Fig. 2. Photograph of incision made for exposure of the neurovascular bundle. **H** marks direction of head. **T** marks direction of tail.

microscissors in the artery, measuring approximately one-quarter of its circumference.

MODELS OF INJURY

Balloon Injury

Using a vein lifter, a three French Fogarty balloon catheter is introduced in the uninflated state (Fig. 4). The proximal loop is then loosened with the aid of the shorter suture inserted through the loop earlier. With gentle back retraction, the catheter can be advanced well into the abdominal aorta. The catheter is then expanded with 0.55 cc of air and withdrawn in the inflated state. When the catheter is pulled to the level of the iliac bifurcation, resistance may be felt. A small amount of air can be released from the balloon in order to allow it to be pulled into the iliac artery. This procedure is repeated three times. A characteristic rubbing sensation can be felt through the catheter as the endothelium is denuded. The injury produced must be reproducible from animal to animal, and we therefore suggest that one person perform all of the injuries in the same manner. Alternatively, the artery may be injured by inflating an oversize balloon in the vessel, causing injury through stretching and often rupture of the internal elastic membrane (2.5–3.5-mm balloons inflated at 8–12 atmospheres pressure).

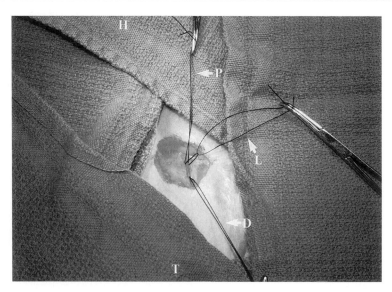

Fig. 3. Photograph of artery after dissection is completed and ties attached. **H** marks direction of head. **T** marks direction of tail. **P** marks proximal tie. **D** marks distal tie. **L** marks the loosening loop inserted through the proximal tie.

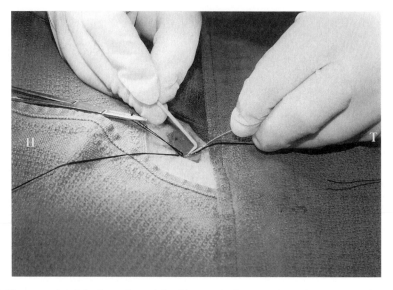

Fig. 4. Photograph of the insertion of the Fogarty balloon catheter into the arteriotomy. **H** marks direction of head. **T** marks direction of tail.

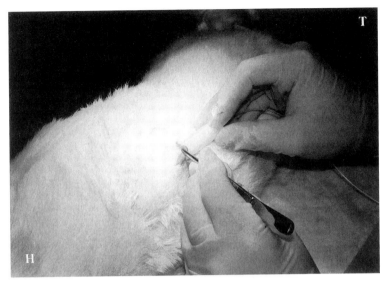

Fig. 5. Photograph of an osmotic minipump being inserted into a subcutaneous pouch created on the animal's flank. **H** marks direction of head. **T** marks direction of tail.

Stents

Stents may be deployed following injury or as a primary form of injury, leaving the endothelium intact. They can be introduced in the same fashion as the balloon catheters. Depending on the stent design, struts may catch on the edge of the arteriotomy, complicating attempts to pass the stent. If this occurs, a 6F sheath can be inserted with minimal difficulty into the artery, which can facilitate entry of the stent. Once the stent is introduced, we insert a finger in the incision and feel the artery where it passes under the inguinal ligament. We adjust the position of the balloon upon which the stent is mounted so that we can feel the distal portion of the balloon at the level of the inguinal ligament. The stent is then deployed according to protocol, just proximal to the inguinal ligament. If desired, the stent may be positioned fluoroscopically. Dye may be injected through a catheter inserted in the contralateral artery in order to position the stent. We administer aspirin in water beginning the day before stenting, as well as an IV bolus of heparin (100 U/kg) at the time of stenting in order to minimize acute thrombosis.

Double Injury

Double injury is an alternative method that some investigators feel more accurately models angioplasty. In this model, an initial injury is made with balloon dilatation or overstretching of the vessel, and the animal is allowed to recover for a period of time (typically 14 d). At this stage a second angioplasty

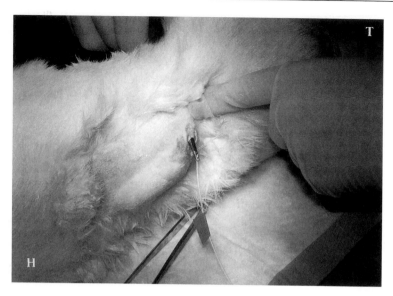

Fig. 6. Photograph demonstrating the use of Kelly clamps to dissect bluntly through the subcutaneous space and pull the pump tube into the groin from the flank. **H** marks direction of head. **T** marks direction of tail.

is performed, usually with fluoroscopic guidance to allow assessment of initial lesion location and severity.

Osmotic Pump Placement

Osmotic pumps (Alza Corp., Palo Alto, CA) are available in a variety of sizes which can deliver substances intravenously for up to 4 wk after placement. After the substance is placed within the pump and the pump line is primed with the same solution, the pump is allowed to equilibrate overnight in normal saline at 37°C. Before surgery, a patch is shaved on the animal's flank (approx 5 × 10 cm in size and 5 cm rostral to the hip) and prepped in a sterile fashion as described in the previous section (Fig. 1). After arterial injury is performed, an incision large enough to insert the pump subcutaneously is made on the animal's flank (Fig. 5). A straight Kelly clamp is then used to bluntly dissect from the groin to the flank incision along the subcutaneous plane. The end of the pump tube is grasped with the Kelly clamp and pulled through to the groin (Fig. 6). Two ligatures are placed around the femoral vein. To prevent the pump tube from kinking, we run the tube through 2- to 3-cm pieces of 0.125-inch internal diameter Tygon tubing, and secure it with 3-0 Maxon suture to the femoral muscles, carefully guiding the tube so that it can be easily placed into the femoral vein (Fig. 7). The tube should be cut with a beveled edge to a length that will

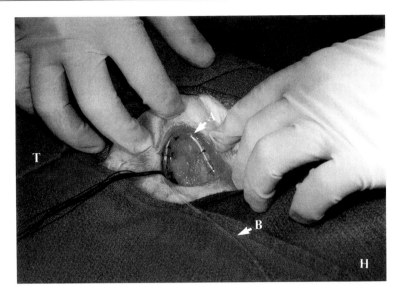

Fig. 7. Photograph of the insertion of the pump tubing into the femoral vein. The position of the Tygon tubes (**A**) used to secure and guide the pump tubing (**B**) can be seen. **H** marks direction of head. **T** marks direction of tail.

reach to a point below the iliac bifurcation. The tube is carefully inserted into a femoral venotomy. The tube must advance with ease and must not be forced in order to prevent damage to the vein. The silk ligature is used to secure the pump line proximally tight enough to hold the tube in place, but not tight enough to obstruct the pump tube. The distal ligature is then used to tie off the vein distal to the pump tube. The pump is secured on the flank with 0.125-inch internal-diameter Silastic tubing. As shown completed in Fig. 8, a small hole is cut through the middle of the Silastic tubing, and a piece of 2-0 silk suture on a straight needle is passed through the hole and out the end of the tube. It is placed through the animal's skin and under the pump, exiting on the opposite side, and then placed back through the Silastic tubing, through the middle hole, and tied to secure the pump against the animal's side. The procedure is repeated twice, and the entry incision is closed. A smaller piece of Silastic tubing may be placed to act as a barrier to the pump migrating towards the tail.

Closure

We typically use 3-0 Dacron suture to close the groin incisions, which can be closed with interrupted, running or subcutaneous stitches. If subcutaneous stitches are not used, we recommend the use of collars to prevent the animals from opening their wounds.

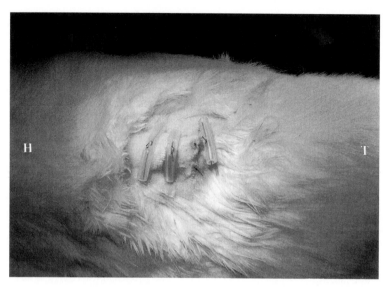

Fig. 8. Photograph of the osmotic pump secured in place with two Silastic tubes used to secure the pump and a separate piece of tubing placed more caudal, used as a barrier to migration of the pump. **H** marks direction of head. **T** marks direction of tail.

HARVEST

At the time of harvest, the animal is sedated with xylazine and ketamine. An iv catheter is placed within the ear vein. At this point, 5-Bromo- 2'-deoxyuridine (BrdU) can be given at a dose of 50 mg/kg to allow later quantification of cellular proliferation. After allowing circulation of BrdU for approx 1 hr, the animal is deeply anesthetized with nembutal (1–2 cc). The animal will often lose spontaneous respiration with this dose of nembutal, but should retain a heartbeat. An incision is made extending from the groin to the thoracic cavity. The diaphragm is cut transversely to expose the heart, and the inferior vena cava is identified and incised. A 14-gauge catheter is inserted into the left ventricle, and 0.9% NaCl is allowed to flow wide open until the blood emerging from the inferior vena cava incision is essentially clear (approx 300–500 cc). At this point, one can dissect and recover the iliac arteries, or a fixative can be used to fix the arteries *in situ* through infusion via the left ventricular puncture. Methods of fixation and specimen handling are discussed in Chapter 22.

REFERENCES

1. Finking G, Hanke H. Nikolaj Nikolajewitsch Anitschkow (1885–1964) established the cholesterol-fed rabbit as a model for atherosclerosis research. Atherosclerosis 1997; 135:1–7.
2. Anitschkow N, Chalatow S. Ueber experimetelle cholesteringsteatose und ihre bedeutun fur die entstehung einiger pathologischer prozesse. Centrbl Allg Pathol Pathol anat 1913; 24:1–9.

3. Baumgartner HR, Studer A. Effects of vascular catheterization in normo- and hypercholesteremic rabbits. Pathol Microbiol 1966; 29:393–405.
4. Weidinger FF, McLenachan JM, Cybulsky MI, et al. Hypercholesterolemia enhances macrophage recruitment and dysfunction of regenerated endothelium after balloon injury of the rabbit iliac artery. Circulation 1991; 84:755–767.
5. Faxon DA, Weber VJ, Haudenschild C, Gottsman SB, McGovern WA, Ryan TJ. Acute effects of transmural angioplasty in three experimental models of atherosclerosis. Arteriosclerosis 1982; 2:125–133.
6. The National Research Council. Guide for the Care and Use of Laboratory Animals. Washington, DC: National Academy Press, 1996:123.
7. Rogers C, Welt FGP, Karnovsky MJ, Edelman ER. Monocyte recruitment and neointimal hyperplasia in rabbits: coupled inhibitory effects of heparin. Arterioscler Thromb Vasc Biol 1996; 16:1312–1318.
8. Bocan TM, Mueller SB, Mazur MJ, Uhlendorf PD, Brown EQ, Kieft KA. The relationship between the degree of dietary-induced hypercholesterolemia in the rabbit and atherosclerotic lesion formation. Atherosclerosis 1993; 102:9–22.
9. Rogers C, Karnovsky MJ, Edelman ER. Inhibition of experimental neointimal hyperplasia and thrombosis depends on the type of vascular injury and the site of drug administration. Circulation 1993; 88:1215–1221.
10. Saso Y, Kitamura K, Yasoshima A, et al. Rapid induction of atherosclerosis in rabbits. Histol Histopathol 1992; 7:315–320.
11. Buja LM, Kita T, Goldstein JL, Watanabe Y, Brown MS. Cellular pathology of progressive atherosclerosis in the WHHL rabbit. An animal model of familial hypercholesterolemia. Arteriosclerosis 1983; 3:87–101.
12. Kohn DF, Wixson SK, White WJ, Benson GJ. Anesthesia and Analgesia in Laboratory Animals. Academic Press, New York, 1997:426.

2

The Porcine Model of Coronary Restenosis

Robert S. Schwartz, MD, Birgit Kantor, MD, and David R. Holmes Jr., MD

INTRODUCTION

Human coronary restenosis remains an elusive problem, and a major limitation of all percutaneous interventional coronary revascularization procedures, despite intracoronary stenting *(1–9)*. Restenosis has recently gained even greater importance, since trials comparing PTCA with coronary bypass surgery (BARI, EAST, CABRI) suggest that angioplasty is comparable therapy for cardiac events and symptoms, but the two differ strikingly regarding the need for repeat interventions and cost *(10–12)*. Restenosis lies at the center of these problematic differences.

A wide spectrum of pharmacologic strategies have demostrated either complete failure, or at best equivocal success *(13–27)*. New devices have also failed to show substantial effect *(28)*. The incidence, clinical time course, and angiographic correlates of coronary restenosis have been well described, yet a limited understanding of its pathophysiology has prevented the formulation of

From: *Contemporary Cardiology: Vascular Disease and Injury: Preclinical Research*
Edited by: D. I. Simon and C. Rogers © Humana Press Inc., Totowa, NJ

Table 1
Clinical Problems Involving Exuberant
Neointimal Hyperplasia

Small-diameter vascular grafts
Prosthetic grafts
Vasculitis
Transplant coronary artery disease
Atherosclerosis

a truly effective therapy. Only recently has vascular brachytherapy with β or γ radiation suggested that neointimal hyperplasia may be limited.

While many animal arterial injury models have been developed and extensively studied to test potential therapies, a limited knowledge of the relevance of such models to human restenosis poses a major drawback. These models have been used to test preclinical therapies, and to provide a better understanding of the pathophysiology of the restenosis problem. Studies using such models have provided a framework for a better knowledge of the arterial response to injury (29–31).

Published results from many animal studies often fail to translate to clinical trials, resulting in confusion about the models, restenosis mechanisms, and potential solutions. However, in most instances, a careful review and consideration of such studies frequently reveals that the interpretation of the results, and not the models themselves, have failed. In general, the porcine model of restenosis seems practical, and substantially representative of human remodeling and neointimal formation. We must formulate a better understanding of this useful model to determine when and how far to apply it in understanding the restenosis problem.

Restenosis in its simplest form is the healing response following arterial injury caused by revascularization (32–38). It is commonly attributed to several factors, including acute and chronic remodeling, (39–42) thrombus at the injury site, medial smooth-muscle-cell (SMC) migration and proliferation, and extracellular matrix production (43–49). In these times, when coronary stent placement is ubiquitous, remodeling at the angioplasty site is minimized. However, the stent itself enhances neointimal hyperplasia, reducing the problem to understanding and limiting neointimal thickening (50). Neointima plays an important role in many arterial diseases (see Table 1).

PORCINE CORONARY ARTERY INJURY MODELS

The coronary arteries of domestic crossbred pigs respond in a very similar fashion to human coronary arteries after sustaining deep injury (51). A hyper-

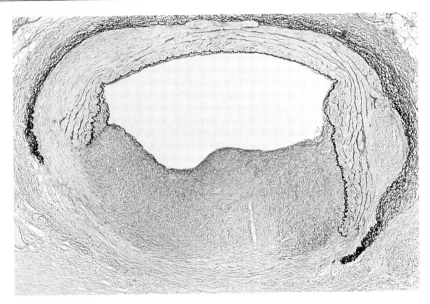

Fig. 1. Photomicrograph of a porcine coronary artery 28 d after oversized balloon injury. Not all wires penetrated into the vessel media. The balloon lacerated the media and created a large dissection *(bottom)* that filled with neointima. The neointima grows only at sites of internal elastic lamina and medial rupture. The amount of neointimal formation is variable, and in general is proportional to the size of the fracture length. A typical response index is intimal area/fracture length. Elastic van Gieson's stain, magnification × 10.

cholesterolemic diet produces lesions which are histopathologically identical, but more severe than those produced by standard laboratory diets *(52)*.

The carotid arteries are typically used for arterial access in this model, although the femoral arteries may also be used without difficulty. Standard human coronary-guide catheters and curves for human coronary angioplasty fit the porcine aortic root well (20–40 kg animals) for engagement of the left main or right coronary arteries.

Severe mechanical arterial injury is done to the coronary arteries either by a coronary angioplasty balloon alone, *(30,53,54)* or by delivering an oversized metal coronary stent to the artery for chronic implant. Both methods create an injury that results in a thick neointima within 20–28 d (*see* Figs. 1–3). The histopathologic features of this neointima are identical to human restenotic neointima (Fig. 4), and the neointima is often voluminous enough to cause relevant luminal narrowing.

Specimens from balloon-injured vessels without stents typically show a single laceration of media, filled at 28 d by a variable amount of neointima. Oversized stent placement in arteries show multiple injuries in each section.

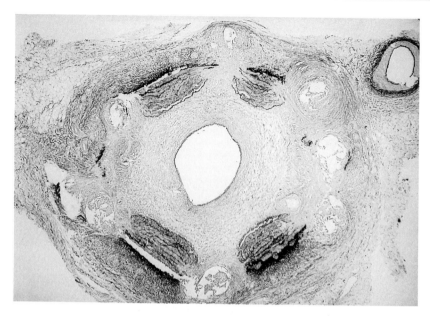

Fig. 2. Section showing severe injury in a normal porcine coronary artery at 28 d after coronary artery injury. All wires have produced severe damage, as evidenced by voluminous neointimal thickening at all sites circumferentially around the lm. The lm is markedly compromised by this injury. Elastic van Gieson's stain, magnification × 10.

Each injury site is characterized in the porcine oversized stent-injury model as a mean injury score (Table 2) that is ordinally proportional to injury depth *(53,54)*. The amount of neointimal thickening is directly proportional to this score (Fig. 5). This permits creation of an injury-response regression line that can be used to quantitate the response to potential therapies *(55)*.

An interesting consideration is whether neointimal formation resulting from injury by balloon alone differs from that caused by oversized stents, and several considerations are important to answering to this question. The first is whether the stent alters the mechanism of neointimal formation. Neointimal thickness is strongly related to the depth of injury in the stented injuries—an observation which has important implications. At low or zero levels of arterial injury, neointima at stent-wire sites is quite thin—essentially the same as that of "appropriately sized" stents. It is only when stent wires fracture the internal elastic lamina, lacerate media, or perforate through the external elastic lamina that neointimal thickness grows substantially to the point of creating macroscopic stenoses. This set of observations suggests that it is the *injury* from the stent wires, rather than the wires themselves, that is responsible for neointimal generation. The stent is thus a means of reliably producing injury to the arterial

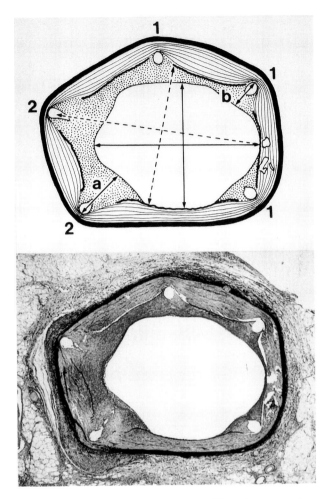

Fig. 3. Photomicrograph of a porcine coronary artery 28 d after severely oversized coil injury. Not all wires penetrated into the vessel media. In this section, the two coils at the bottom of the vessel lacerated the media and resulted in substantial neointimal thickening. Conversely, the farthest right wire did not, and less thickening resulted. A short segment of vessel media at the bottom-most portion of the figure is entirely normal, without any neointima, although this segment was stretched by the balloon. This normal-appearing segment has the farthest distance between any coil wires. The top image shows the method of quantitating injury produced by the stent wires. The Elastic van Gieson's stain, magnification × 10.

wall. When the stent itself is not a cause of injury, it does not produce substantial neointimal thickening. Evidence from studies with rabbit femoral arteries indicates that oversized, injurious stent wires provide a strong, prolonged stimulus to mitosis in the intima of the vessel. It is also clear that the stent metal

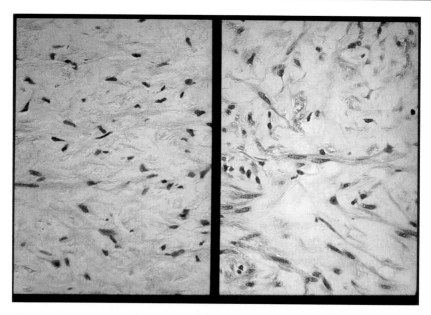

Fig. 4. High-power side-by-side comparison of a representative sample of human restenotic neointima *(left)* and tissue from the porcine restenosis model *(right)*. The character of cells and proportion of ground substance is histopathologically identical. Hematoxylin Eosin stain, magnification × 300.

Table 2
Ordinal Arterial Injury Score

Score	Injury
0	Internal elastic lamina intact; endothelium typically denuded; media compressed but not lacerated
1	Internal elastic lamina lacerated; media typically compressed but not lacerated
2	Internal elastic lacerated; media visibly lacerated; external elastic lamina intact but compressed
3	External elastic lamina lacerated; typically large transluminal lacerations of media; coil wires sometimes residing in adventitia

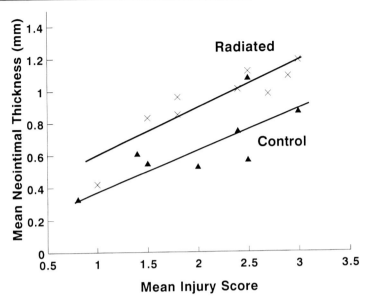

Fig. 5. Regression lines of mean neointimal thickness vs mean injury score for porcine 26 coil-injured coronary-artery segments. The two regression lines are from a study comparing external-beam radiation with control, no radiation. The external radiation exacerbated the injury, and worsened the neointimal thickening. This is shown by a parallel regression line, but with a larger y-intercept.

causes essentially no foreign-body reaction, since many studies have shown little or no chronic inflammatory cellular response at wire sites (i.e., no giant cells). Most importantly, the stent in this model assumes even greater importance when considering that a majority of patients receiving angioplasty also receive stents.

One reason for the greater neointimal thickening with oversized stent placement is that typically, five or more injury sites result in a localized region around the vessel circumference, each generating neointima. This type of injury pattern differs from the inflation-only injuries, where a single large dissection is typical (Fig. 1). This injured location is the site of neointimal development.

In the oversized stent model, quantitation of vessel injury is facilitated by the discrete stent injury points, and the exact size and extent of injury can be measured and compared directly with the neointimal thickening response using regression methods. A similar proportional response between injury and neointimal thickness has been shown by Bonan for the inflation-only injury method (56). This consistency with the injury-neointimal-thickness response found for the oversized stent injury method is reassuring; the neointima of both models is likely formed by similar mechanisms. It is possible that thrombus volume differs at the injury sites for inflation-only and oversized stent-injury models. This may be caused either by the stent itself, or the increased injury present in the vessel wall that in turn causes increased thrombus deposition. It is likely that increased thrombus is partially responsible for the greater amount of neointima occurring in the stented model. The mechanisms of healing—whether from balloon inflation only or oversized stent—are the same. These photomicrographs, (Fig. 1) from a balloon-only coronary artery injury, show a typical single medial dissection beginning to heal. Thrombus is present early, and is heals from the *luminal* side toward the adventitial surface. A thin cap of SMCs is present on the luminal surface of the thrombus. This finding should not be surprising—it would be unusual to find stented arterial injuries healing through different mechanisms than inflation-only injuries. Recent findings from irradiated arteries in both human patients and pigs suggest that mural thrombus attached to and covering the stent struts and the injury site is the earliest response in the healing process. In cases of irradiated vessels, healing is halted and only such layers of thrombus are present, without cellular organization.

The oversized stent and inflation-only porcine coronary-injury models are thus quite comparable. Reliability of lesion generation depends primarily on the operator's ability to cause enough arterial injury to generate neointima in either model, but not so much that acute vessel thrombosis occurs with resultant animal death. This finite incidence of thrombosis is considered a problem by investigators, but is in fact a representation of stent thrombosis that occurs in human patients.

Quantitation of vessel injury and the neointimal thickening response is facilitated in the oversized stent model, because discrete injury points are observed and quantitated. The differences and similarities of these two models are summarized in Table 3. The importance of proper, blinded quantitation cannot be overemphasized in this context.

ANIMAL RESTENOSIS MODEL TESTING: DIVERGENT RESULTS FROM CLINICAL TRIALS

Many pharmacologic agents have been tested in the animal models described above, and representative results are summarized in Table 4. These data indicate that many agents are effective in animal models, yet these same agents are *ineffective* when tested in human clinical trials. Examples are antiplatelet drugs, *(27,57–61)* anticoagulants, *(62)* calcium-channel blockers, *(63,64)* angiotensin converting enzyme inhibitors, *(15,65)* and antiproliferatives *(13).* The disparity of results between animal-model research and clinical trials has led to skepticism about the validity of animal models in restenosis research.

Table 3
Comparison of Oversized Stent and Inflation-Only Porcine Model

	Oversized stent	Balloon injury only
Number of injury sites	Multiple	Single
Size of injury sites	Smaller, constant	Larger, variable
Injury quantitation	Easier (injury score)	More difficult (fracture length)
Response variables	Neointimal thickness Neointimal area Lumen area Injury-NI thickness Regression	Intimal area (IA) Fracture length (FL) Quotient IA/FL
Neointimal response to injury	Proportional	Proportional
Thrombus at injury site	Present	Present

Many therapies effectively limit proliferation and migration in rat carotid arteries. Why do the results of so many animal studies not reflect those seen in clinical trials of the same agents? A number of interpretations explain this observation. One consideration is that the rat carotid model is the oldest. More agents have been tried, and thus more have been found successful in this model. The rabbit iliac model has also been extensively studied and tested. Since the porcine models are newer, fewer agents have been tested and found effective. Are the mechanisms of neointimal formation different among these animal models and in human patients? Are other factors in the models themselves or their analysis methods responsible for the discrepancies? The answers to these questions are unknown, but are essential for developing solutions based on animal-model data.

In the rat carotid model, proliferation of SMCs has been documented in detail (66–68). Yet neointimal volume in these injured arteries is small, and rarely causes arteriographically detectable luminal stenoses. The porcine model also shows cellular proliferation, but hemodynamically significant stenoses regularly occur. Are the pathophysiologic mechanisms different across species? Strong teleologic arguments must be raised against the hypothesis that the arterial response to injury occurs differently across species. The apparent disparity in animal-model results must be examined if they are to be reconciled by a unifying hypothesis of restenosis pathophysiology.

Table 4
Porcine Coronary Model

Agent	Efficacy	References
Angiopeptin	++	95–97
Lovastatin	+/-	98, 99
Hirudin	+	100, 101
Methotrexate	N	102
Probucol	++	103
Trandolapril/Captopril	N	104
Enalapril	N	105
AII Inhibition	N	106
X-Irradiation	N/++	73, 107–117
Endothelin Inhibition	+/-	118
Antisense: CDC2/PCNA	N	119
Vitamins C/E	N	120

Key: ++   Effective in Neointimal Reduction
      N   Not Effective

TRANSLATING RESULTS OF ANIMAL MODELS TO CLINICAL TRIALS

The porcine coronary models using either the stent or overstretch injury alone have increasingly become the standard by which potential restenosis therapies are applied. In the past, negative trials in the pig have corresponded to negative clinical trials, suggesting that this model has specificity. Since there were few or no therapies available that showed positive results in human patients, the effective sensitivity of the model was uncertain. Recent clinical trials suggest that ionizing radiation may limit neointimal hyperplasia in human patients (69–72). Interestingly, the pig model showed that external-beam radiation was not only ineffective against neointima—it actually *stimulated* growth (73). More recently, other investigators have examined intravascular radiation and found this modality effective against neointima. Interestingly, subsequent clinical trials suggest the efficacy of intravascular radiation in human patients. This seminal observation—if demonstrated with subsequent larger randomized trials—will add useful data to our understanding of precisely how the porcine model will translate when applied to human patients. Specifically, the multiple methods of assessing efficacy in the pig coronary (percent stenosis and reduction, neointimal thickness, remodeling) (*see* Fig. 6A–C) will be considered, and the best correlate of human data determined. Subsequent new or modified therapeutic modalities may then be tested to rapidly converge on the best treatments for the problem.

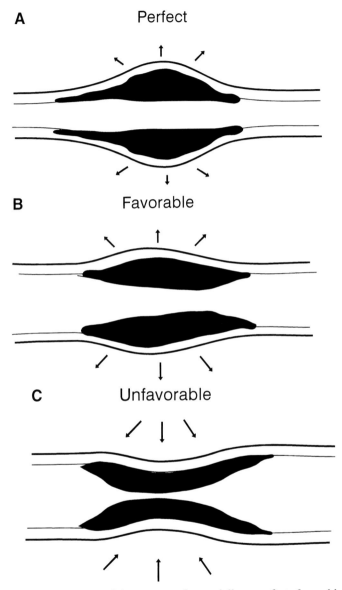

Fig. 6. Schematic representation of three types of remodeling: perfect, favorable, and un-favorable. (**A**) In perfect remodeling, the artery expands its diameter perfectly to compensate exactly for the vol of neointima that grows. The lumen is not compromised in this situation. (**B**) This figure shows favorable remodeling. In this case, the artery cannot perfectly remodel, but is able to partially expand in an attempt to accommodate neointimal thickening. The lumen is only partially compromised by the neointimal thickening, while expanding outwardly and incompletely. (**C**) In unfavorable remodeling, the artery either does not expand at all, or actually contracts. The artery develops a severe stenosis as a result.

The thrombotic response to arterial injury may differ substantially across species. In the rat carotid model, a thin layer of platelets accumulates at the endothelial denudation site. However, significant fibrin-rich thrombus is virtually never found in this model. Conversely, in the rabbit iliac model, macroscopic thrombus does occur, as characterized in a preliminary report (74,75). In the porcine carotid and coronary models, fibrin-rich mural thrombus also plays a significant role in the response to injury. In the coronary arteries, fibrin-rich thrombus provides a framework for colonization by medial SMCs. This foundation eventually forms the organized neointima, a mechanism also suggested in the rabbit. The question of mural thrombus vol and its relation to eventual neointimal vol is critical, and is under investigation. Differences in mural thrombus vol formed in the days and weeks following angioplasty could govern the occurrence of restenosis, as suggested by the rabbit and porcine models. Differences of native thrombolytic potential across species might partially explain differences in mural thrombus. The distinction between "proliferation" and "thrombus" may be blurred, since proliferation may be occurring within thrombus. The rat carotid artery may not generate substantial neointimal vol (and macroscopic stenoses), because it does not form macroscopic thrombus. This suggests an explanation for agents effective in the rat carotid model, yet ineffective in human clinical trials. These agents might be very effective in reducing SMC migration and proliferation, yet exhibit little effect on chronic mural thrombus deposition. Only a part of restenotic neointimal formation may be addressed by these strategies, resulting in clinical failures.

REASONS FOR THE FAILURE OF ANIMAL MODELS TO PREDICT CLINICAL RESULTS

Questions remain about why certain therapeutic strategies which successfully inhibit neointima in some animal models fail to predict clinical trial results. Several potential explanations exist for these discrepancies.

There is still uncertainty regarding how doses of pharmacologic agents given to rodents and other small animals translate to comparable human doses. Two examples from the literature are noteworthy. Studies have shown that Angiotensin Converting Enzyme (ACE) inhibition effectively limits neointimal formation in the rat (76–81). In a key study, (77) the common carotid arteries of rats were denuded of endothelium in the usual fashion, and animals were treated with either captopril 100 mg/kg or cilazapril 10 mg/kg body weight per d beginning 6 d before arterial injury and continuing until the time of euthanasia. An impressive reduction in the percentage of neointimal coverage of the internal elastic lamina was found in both drug treatment groups ($42 \pm 11\%$ captopril treated vs $111 \pm 10\%$ control, and $35 \pm 9\%$ cilazapril treated vs $93 \pm 5\%$ control). This important study provided the stimulus for two large, well-executed clinical trials of cilazapril in Europe (MERCATOR) and the United States (MARCATOR).

Both clinical trials showed this agent had essentially no impact on restenosis *(65,82)*. The highest cilazapril dose used in MARCATOR was 20 mg/d for 24 wk. In a 70-kg patient, this dose corresponds to 0.29 mg/kg body weight, or 2.5% of the dose reported effective in rats on a body weight basis. In patients, even 20 mg/d was high, because many patients were intolerant as a result of orthostatic hypotension and other side effects. A marked discrepancy thus existed between the effective dose in rats compared to humans. Furthermore, the most effective regimen in rats involved 6 d of drug pretreatment before injury. This pretreatment regimen was not used in either the MERCATOR or MARCATOR trials.

A similar situation is found in a study of colchicine in the rabbit iliac artery model *(83,84)*. Colchicine was administered to rabbits at either 0.02 mg/kg-d or 0.2 mg/kg-d. The endpoints of this study were angiographic luminal diameter. Neointimal thickening in the control group changed from a mean of 1.7 ± 0.3 mm immediately following angioplasty to 0.6 ± 0.4 mm. In the group receiving colchicine (0.2 mg/kg), mean luminal diameter was reduced from a mean of 1.7 ± 0.3 mm following angioplasty to 1.1 ± 0.6 mm. In the 0.02 mg/kg-d colchicine group, mean luminal diameter dropped from 1.7 ± 0.3 mm following angioplasty to 0.9 ± 0.5 mm—a result not statistically different from control. In the high-dose colchicine group, the incidence of restenosis was reduced by 50%. However, studies of colchicine in patients have shown no evidence of clinical benefit when used in doses of 1.2 mg/d or 1 mg/d, with angiography or exercise thallium scintigraphy as endpoints *(26,85,86)*. The equivalent doses in a 70-kg human were 0.01 mg/kg-d, or only 5% of the most effective dose in rabbits. The side-effect profile of colchicine is well-known. Colchicine doses as high as 0.2 mg/kg-d in patients would be impossible to achieve without severe side effects.

In the pharmacology of drug testing across sppeies (including human patients), dosing is generally begun at comparable weight-adjusted (mg/kg) levels. It is possible, but unlikely, that the high doses used in rats and rabbits were comparable in efficacy to the doses used in the clinical human trials.

The normal coronary artery of a young rat, rabbit, or pig differs markedly from the atherosclerotic coronary artery of an older human patient. The arteries of these animal models—even those of the hyperlipidemic rabbit (developing over a period of 4 wk instead of decades as in humans)—do not show densely fibrous and acellular plaques with ulceration, calcification, thrombosis, and hemorrhage into the vessel wall. The impact of this atherosclerotic environment on restenosis is unknown. Whether the use of models that produce atherosclerosis will have advantages over nonatherosclerotic models is unknown. Yet, considering that restenosis is a response to arterial injury, there are only minimal differences in healing time as a function of age.

The positive relationship between arterial injury and neointimal thickness has been documented in the porcine coronary and carotid arteries. Clinical patient studies are emerging that also support a proportionality between increased vessel injury during revascularization and increased neointimal thickness. This proportional response in patients must be inferred only indirectly, since arterial injury cannot be assessed angiographically. Surrogate parameters for vessel injury include balloon:artery ratio, severity of initial stenosis (i.e., more severe stenoses undergo a larger relative dilation), acute complications, and the size of the initial lumen immediately following angioplasty. Most have correlated with increased restenosis risk in clinical studies (87,88). A major advantage of histopathologic assessment in animal models is that vessel injury can be directly and semiquantitatively assessed. If a proportionality exists between depth of injury and neointimal response in animal models other than the porcine coronary model, it might be of substantial benefit in the models. Typically, artifact results when vessel injury is not accounted for as a covariate in animal studies, since conclusions regarding differences in efficacy might result from differences in injury among the treated and control groups.

The methods used to determine biologic response play a pivotal role in the outcome of any study. The most quantifiable and tangible outcome of clinical trials is quantitative coronary angiographic measurement of absolute lm size, or percent luminal stenosis. The issue of defining restenosis has been fully explored in published studies (89). Restenosis rates using quantitative coronary angiography vary widely even within the same patient data set, depending on the definition used.

In animal-model studies, quantitative histopathologic measurements are generally the endpoints used to determine efficacy. Much quantifiable information is available from microscopic examination of histopathologic specimens. The area of neointima, media, and residual lumen size can be measured precisely and compared across treatment groups using digital microscopic methods.

The study of cilazapril in rats would have reported a negative conclusion if the accepted angiographic criteria of 0.72 mm minimum luminal diameter change had been applied to the histologic lumen diameter data. Data from this study were analyzed using three measurements: neointimal area, the quotient of (neointimal/medial area), and percent coverage of the internal elastic lamina by neointima. Since the media is typically 50 μ in the rat, neointimal formation is typically 50–100 μ thick. Although the inhibition of neointimal thickness by cilazapril was 80%, the *absolute* inhibition was only 90 μ (0.09 mm). Inhibition of neointimal thickness must be at least 0.36 mm to be minimally detectable using angiography (90–93).

In another example, lovastatin was studied for its ability to reduce neointimal thickening in the nitrogen-desiccated hypercholesterolemic rabbit iliac artery, using angiographic endpoints (94). The mean angiographic arterial diameter in the control group immediately following angioplasty was 1.73 mm. At follow-up it was 0.91 mm—a difference of 0.82 mm. In the lovastatin-treated group, the immediate postangioplasty result was 1.44 mm, decreasing at follow-up to 1.16 mm—a change of 0.28 mm. Although statistically significant, these changes (1.82–0.28, or 0.54 mm) would not be discernable within angiographic definitions of clinical trials. While the data from this study clearly demostrate a modestly beneficial effect from lovastatin, the identical angiographic result in a human trial would be interpreted as having no effect.

The assessment of histopathologic efficacy is important, and should be performed in all animal studies. However, to better predict results in human trials when performing animal studies, microscopically planimetered minimal luminal diameters and percent stenoses should be measured. These measurements more accurately represent surrogate parameters for what would be found in a human angiographic restenosis trial. Variability of efficacy measurement may thus be a major factor in explaining why successful animal-trial results have not translated to clinical efficacy.

CONSISTENCY AMONG ANIMAL RESTENOSIS MODELS: A UNIFIED APPROACH

Many similarities exist among the animal restenosis models. Neointima forms through SMC migration, proliferation, and matrix synthesis in response to injury in all models. How can the apparent differences be reconciled?

The primary differences among animal models lie in the *volume* of neointima from a certain amount of arterial injury. As noted previously, studies of neointimal formation over time in both porcine and rabbit models suggest that mural thrombus at the injury site is a major determinant of neointimal vol. The healing process occurs from the *luminal side outward toward adventitia*. Smooth-muscle-cell migration from nearby medial sites has been documented in the porcine model, both for balloon inflation-only injuries and oversized stent injuries.

CONCLUSION

The importance of using analysis methods comparable to clinical trials (angiography, intravascular ultrasound) should be applied to animal trials. The many response variables to injury for the artery should be studied to determine which can best predict results in human trials. Different data analysis methods may play a major role in the variability of studies. Coronary angiography is the "gold standard" in patients against which all treatments will eventually be tested; thus arterial lm size (absolute and relative or percent stenosis) must be evaluated when analyzing data from animal-model studies.

The importance of using similar drug doses and timing for animal models and clinical trials cannot be overstated. Effective agents may have already been tested in the wrong doses or timing, with false-negative results. If concentration is a problem because of side effects, local delivery to the angioplasty site may be considered.

The variability of restenotic neointimal formation in different species is substantial. At either end of the spectrum of neointimal vol, species should be carefully analyzed for clues explaining why some species generate very little neointima following coronary-artery injury. The current animal models may be far more alike than at first apparent from the divergent results in published studies.

A stratified approach to testing potentially effective agents in multiple animal models should be implemented *before* clinical trials to minimize the possibility of negative results. Agents may be screened in the rat carotid-artery model before testing in other animal restenosis models and before human trials.

While there may be no perfect animal model for human restenosis, modeling a biologic process should be conducted to first understand the mechanisms of that process, followed by formulating and testing therapeutic strategies based on well-founded hypotheses. Strategies should be designed and tested to verify or refute these individual hypotheses. For restenosis, this process has been reversed: in the rush to solve the problem, understanding the biologic process is far from complete. Numerous pharmacologic agents and new device technologies have been tested in models without firm hypotheses for mechanisms. The limitations of these models are poorly understood, because of the markedly divergent results in human studies.

A solution to restenosis will result from the continued, meticulous study of neointimal formation in many models, leading to a full understanding of the limitations of the models and preventing erroneous conclusions from those models when applied to clinical trials.

REFERENCES

1. Holmes D, Fitzgerald P, Goldberg S, LaBlanche J, Lincoff AM, Savage M, et al. The PRESTO (Prevention of restenosis with tranilast and its outcomes) protocol: a double-blind, placebo-controlled trial. Am Heart J 2000; 139:23–31.
2. Ruygrok PN, Melkert R, Morel MA, Ormiston JA, Bar FW, Fernandez-Aviles F, et al. Does angiography six months after coronary intervention influence management and outcome? Benestent II Investigators. J Am Coll Cardiol 1999; 34:1507–1511.
3. de Feyter PJ, Kay P, Disco C, Serruys P. Reference chart derived from post-stent-implantation intravascular ultrasound predictors of 6–month expected restenosis on quantitative coronary angiography. Circulation 1999; 100:1777–1783.
4. van Domburg RT, Foley DP, de Jaegere PP, de Feyter P, van den Brand M, van der Giessen W, et al. Long term outcome after coronary stent implantation: a 10 year single centre experience of 1000 patients. Heart 1999; (Suppl 2)II82:27–34.

5. Di Luzio V, De Remigis F, De Curtis G, Paparoni S, Pecce P, Di Emidio L, et al. Coronary restenosis after optimal (stent-like) initial angiographic results obtained by traditional balloon angioplasty. (Review). Giornale Ital Cardiol 1997; 27:645–653.

6. Kastrati A, Schuhlen H, Hausleiter J, Walter H, Zitzmann-Roth E, Hadamitzky M, et al. Restenosis after coronary stent placement and randomization to a 4–week combined antiplatelet or anticoagulant therapy: six-month angiographic follow-up of the Intracoronary Stenting and Antithrombotic Regimen (ISAR) Trial (see comments). Circulation 1997; 96:462–467.

7. Kastrati A, Schomig A, Elezi S, Schuhlen H, et al. —Predictive factors of restenosis after coronary stent placement J Am Coll Cardiol 1997; 30:1428–1436.

8. Hoffmann R, Mintz G, Dussaillant G, Popma J, Pichard A, Satler L, et al. Patterns and mechanisms of in-stent restenosis. A serial intravascular ultrasound study. Circulation 1996; 94:1247–1254.

9. Shiran A, Mintz GS, Waksman R, Mehran R, Abizaid A, Kent KM, et al. Early lumen loss after treatment of in-stent restenosis: an intravascular ultrasound study. Circulation 1998; 98:200–203.

10. BARI, CABRI, EAST, GABI, and RITA: coronary angioplasty on trial. Lancet 1990; 335:1315–1316 (editorial).

11. Alazraki NP, Krawczynska EG, Kosinski AS, DePuey EG, 3rd, Ziffer JA, Taylor AT, Jr., et al. Prognostic value of thallium-201 single-photon emission computed tomography for patients with multivessel coronary artery disease after revascularization (the Emory Angioplasty versus Surgery Trial [EAST]). Am J Cardiol 1999; 84:1369–1374.

12. Dagres N, Erbel R. Comparison between PTCA and bypass operation. Results of large randomized studies. Med Klin 1998; 93:22–26, 58.

13. Freed M, Safian RD, O'Neill WW, Safian M, Jones D, Grines CL. Combination of lovastatin, enalapril, and colchicine does not prevent restenosis after percutaneous transluminal coronary angioplasty. Am J Cardiol 1995; 76:1185–1188.

14. Schulman SP, Goldschmidt-Clermont PJ, Topol EJ, Califf RM, Navetta FI, Willerson JT, et al. Effects of integrelin, a platelet glycoprotein IIb/IIIa receptor antagonist, in unstable angina. A randomized multicenter trial. Circulation 1996; 94:2083–2089.

15. Faxon DP. Effect of high dose angiotensin-converting enzyme inhibition on restenosis: final results of the MARCATOR Study, a multicenter, double-blind, placebo-controlled trial of cilazapril. The Multicenter American Research Trial With Cilazapril After Angioplasty to Prevent Transluminal Coronary Obstruction and Restenosis (MARCATOR) Study Group. J Am Coll Cardiol 1995; 25:362–369.

16. Califf RM, Lincoff AM, Tcheng JE, Topol EJ. An overview of the results of the EPIC trial. Eur Heart J 1995; 16:43–49.

17. Ohman EM, Harrington RA, Lincoff AM, Kitt MM, Kleiman NS, Tcheng JE. Early clinical experience with integrelin, an inhibitor of the platelet glycoprotein IIb/IIIa integrin receptor. Eur Heart J 1995; 16:50–55.

18. Schafer AI. Antiplatelet therapy with glycoprotein IIb/IIIa receptor inhibitors and other novel agents. Tex Heart Inst J 1997; 24:90–96.

19. Gapinski JP, VanRuiswyk JV, Heudebert GR, Schectman GS. Preventing restenosis with fish oils following coronary angioplasty. A meta-analysis. Arch Intern Med 1993; 153:1595–1601.

20. Austin GE. Lipids and vascular restenosis. Circulation 1992; 85:1613–1615.

21. Bell L, Madri JA. Original Contributions: effect of Platelet Factors on Migration of Cultured Bovine Aortic Endothelial and Smooth Muscle Cells. Circ Res 1989; 65:1057–1065.

22. Bowles MH, Klonis D, Plavac TG, Gonzales B, Francisco DA, Roberts RW, et al. EPA in the prevention of restenosis post PTCA. Angiology 1991; 42:187–194.

23. Califf R, Ohmann E, Frid D, Fortin D, Mark D, Hlatky M, et al. Restenosis: the clinical issues. In: Topol E., ed. Textbook of Interventional Cardiology. W.B. Saunders, Philadelphia, 1990, pp. 363–394.

24. Finci L, Hofling B, Ludwig B, Bulitta M, Steffenino G, Etti H, et al. Sulotroban during and after coronary angioplasty. A double-blind, placebo controlled study. Z Kardiol 1989; 3: 50–54.

25. Israel DH, Gorlin R. Fish oils in the prevention of atherosclerosis. J Am Coll Cardiol 1992; 19:174–185.

26. OKeefe JHJ, McCallister BD, Bateman TM, Kuhnlein DL, Ligon RW, Hartzler GO. Ineffectiveness of colchicine for the prevention of restenosis after coronary angioplasty. J Am Coll Cardiol 1992; 19:1597–1600.

27. Taylor R, Gibbons F, Cope G, Cumpston G, Mews G, Luke P. Effects of low dose aspirin on restenosis after coronary angioplasty. Am J Cardiol 1991; 68:874–878.

28. Kimura T, Kaburagi S, Tamura T, Yokoi H, Nakagawa Y, Hamasaki N, et al. Remodeling of human coronary arteries undergoing coronary angioplasty or atherectomy. Circulation 1997; 96:475–483.

29. Schwartz RS, Murphy JG, Edwards WD, Camrud AR, Vlietstra RE. Restenosis occurs with internal elastic lamina laceration and is proportional to severity of vessel injury in a porcine coronary artery model. [abstract]. Circulation 1990; 82:III–656.

30. Schwartz RS, Murphy JG, Edwards WD, Camrud AR, Vlietstra RE, Holmes DR. Restenosis after balloon angioplasty: a practical proliferative model in porcine coronary arteries. Circulation 1990; 82:2190–2200.

31. Schwartz RS, Murphy JG, Edwards WD, Camrud AR, Garratt KN, Vlietstra RE, et al. Coronary artery restenosis and the "virginal membrane": smooth muscle cell proliferation and the intact internal elastic lamina. J Inv Card 1991; 3:3–8.

32. Bonan R, Paiement P, Scortichini D, Cloutier MJ, Leung TK. Objective Evaluation of a restenosis-injury index in porcine arteries. Proceedings of the Restenosis Summit IV, Cleveland, OH, 1992.

33. Bonan R, Paiement P, Scortichini D, Cloutier MJ, Leung TK. Coronary restenosis: evaluation of a restenosis injury index in a swine model. Am Heart J 1993; 126:1334–1340.

34. Bonan R, Paiement P, Leung TK. Swine model of coronary restenosis: effect of a second injury. Catheterization Cardiovasc Diagn 1996; 38:44–49.

35. Ellis SG, Muller DW. Arterial injury and the enigma of coronary restenosis. J Am Coll Cardiol 1992; 19:275–277.

36. Ferns GA, Stewart LAL, Anggard EE. Arterial response to mechanical injury: balloon catheter de-endothelialization. Atherosclerosis 1992; 92:89–104.

37. Indolfi C, Esposito G, Di Lorenzo E, Rapacciuolo A, Feliciello A, Porcellini A, et al. Smooth muscle cell proliferation is proportional to the degree of balloon injury in a rat model of angioplasty. Circulation 1995; 92:1230–1235.

38. Karas SP, Gravanis MB, Santoian EC, Robinson KA, Anderberg KA, King SB, 3d. Coronary intimal proliferation after balloon injury and stenting in swine: an animal model of restenosis. J Am Coll Cardiol 1992; 20:467–474.

39. Back MR, White RA, Kwack EY, Back LH. Hemodynamic consequences of stenosis remodeling during coronary angioplasty. Angiology 1997; 48:99–109.

40. Mintz GS, Kent KM, Pichard AD, Satler LF, Popma JJ, Leon MB. Contribution of inadequate arterial remodeling to the development of focal coronary artery stenoses. An intravascular ultrasound study. Circulation 1997; 95:1791–1798.

41. Schwartz RS, Topol EJ, Serruys PW, Sangiorgi G, Holmes DR, Jr. Artery size, neointima, and remodeling: time for some standards. J Am Coll Cardiol 1998; 32:2087–2094.

42. Sabate M, Serruys PW, van der Giessen WJ, Ligthart JM, Coen VL, Kay IP, et al. Geometric vascular remodeling after balloon angioplasty and beta-radiation therapy: a three-dimensional intravascular ultrasound study. Circulation 1999; 100:1182–1188.

43. Strauss BH, Chisholm RJ, Keeley FW, Gotlieb AI, Logan RA, Armstrong PW. Extracellular matrix remodeling after balloon angioplasty injury in a rabbit model of restenosis. Circ Res 1994; 75:650–658.

44. Chesebro JH, Badimon L, Fuster V. Importance of antithrombin therapy during coronary angioplasty. J Am Coll Cardiol 1991; (suppl B): 96B-100B.

45. Clowes A, Reidy M, Clowes M. Kinetics of cellular proliferation after arterial injury: I. Smooth muscle growth in absence of endothelium. Lab Investig 1983; 49:327–332.

46. Foley DP, Hermans WM, Rensing BJ, de Feyter PJ, Serruys PW. Restenosis after percutaneous transluminal coronary angioplasty. Herz 1992; 17:1–17.

47. Lam JYT, Chesebro JH, Steele PM, Dewanjee MK, Badimon L, Fuster V. Deep arterial injury during experimental angioplasty: relationship to a positive Indium-111 labeled platelet scintigram, quantitative platelet deposition and mural thrombus. J Am Coll Cardiol 1986; 8:1380–1386.

48. Liu MW, Roubin GS, King SB, 3rd. Restenosis after coronary angioplasty. Potential biologic determinants and the role of intimal hyperplasia. Circulation 1989; 79:1374–1387.

49. Zijlstra F, den Boer A, Reiber JH, van Es GA, Lubsen J, Serruys PW. Assessment of immediate and long-term functional results of percutaneous transluminal coronary angioplasty. Circulation 1988; 78:15–24.

50. Mintz G, Kent K, Pichard A, Popma J, Satler L, Leon M. Intravascular ultrasound insights into mechanisms of stenosis formation. Cardiol Clin 1997; 15:17–29.

51. Schwartz R, Holmes DJ. Pigs, Dogs, Baboons, and Man: lessons for Stenting from Animal Studies. J Interven Cardiol 1994; 7:355–368.

52. Carter AJ, Laird JR, Farb A, Kufs W, Wortham DC, Virmani R. Morphologic characteristics of lesion formation and time course of smooth muscle cell proliferation in a porcine proliferative restenosis model. J Am Coll Cardiol 1994; 24:1398–1405.

53. Schwartz R, Huber K, Murphy J, Edwards W, Camrud A, Vlietstra R, et al. Restenosis and the proportional neointimal response to coronary artery injury: results in a porcine model. J Am Coll Cardiol 1992; 19:267–274.

54. Schwartz RS, Murphy JG, Edwards WD, Camrud AR, Vlietstra RE, Holmes DR, Jr. Restenosis and the Proportional Neointimal Response to Coronary Artery Injury: results in a Porcine Model. J Am Coll Cardiol 1991.

55. Huber KC, Schwartz RS, Edwards WD, Camrud AR, Murphy JG, Jorgenson MA, et al. Restenosis and angiotensin converting enzyme inhibition: effects on neointimal proliferation in a porcine coronary injury model. Circulation 1991; 84:II–298.

56. Bonan R, Paiement P, Leung TK. Swine model of coronary restenosis: effect of a second injury. Catheterization Cardiovasc Diagn 1996; 38:44–49.

57. Barnathan E, Schwartz J, Taylor L, Laskey W, Kleavland J, Kussmaul W, et al. Aspirin and dipyridamole in the prevention of acute coronary thrombosis complicating coronary angioplasty. Circulation 1987; 76:125–134.

58. Grigg LE, Kay TW, Valentine PA, Larkins R, Flower DJ, Manolas EG, et al. Determinants of restenosis and lack of effect of dietary supplementation with eicosapentaenoic acid on the incidence of coronary artery restenosis after angioplasty. J Am Coll Cardiol 1989; 13:665–672.

59. Koster JK Jr., Tryka AF, H'Doubler P, Collins JJJ. The effect of low-dose aspirin and dipyridamole upon atherosclerosis in the rabbit. Artery 1981; 9:405–413.
60. Riess H, Hofling B, von Arnim T, Hiller E. Thromboxane receptor blockade versus cyclooxygenase inhibition: antiplatelet effects in patients. Thromb Res 1986; 42:235–245.
61. Schwartz L, Bourassa MG, Lesperance J, Aldridge HE, Kazim F, Salvatori VA, et al. Aspirin and dipyridamole in the prevention of restenosis after percutaneous transluminal coronary angioplasty. N Engl J Med 1988; 318:1714–1719.
62. Thornton MA, Gruentzig AR, Hollman J, King SB, 3rd, Douglas JS, Jr. Coumadin and aspirin in prevention of recurrence after transluminal coronary angioplasty: a randomized study. Circulation 1984; 69:721–727.
63. Corcos T, David PR, Bal PG, Renkin J, Dangoisse V, Rapold HG, et al. Failure of diltiazem to prevent restenosis after percutaneous transluminal coronary angioplasty. Am Heart J 1985; 109:926–931.
64. O'Keefe JHJ, Giorgi LV, Hartzler GO, Good TH, Ligon RW, Webb DL, et al. Effects of diltiazem on complications and restenosis after coronary angioplasty. Am J Cardiol 1991; 67:373–6.
65. Anonymous. Does the new angiotensin converting enzyme inhibitor cilazapril prevent restenosis after percutaneous transluminal coronary angioplasty? Results of the MER-CATOR study: a multicenter, randomized, double-blind placebo-controlled trial. Circulation 1992; 86:100–110.
66. Fingerle J, Johnson R, Clowes AW, Majesky MW, Reidy MA. Role of platelets in smooth muscle cell proliferation and migration after vascular injury in rat carotid artery. Proc Natl Acad Sci USA 1989; 86:8412–8416.
67. Hanke H, Strohschneider T, Oberhoff M, Betz E, Karsch K. Time course of smooth muscle cell proliferation in the intima and media of arteries following experimental angioplasty. Circ Res 1990; 67:651–659.
68. Hanke H, Haase KK, Hanke S, Oberhoff M, Hassenstein S, Betz E, et al. Morphological changes and smooth muscle cell proliferation after experimental excimer laser treatment. Circulation 1991; 83:1380–9.
69. Williams DO. Radiation vascular therapy: a novel approach to preventing restenosis. Am J Cardiol 1998; 81:18E-20E.
70. Kay IP, Sabate M, Van Langenhove G, Costa MA, Wardeh AJ, Gijzel AL, et al. Outcome from balloon induced coronary artery dissection after intracoronary beta radiation. Heart 2000; 83:332–337.
71. Meerkin D, Tardif JC, Crocker IR, Arsenault A, Joyal M, Lucier G, et al. Effects of intracoronary beta-radiation therapy after coronary angioplasty: an intravascular ultrasound study. Circulation 1999; 99:1660–1665.
72. Teirstein PS. Prevention of vascular restenosis with radiation. Tex Heart Inst J 1998; 25: 30–33.
73. Schwartz R, Koval T, Edwards W, Camrud A, Bailey K, Browne K, et al. Effect of external beam irradiation on neointimal hyperplasia after experimental coronary artery injury. J Am Coll Card 1992; 19:1106–1113.
74. Preisack MB, Karsch KR. The paradigm of restenosis following percutaneous transluminal coronary angioplasty. Eur Heart J 1993; 14(1):187–192.
75. Bauters C, Labalanche J, McFadden E, Hamon M, Bertrand M. Angioscopic thrombus is associated with a high risk of restenosis. Circulation 1995; 92:1912.
76. Powell J, Muller R, Baumgartner H. Suppression of the vascular response to injury: the role of angiotensin-converting enzyme inhibitors. J Am Coll Cardiol 1991; 17:137B-142B.

77. Powell J, Clozel J, Muller R, Kuhn H, Hefti F, Hosang M, et al. Inhibitors of angiotensin-converting enzyme prevent myointimal proliferation after vascular injury. Science 1989; 245:186–188.

78. Bilazarian S, Currier J, Haudenschild C, Heyman D, Powell J, Ryan T, et al. Angiotensin converting enzyme inhibition reduces restenosis in experimental angioplasty. J Am Coll Cardiol 1991; 17:268A.

79. Berk B, Vekshtein V, Gordon H. Angiotensin II-stimulated protein synthesis in cultured vascular smooth muscle cells. Hypertension 1989; 13:305–314.

80. Brozovich FV, Morganroth J, Gottlieb NB, Gottlieb RS. Effect of angiotensin converting enzyme inhibition on the incidence of restenosis after percutaneous transluminal coronary angioplasty. Catheterization Cardiovasc Diagn 1991; 23:263–267.

81. Daemen MJ, Lombardi DM, Bosman FT, Schwartz SM. Angiotensin II induces smooth muscle cell proliferation in the normal and injured rat arterial wall. Circ Res 1991; 68: 450–456.

82. Faxon DP. Angiotensin converting Enzyme Inhibition and restenosis: the final results of the MARCATOR Trial [abstract]. Circulation 1992; 86:I–53.

83. Bauriedel G, Heimerl J, Beinert T, Welsch U, Hofling B. Colchicine antagonizes the activity of human smooth muscle cells cultivated from arteriosclerotic lesions after atherectomy. Coron Artery Dis 1994; 5:531–539.

84. Gradus-Pizlo I, Wilensky RL, March KL, Fineberg N, Michaels M, Sandusky GE, et al. Local delivery of biodegradable microparticles containing colchicine or a colchicine analogue: effects on restenosis and implications for catheter-based drug delivery. J Am Coll Cardiol 1995; 26:1549–1557.

85. O'Keefe J, McCallister B, Bateman T, Kuhnlein D, Ligon R, Hartzler G. Colchicine for the prevention of restenosis after coronary angioplasty. J Am Coll Cardiol 1991; 17:181A.

86. Grines C, Rizik D, Levine A, Schreiber T, Gangadharan V, Ramos R, et al. Colchicine angioplasty restenosis trial (CART) [abstract]. Circulation 1991; 84:II–365.

87. Roubin GS, Douglas JS, Jr, King SB, 3rd, Lin SF, Hutchison N, Thomas RG, et al. Influence of balloon size on initial success, acute complications, and restenosis after percutaneous transluminal coronary angioplasty. A prospective randomized study. Circulation 1988; 78:557–565.

88. Nichols A, Smith R, Berke A, Shlofmitz R, Powers E. Importance of balloon size on initial success, acute complications, and restenosis after percutaneous transluminal coronary angioplasty. A prospective randomized study. J Am Coll Cardiol 1989; 13:1094–2000.

89. van der Giessen WJ, Hermans WRM, Rensing BJ, Foley DP, Serruys PW. Clinical and angiographic definitions of restenosis: recommendations for clinical trials. In Schwartz RS, ed. Coronary Restenosis. Blackwell Scientific, Boston, 1992, pp 169–191.

90. Serruys PW, Luijten HE, Beatt KJ, Geuskens R, de Feyter PJ, van den Brand M, et al. Incidence of restenosis after successful coronary angioplasty: a time-related phenomenon. A quantitative angiographic study in 342 consecutive patients at 1, 2, 3, and 4 months. Circulation 1988; 77:361–371.

91. Serruys PW, Juilliere Y, Bertrand ME, Puel J, Rickards AF, Sigwart U. Additional improvement of stenosis geometry in human coronary arteries by stenting after balloon dilatation. Am J Cardiol 1988; 61:71G-76G.

92. Serruys P, Hermans R. The new angiotensin converting enzyme inhibitor cilazapril does not prevent restenosis after coronary angioplasty: the results of the MERCATOR trial [abstract]. J Am Coll Cardiol 1992; 19:258A.

93. Strauss BH, Juilliere Y, Rensing BJ, Reiber JH, Serruys PW. Edge detection versus densitometry for assessing coronary stenting quantitatively. Am J Cardiol 1991; 67:484–490.

94. Gellman J, Ezekowitz MD, Sarembock IJ, Azrin MA, Nochomowitz LE, Lerner E, et al. Effect of lovastatin on intimal hyperplasia after balloon angioplasty: a study in an atherosclerotic hypercholesterolemic rabbit. J Am Coll Cardiol 1991; 17:251–259.

Additional Reading and Background

95. Hong MK, Kent KM, Tio FO, Foegh M, Kornowski R, Bramwell O, et al. Single-dose intramuscular administration of sustained-release Angiopeptin reduces neointimal hyperplasia in a porcine coronary in-stent restenosis model. Coron Artery Dis 1997; 8:101–104.
96. Howell MH, Adams MM, Wolfe MS, Foegh ML, Ramwell PW. Angiopeptin inhibition of myointimal hyperplasia after balloon angioplasty of large arteries in hypercholesterolaemic rabbits. Clin Sci 1993; 85:183–188.
97. Santoian ED, Schneider JE, Gravanis MB, Foegh M, Tarazona N, Cipolla GD, et al. Angiopeptin inhibits intimal hyperplasia after angioplasty in porcine coronary arteries. Circulation 1993; 88:11–14.
98. Veinot JP, Edwards WD, Camrud AR, Jorgenson MA, Holmes DR, Jr., Schwartz RS. The effects of lovastatin on neointimal hyperplasia following injury in a porcine coronary artery model. Can J Cardiol 1996; 12:65–70.
99. Ragosta M, Barry WL, Gimple LW, Gertz SD, McCoy KW, Stouffer GA, et al. Effect of thrombin inhibition with desulfatohirudin on early kinetics of cellular proliferation after balloon angioplasty in atherosclerotic rabbits. Circulation 1996; 93:1194–2000.
100. Meyer BJ, Fernandez-Ortiz A, Mailhac A, Falk E, Badimon L, Michael AD, et al. Local delivery of r-hirudin by a double-balloon perfusion catheter prevents mural thrombosis and minimizes platelet deposition after angioplasty. Circulation 1994; 90:2474–2480.
101. Schwartz R, Holder D, Holmes DJ, Veinot J, Camrud A, Jorgenson M, et al. Neointimal thickening after severe coronary artery injury is limited by short term administration of a factor Xa inhibitor: results in a porcine model. Circulation 1996; 83:1542–1548.
102. Muller DWM, Topol EJ, Abrams GD, Gallagher KP, Ellis SG. Intramural methotrexate therapy for the prevention of neointimal thickening after balloon angioplasty. J Am Coll Cardiol 1992; 20:460–462.
103. Schneider J, Berk B, Santoian E, Gravanis M, Cipolla G, Tarazona N, et al. Oxidative stress is important in restenosis: reduction of neointimal formation by the antioxidant probucol in a swine model of restenosis. Circulation 1992; 86:I–186.
104. Huber KC, Schwartz RS, Edwards WD, Camrud AR, Bailey KR. Effects of angiotensin converting enzyme inhibition on neointimal hyperplasia in a porcine coronary injury model. Am Heart J 1993; 125:695–701.
105. Churchill DA, Siegel CO, Dougherty KG, Raizner AE, Minor ST. Failure of enalapril to reduce coronary restenosis in a swine model [abstract]. Circulation 1991; 84:II–297.
106. Huckle WR, Drag MD, Acker WR, Powers M, McFall RC, Holder DJ, et al. Effects of subtype-selective and balanced angiotensin II receptor antagonists in a porcine coronary artery model of vascular restenosis. Circulation 1996; 93:1009–1119.
107. Waksman R, Robinson KA, Crocker IR, Wang C, Gravanis MB, Cipolla GD, et al. Intracoronary low-dose beta-irradiation inhibits neointima formation after coronary artery balloon injury in the swine restenosis model. Circulation 1995; 92:3025–3031.
108. Waksman R, Robinson KA, Crocker IR, Gravanis MB, Palmer SJ, Wang C, et al. Intracoronary radiation before stent implantation inhibits neointima formation in stented porcine coronary arteries. Circulation 1995; 92:1383–1386.
109. Waksman R, Robinson KA, Crocker IR, Gravanis MB, Cipolla GD, King SB, 3rd. Endovascular low-dose irradiation inhibits neointima formation after coronary artery balloon injury in swine. A possible role for radiation therapy in restenosis prevention. Circulation 1995; 91:1533–1539.

110. Waksman R, Robinson KA, Crocker IR, Wang C, Gravanis MB, Cipolla GD, et al. Intracoronary low-dose beta-irradiation inhibits neointima formation after coronary artery balloon injury in the swine restenosis model. Circulation 1995; 92:3025–3031.

111. Waksman R, Robinson KA, Crocker IR, Gravanis MB, Palmer SJ, Wang C, et al. Intracoronary radiation before stent implantation inhibits neointima formation in stented porcine coronary arteries. Circulation 1995; 92:1383–1386.

112. Waksman R, Robinson KA, Crocker IR, Gravanis MB, Cipolla GD, King SB, 3rd. Endovascular low-dose irradiation inhibits neointima formation after coronary artery balloon injury in swine. A possible role for radiation therapy in restenosis prevention. Circulation 1995; 91:1533–9.

113. Waksman R, Robinson KA, Crocker IR, Wang C, Gravanis MB, Cipolla GD, et al. Intracoronary low-dose beta-irradiation inhibits neointima formation after coronary artery balloon injury in the swine restenosis model. Circulation 1995; 92:3025–3031.

114. Waksman R, Kosinski AS, Klein L, Boccuzzi SJ, King SB, 3rd, Ghazzal ZM, et al. Relation of lumen size to restenosis after percutaneous transluminal coronary balloon angioplasty. Lovastatin Restenosis Trial Group. Am J Cardiol 1996; 78:221–224.

115. Wilcox JN, Waksman R, King SB, 3rd, Scott NA. The role of the adventitia in the arterial response to angioplasty: the effect of intravascular radiation. Int J Radiat Oncol Biol Phys 1996; 36:789–796.

116. Wiedermann JG, Marboe C, Amols H, Schwartz A, Weinberger J. Intracoronary irradiation markedly reduces restenosis after balloon angioplasty in a porcine model. J Am Coll Cardiol 1994; 23:1491–1498.

117. Weinberger J, Amols H, Ennis RD, Schwartz A, Wiedermann JG, Marboe C. Intracoronary irradiation: dose response for the prevention of restenosis in swine. Int J Radiat Oncol Biol Phys 1996; 36:767–775.

118. Burke SE, Lubbers NL, Gagne GD, Wessale JL, Dayton BD, Wegner CD, et al. Selective antagonism of the ET(A) receptor reduces neointimal hyperplasia after balloon-induced vascular injury in pigs. J Cardiovasc Pharmacol 1997; 30:33–41.

119. Robinson KA, Chronos NA, Schieffer E, Palmer SJ, Cipolla GD, Milner PG, et al. Endoluminal local delivery of PCNA/cdc2 antisense oligonucleotides by porous balloon catheter does not affect neointima formation or vessel size in the pig coronary artery model of postangioplasty restenosis. Catheterization Cardiovasc Diagn 1997; 41:348–353.

120. Nunes GL, Sgoutas DS, Redden RA, Sigman SR, Gravanis MB, King SB 3rd, et al. Combination of vitamins C and E alters the response to coronary balloon injury in the pig. Arterioscler Thromb Vasc Biol 1995; 15:156–165.

3

Atherosclerotic Porcine Coronary Stent Model

Technical Methods for Preclinical Studies

Andrew J. Carter, DO

CONTENTS

INTRODUCTION
TECHNICAL METHODS
INTERPRETATION OF DATA
LIMITATIONS AND RELEVANCE TO CLINICAL INVESTIGATION
REFERENCES

INTRODUCTION

Preclinical testing of interventional cardiovascular devices such as endovascular stents requires an appropriate animal model to test the performance characteristics and blood and chronic tissue biocompatibility. The United States Food and Drug Administration has proposed guidelines that require evaluation of coronary angioplasty devices in an atherosclerotic model prior to approval for clinical investigations *(1)*. Unfortunately, large animal models of spontaneous atherosclerosis have limited availability, and their cost is prohibitive for most experimental applications. Porcine coronary models have been developed that use dietary manipulation and arterial injury to produce an accelerated atherosclerotic lesion *(2–5)*.

The porcine model offers advantages over some experimental models because of animal availability, cost, and similarities to human coronary anatomy and platelet coagulation systems *(4–11)*. Pigs also spontaneously develop coronary atherosclerosis that can be accelerated by experimental conditions and genetic manipulation of the species. *(2,3,5,12)*. The morphology of the porcine coronary atheroslcerotic plaque can be modulated by the type of dietary manipulation as well as the method of injury to induce the lesion *(13)*.

From: *Contemporary Cardiology: Vascular Disease and Injury: Preclinical Research*
Edited by: D. I. Simon and C. Rogers © Humana Press Inc., Totowa, NJ

The purpose of this chapter is to provide a description of the atherosclerotic porcine coronary stent model used in preclinical cardiovascular device and drug research. The chapter is structured to serve as a practical reference for investigators with a focus on basic supplies, instrumentation, surgical methods, and histologic analysis. Ultimately, the successful completion of experimental studies in this porcine model and other animal models requires a careful team approach with the clinician scientist, veterinarian, and technical support staff.

TECHNICAL METHODS

Supplies and Sources

- 25-to-35-kg castrated male or female Yucatan miniature swine (Lone Star Laboratory Swine, Seguin, TX; Charles River Farms, Southbridge, MA).
- 20% fat and 2–4% cholesterol diet (Purina Mills, Richmond, IN).
- Endotracheal tube with inflatable cuff, laryngoscope, blade, and styles.
- Anesthesia machine adapted for isoflurane with mechanical ventilator (J. A. Webster Veterinary Supply, Brookline, MA).
- Physiologic monitor for electrocardiogram, invasive arterial blood pressure, and pulse oximetry (J. A. Webster Veterinary Supply, Brookline, MA; Datascope, Paramus, NJ).
- Intravenous tubing, 18- or 21-gauge angiocath, 18- and 21-gauge needles, suture (0 silk, 3–0 dexon, 4–0 polydek), silicone elastomer surgical or umbilical tape and skin staples.
- Aseptic surgical instruments and supplies for vascular access.
- 6, 7, or 8 F introducer sheaths (Cordis, Miami Lakes, FL; USCI, Billerica, MA).
- Manifold with ports for invasive BP monitoring, saline flush, and contrast injection.
- Hypaque 76 or equivalent iv contrast.
- Fluoroscopic or cineangiographic equipment with cine film and digital or VCR recorder.
- Cardiac defibrillator.
- Angioplasty catheters, guide wires and accessories (guiding catheter, balloon inflation device, Y-adapter) (Cordis, Miami Lakes, FL; Scimed Boston Scientific, Maple Grove, MN; Guidant, Inc., Santa Clara, CA).
- Histology tissue-perfusion equipment and fixative solutions.

Material and Drug Preparation

- Heparin soln (1,000 U/cc USP) 150 U/Kg iv to be administered following introducer sheath insertion for angioplasty/stent deployment. Confirm activated clotting time >300 s prior to angioplasty or stent deployment.
- Saline flush for injection manifold: 0.45N saline sterile solution iv, with 10 U/cc heparin.

- Nitroglycerin: injected intracoronary 1.0 to 2.0 cc of 100–200 mg/cc solution prior to and after balloon injury or stent placement.
- Anesthetic: 1) fentanyl 50 mg/mL; 2) standard concentrations of ketamine 50 mg/mL; and 3) xylazine 20 mg/mL mixed 20 to 1 in solution.
  Ketamine 20 mg/kg and xylazine 1 mg/kg im for induction.
  Ketamine 50 mg/mL administered iv via the ear vein with a 24-gauge needle or angiocath, 0.5–1.0 cc to induce and maintain anesthesia with 0.25–0.5 cc boluses as required.
  Maintenance with iv fentanyl 75–150 μg/kg per h.
  Inhalant anesthesia isoflurane 1–2% (13).
- Antibiotic: cefazolin sodium 1 g prepared by suspending in 2.5 cc saline. Administer 500 mg iv (1.25 cc) prior to recovery. Alternative: Penicillin 600,000 U/im.
- Antiplatelet: Aspirin 81-mg tablet per Os daily after balloon injury or stent implant. Premedicate with 650 mg (use two 325 mg tablets with food) per Os the day prior to balloon injury or stent implant. Optional: Ticlopidine 250 mg per Os the day prior to stent implant and for the first 28 d postop.
- Calcium channel blocker: nifedipine XL 30 mg per Os with food the day prior to balloon angioplasty or stent implant to reduce coronary spasm (15).
- Other drugs: Amiodarone 150 mg iv, bretylium tosylate 100 mg iv, naloxone 0.5 mg iv or im (14,15).

Coronary Arterial Overstretch Injury after 2 Wk on the High-Fat and Cholesterol Diet

- Record animal and date. Restrain the animal and anesthetize, either via iv or inhalant anesthesia. Establish iv access via a marginal ear vein. Shave the midline neck and prepare for surgery in accordance with sterile technique.
- Isolate the right carotid artery, obtain arterial access by puncture with an 18-gauge thin-wall needle, insert a 0.035" guide wire, and cannulate vessel with an 8 F sheath.
- Engage left main coronary with a 6, 7, or 8 F Judkins Left 3.5 or Judkins Right 4 guiding catheter. Complete coronary angiography by injection of 5–7 cc angiographic contrast material via manifold syringe and record.
- Place a 3.0-to-4.0-mm-diameter standard angioplasty balloon catheter over a 0.014" coronary guide wire at the intended site in the target coronary vessel. The balloon inflated diameter should be approx 1.25 to 1.5 times the baseline vessel diameter. Inflate the balloon to 8–10 ATM 2 times for 30 s.
- Remove angioplasty balloon and guide wire. Complete angiography to document the anatomic location and overstretch coronary injury. Remove the guiding catheter, repair the arteriotomy with suture, close the wound with subcutaneous suture, and approximate the skin with surgical staples. Recover from anesthesia.
- 20% fat and 2–4% cholesterol diet for 4 wk (Figs. 1 and 2).

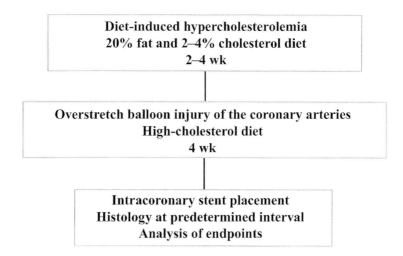

Fig. 1. Overview schematic diagram of the porcine atherosclerotic coronary stent model.

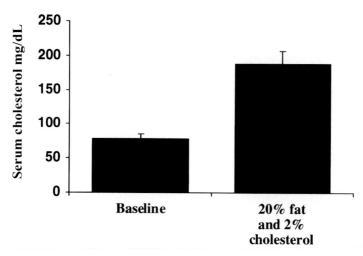

Fig. 2. Bar graph demonstrating the effects of high cholesterol feeding for 4 wk on serum cholesterol levels in Yucatan miniature swine.

Angioplasty and Stent Deployment Procedure

- After 4–6 wk on the high-cholesterol diet, return the animal to the research cath lab.
- Obtain arterial access and administer heparin 150 U/kg iv, measure the activated clotting time. Administer additional heparin if activated clotting

time <300 s. Complete coronary angiography as described in the previous section.

- Flush an 8F Judkins Right 4 guiding catheter with heparinized saline. Insert via the sheath under fluoroscopy into the ascending aorta. Record baseline aortic pressure. Engage the left main coronary ostium with the catheter.
- Perform an angiogram to visualize the left coronary arteries in at least two projections by injecting contrast media through the guiding catheter.
- Select the target arteries for angioplasty and stent implantation, preferably in the proximal (or mid) left anterior descending, circumflex, or right coronary artery.
- Prepare a 3.0-to-4.0-mm (20-mm length) angioplasty balloon catheter or stent delivery system with contrast media according to instructions for use. Preload a 0.014" coronary guide wire in the wire lumen of the angioplasty balloon.
- Advance the guide wire to the distal aspect of the target coronary artery using flouroscopic guidance. Track the angioplasty balloon over the guide wire and center on the lesion. Inflate the balloon to nominal pressure for 60 s. For stent placement, inflate the balloon to the recommended pressure for 15–30 s. Withdraw the angioplasty catheter and guide wire into the guiding catheter. Repeat this sequence in the circumflex or right coronary artery as indicated.
- Administer the nitroglycerin 200 µg IC, complete coronary angiography.
- At study completion, remove all equipment, and repair the carotid artery and skin incision site. Administer antibiotic and recover the animal.
- Chronic maintenance care:
    Aspirin 81 mg per Os with food daily;
    Ticlopidine 250 mg per Os daily for the first 28 d after stent placement; and
    Maintain animal on normal pig chow diet.

Histology

- At the designated study interval the animal should be returned to the lab and prepared as described in the Coronary Arterial Overstretch Injury section.
- Complete coronary angiography as noted in the Coronary Arterial Overstretch Injury Section.
- After euthanasia with a lethal dose of barbiturates, prepare for perfusion fixation of tissue per standard laboratory operating procedures.
- Technique for perfusion fixation of vessels:
    Cannulate ascending aorta, flush with lactated ringers at 80–100 mm Hg pressure for 15–20 min.
    Perfuse with fixative (McDowell Trump soln, formalin, paraform-aldehyde) at 80–100 mm Hg pressure for 30–60 min.
- Preparation of tissue for histology: dissect from the epicardial surface, embed in methylmethacrylate, and cut with a stainless steel carbide knife at 4–5 µM. Stain histologic sections with hematoxylin-eosin and Movat pentachrome stains.
- Vessel morphometry: Measure the cross-sectional area of the proximal edge, proximal body, distal body, and distal edge stent sections with PC or

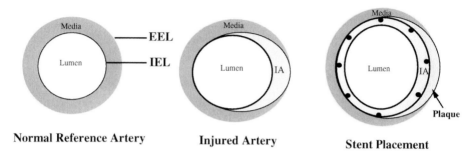

Fig. 3. Illustration of serial histomorphometric analysis of atherosclerotic porcine coronary arteries. Serial analysis of perfusion-fixed tissue allows comparison of the stented coronary arterial segment with nonstented diseased and normal arterial cross-sections. (IA-intimal area)

Macintosh-based computerized digital morphometry system to determine the areas within the external elastic lamina, internal elastic lamina (EL), stent and the vessel lumen. The area within the stent or internal elastic lamina is considered the normal reference lumen area. The percent area stenosis is defined as: [(stent or IEL area—lumen area)/(stent or IEL area)] × 100. Neointimal area is determined by subtracting the area of the lumen from the area within the stent wires. Neointimal thickness extending perpendicular from above the stent to the lumen surface is measured at each wire site. The extent vessel-wall injury induced by the stent is determined using the methods of Schwartz et al *(9)*. Similar morphometric measurements are completed on the control vessels. The data reported for the control vessels represents the most severely diseased section. The medial fracture length and percent medial fracture are measured in all stented and nonstented balloon-injured segments *(see* Fig. 3).

INTERPRETATION OF DATA

The determinants of neointimal formation after stent placement in atherosclerotic arteries are not well-defined. In animal models of restenosis that employ normal arteries, neointimal formation is proportional to the degree of vascular injury *(6–10)*. Rupture of the internal elastic lamina (IEL) and focal destruction of the media by a stent wire or oversized balloon is associated with significantly greater neointimal formation than in an area of the artery where the EL and media are not disrupted *(7–10)*.

The majority of atherosclerotic plaques have an eccentric morphology *(16,17)*. Stent placement in atherosclerotic arteries with eccentric plaques may cause

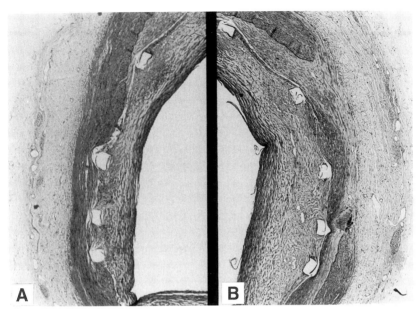

Fig. 4. High-power photomicrographs of an atherosclerotic porcine coronary artery at 2 mo after placement of a balloon expandable stent. In (**A**) the stent struts are embedded in normal media. The struts have caused focal compression of the media, which is associated with a mild neointimal response. In (**B**) the stent struts are embedded in a smooth-muscle-cell rich plaque. The struts have cause focal compression of the plaque. The neointimal thickness is greater than that observed in (**A**). Note the presence of vascular channels, particularly at the base of the neointima. Movat pentachrome, × 40.

injury to both the plaque and normal media (Fig. 4). Therefore, in atherosclerotic arteries the severity of neointimal formation may vary within the artery based on the interface of the stent with the underlying vessel. We reported a 50% increase in neointimal formation after stent placement in atherosclerotic as compared to normal porcine coronary arteries (2,18). Theoretically, both the presence of synthetic type smooth-muscle cells within the atherosclerotic plaque and the absence of the internal elastic lamina to act as a barrier to prevent smooth-muscle-cell (SMC) migration could augment neointimal formation. Thus, analysis of the arterial response to stent placement in atherosclerotic porcine coronary arteries must account for stent interface with the underlying plaque as well as stent-induced arterial injury (Fig. 5). These additional variables require careful consideration when designing experiments and determining an appropriate sample size to identify a significant biologic effect for a particular therapy in an atherosclerotic model.

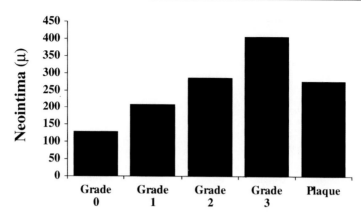

Fig. 5. This bar graph demonstrates the relationship between arterial injury using the grading score of Schwartz et al., *(9)* plaque, and neointimal thickness at 6 mo after placement of Palmaz-Schatz stents in atherosclerotic porcine coronary arteries *(19)*.

LIMITATIONS AND RELEVANCE TO CLINICAL INVESTIGATION

Interpretation of the data obtained in animal models of atherosclerosis and restenosis must be carefully made. Experimental models allow researchers to reproduce specific aspects of a disease state. In the atherosclerotic porcine coronary model, lesions created by balloon injury and high-cholesterol diet differ from the complex atherosclerotic lesions in humans in which focal plaque rupture, necrosis, and calcification are often observed. High-cholesterol feeding and overstretch balloon injury induce a fibrocellular plaque consisting of SMC densely organized in a proteoglycan matrix with only rare macrophages and foam cells *(2)*. Furthermore, the extent of atherosclerotic plaque (10–20% angiographic stenosis) is substantially less in this porcine model than that encountered when stenting diseased human coronary arteries. These factors have significant effects on the biologic response to injury and therapies designed to modulate vascular repair *(13,19)*.

The porcine atherosclerotic coronary stent model can provide useful information about device function, testing local drug or gene therapy, and assessing blood and chronic tissue biocompatibility of endovascular stems. The model may also be useful in elucidating the mechanisms of restenosis and evaluating novel strategies for the prevention of in-stem restenosis.

REFERENCES

1. United States Food and Drug Administration 1994 "Guidelines for the submission of research and marketing applications for interventional cardiology devices."
2. Carter AJ, Laird JR, Kufs WM, Bailey L, Hoopes TG, Reeves T, et al. Coronary stenting with a novel stainless steel balloon expandable stent: determinants of neointimal formation and

changes in arterial geometry after placement in an atherosclerotic model. J Am Coll Cardiol 1996; 27:1270–1277.

3. Gal D, Rongione AJ, Slovenkai GA, DeJesus ST, Lucas A, Fields CD, et al. Atherosclerotic Yucatan microswine: an animal model with high-grade, fibrocalcific, nonfatty lesions suitable for testing catheter-based interevntions. Am Heart J 1990; 119:291–300.

4. White CJ, Ramee SR, Banks AK, Mesa JE, Chokshi S, Isner JM. A new balloon-expandable tantalum coil stent: angiographic patency and histologic findings in an atherogenic swine model. J Am Coll Cardiol 1992; 19:870–876.

5. Muller DOOM, Ellis SG, Topol EJ. Experimental models of coronary restenosis. J Am Coll Cardiol 1992; 19:418–432.

6. Schwartz RS, Murphy JG, Edwards WD, Camrud AR, Vlietstra RE, Holmes DR. Restenosis after balloon angioplasty: a practical proliferative model in porcine coronary arteries. Circulation 1990; 82:2190–2200.

7. Schwartz RS, Huber KC, Murphy JG, et al. Restenosis and the proportional neointimal response to coronary artery injury: results in a porcine model. J Am Coll Cardiol 1992; 19:267–274.

8. Karas SP, Gravanis MB, Santoian EC, Robinson KA, Anderberg KA, King SB, 3rd. Coronary intimal proliferation after balloon injury and stenting in swine: an animal model of restenosis. J Am Coll Cardiol 1992; 20:467–474.

9. Bonan R, Paiement P, Scortichini D, Cloutier M-J, Leung TK. Coronary restenosis: evaluation of a restenosis injury index in a swine model. Am Heart J 1993; 126:1334–1340.

10. Carter AJ, Laird JR, Farb A, Kufs W, Wortham DC, Virmani R. Morphologic characteristics of lesion formation and time course of smooth muscle cell proliferation in a porcine proliferative restenosis model. J Am Coll Cardiol 1994; 24:1398–1405.

11. Grinstead WC, Rogers GP, Mazur W, et al. Comparison of three porcine restenosis models: the relative importance of hypercholesterolemia, endothelial abrasion, and stenting. Coronary Artery Dis 1994; 5:425–434.

12. Prescott MF, Hasler-Rapacz J, Von Linden-Reed J, Rapacz J. Familial hypercholesterolemia associated with coronary atherosclerosis in swine bearing different alleles for apolipoprotein B. Ann NY Acad Sci 1995; 748:283–293.

13. Recchia D, Abendschein DR, Saffitz JE, Wickline SA. The biologic behavior of balloon hyperinflation-induced arterial lesions in hypercholesterolemic pigs depends on the presence of foam cells. Arterioscler Thromb Vasc Biol 1995; 15:924–929.

14. Swindle MM, Horneffer PJ, Gardner TJ, Gott VL, Hall TS, Stuart RS, et al. Anatomic and anesthetic considerations in experimental cardiopulmonary surgery in swine. Lab Anim Sci 1986; 36:357–361.

15. Rodgers GP, Cromeens DM, Minor ST, Swindle MM. Bretylium and diltiazem in porcine cardiac procedures. J Investig Surgery 1988; 1:321–326.

16. Farb A, Virmani R, Atkinson JB, Kolodgie FD. Plaque morphology and pathologic changes in arteries from patients dying after coronary balloon angioplasty. J Am Coll Cardiol 1990; 16:1421–1429.

17. Virmani R, Farb A, Burke AP. Coronary angioplasty from the perspective of atherosclerotic plaque: morphologic predictors of immediate success and restenosis. Am Heart J 1994; 127:163–179.

18. Carter AJ, Farb A, Laird JR, Virmani R. Neointimal formation is dependent on the underlying arterial substrate after coronary stent placement (Abstract). J Am Coll Cardiol 1996; 320A.

19. Carter AJ, Scott D, Bailey L, Fischell DR, Fischell RE, Jones R, et al. High Actvity ^{32}P Stents Promote the Formation of an Atheromatous Neointima in an Atherosclerotic Model. Circulation 1997; 96:I-607.

4

Nonhuman Primate Models of Arterial Injury and Repair

Mark Nedelman, MS,
Christopher Horvath, DVM, MS,
and Campbell Rogers, MD

CONTENTS

INTRODUCTION

The development of new and effective therapies for the prevention of intimal hyperplasia or restenosis and other vascular diseases has relied largely on the use of experimental animal models of vascular injury. The development and use of certain experimental models have been invaluable in the development of new pharmaceuticals in areas such as thrombosis and thrombolysis. The results generated from studies in models of restenosis have suggested that numerous compounds from a wide variety of pharmacological classes appear to be efficacious in inhibiting the proliferative response following acute vascular injury, such as that which occurs during percutaneous coronary interventions. While great strides in elucidating the hematologic, cellular, and molecular response to vascular injury have come from this body of work, no universally accepted pharmacologic treatment or intervention has yet been demonstrated to significantly and reproducibly reduce the incidence of restenosis after acute vascular injury (as caused by balloon angioplasty and/or stent placement) in humans.

From: *Contemporary Cardiology: Vascular Disease and Injury: Preclinical Research*
Edited by: D. I. Simon and C. Rogers © Humana Press Inc., Totowa, NJ

The majority of studies in the field of restenosis have used rat, rabbit, or pig models of vascular injury. Considering the poor track record that each of these experimental models has had to date in predicting efficacy in man, we sought to characterize the pathophysiological response in a nonhuman primate following acute vascular injury. The goal of our studies has been to expand the tools currently available for investigating mechanisms of neointimal formation and ultimately to develop new therapies for treating restenosis and other related pathologies. There is scant published data on vascular injury in nonhuman primate models, *(1)* yet our efforts would not only allow examination in a species closer to clinical settings, but also allow study of novel biotherapeutics developed for human use with limited species cross-reactivity.

MATERIALS AND METHODS

Animals

Male cynomolgus monkeys *(Macaca fascicularis)* were selected for study, and weighed 3.5–4.5 kg at study initiation. Animals were sexually mature and considered to be adults. All animals completed a period of quarantine prior to initiation. During this period, three intradermal tuberculin tests were conducted at approx 2-wk intervals on all monkeys. The monkeys were released from quarantine after the third consecutive negative tuberculin test. Various samples were also collected, including blood for hematology and clinical chemistry, rectal swab for culture, and feces for ova and parasite determinations. A physical examination was also performed prior to release, including ophthalmic examination on all animals. All animals were determined to be in good health as determined by a Test Facility veterinarian. Individual animals were monitored and followed throughout the course of quarantine and study by permanent tattoo and/or collar tag.

The Test Facility is accredited by the Association for Assessment and Accreditation of Laboratory Animal Care (AAALAC) and licensed by the United States Department of Agriculture (USDA) to conduct research in laboratory animals in compliance with the Animal Welfare Act, USDA regulations, and National Research Council (NRC) guidelines. All animal activities described here were subject to review and approval by the Institutional Animal Care and Use Committee (IACUC) of the Test Facility.

Animal Husbandry and Diet

All procedures were performed as described in the Guide for the Care and Use of Laboratory Animals, National Research Council (Revised 1996) and/or in accordance with the Standard Operating Procedures of the Test Facility. Animals were individually housed during quarantine and study periods. All husbandry supplies and environmental conditions were identical at all times. Room temperature in the animal quarters was maintained between 18°C–29°C (64°F–84°F), and the humidity range between 30–70%. Rooms were on a 12–h light/dark cycle with at least 10 air changes per h.

All animals were fed daily and maintained on a diet of LabChows (Purina Mills, Inc. Certified Primate Chow Brand Animal Diet 5048). As part of the Test Facilities primate enrichment program, all animals had their diet supplemented with washed, fresh produce. Tap water was provided to all animals *ad libitum*. Biannual water analyses were conducted by an independent laboratory for analyses including heavy metals, chlorinated hydrocarbons, organophosphates, nitrates, nitrites, standard plate count, total trihalomenthanes, and dissolved minerals—and the possibility that any of these interfering substances may have on study outcome was considered.

In Vivo Procedures

To date, many of the clinical trials investigating new antirestenotic therapies have employed continuous infusion of a drug for a period of time either starting before intervention or at the time of a procedure as a means of maintaining "therapeutic" blood levels. In order for this to occur in an experimental setting, animals should be instrumented so that delivery of a drug by continuous infusion is possible while minimizing stress and the need for frequent tranquilization or anesthesia. Otherwise, repetitive iv, sc, or ip injections have been administered to animals in an attempt to maintain adequate blood concentrations of a drug. With this process, it is difficult, if not impossible, to evaluate drug pharmacokinetics and pharmacodynamics.

We have previously developed and characterized a system whereby animals have vascular access ports (VAPs) placed intravenously, for both continuous infusion and/or blood collection. A drug may then be continuously infused, via a jacket-and-tether system, while animals are "free" within their caging, and/or blood may be obtained for analyses with a minimum of restraint or stress. Two separate VAPs are used when simultaneous drug administration and blood sampling are required.

Anesthesia

The animals were preanesthetized (ketamine HCl, 10 mg/kg im, atropine SO_4, 0.04 mg/kg im) prior to preparation for surgery for VAP placement and or vascular injury, and immediately intubated and maintained in anesthesia with isoflurane inhalant anesthetic. The $ETCO_2$ was maintained within individual physiological ranges. An intravenous catheter was placed in a peripheral vein for administration of fluids during anesthesia (lactated ringers solution) at a rate of 5–10 mL/kg/h.

Antibiotic Therapy

Animals were given a single injection of benzathine/procain penicillin G (42,000 IU/kg, im) prior to surgery and/or interventional procedures.

Surgical Procedures (Vascular Access Ports)

A skin incision measuring approx 2–3 cm is made approx 1 cm cranial to the inguinal ring, and about 1 cm ventral to the iliac crest. The underlying muscles are exposed, and the wound is retracted with a self-retaining retractor. The iliac artery and vein are then exposed by performing a myotomy of the gluteal muscles ventral to where they attach to the iliac crest. The iliac vein is mobilized a distance of about 1 cm prior to its entrance into the abdominal cavity. Two encircling ligatures are then placed around the vein, approx 1 cm apart (the distal one will be tied). A 1- to 2-cm incision is then made in the skin immediately caudal to the last rib, and about 1 cm ventral to the midline. A subcutaneous pocket in this area is made to accommodate the presence of the VAP, and a trocar is passed between this incision and the one overlying the iliac vessels. A 5 Fr coated polyurethane catheter is passed through the trocar from the inguinal incision to the paralumbar one, and the trocar is removed. The catheter is attached to the VAP cranially, and filled with the irrigation solution. A small phlebotomy is then made in the vein between the two ligatures and the catheter is introduced cranially into the vein at a distance of about 5 cm, or to the first "suture bulb" on the catheter. The ligatures are tied, securing the catheter within the vein. The cranial portion of the catheter is then cut to length, and attached to the VAP, which is finally positioned in the previously created subcutaneous pocket. The VAP is immobilized to the underlying muscle with two sutures of 2/0 monofilament nylon, and the wound closed in at least two layers with appropriately sized absorbable suture material. The skin is closed in a subcuticular pattern with appropriately sized absorbable suture material. The inguinal incision is also closed in layers, and the skin is approximated with absorbable suture material in a subcuticular pattern. Animals are allowed to recover for a minimum of 7 d post-VAP surgery before subsequent vascular injury procedures.

Experimental Model (Balloon Denudation and Stent Implantation)

A number of studies employing the same basic procedures have been conducted in the development and characterization of this model. Animals are anesthetized as previously described and positioned in dorsal recumbency on a fluoroscopy table. All sites for vascular access are clipped and prepared for aseptic surgery. The right carotid artery is surgically exposed and isolated, and a 6F percutaneous vascular introducer sheath (CP-07711, Arrow International, Reading, PA, or equivalent) is inserted and secured into the carotid artery to

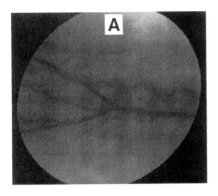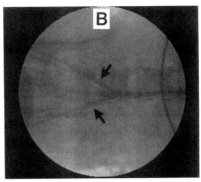

Fig. 1. Angiograms of monkey aorta and iliac arteries before (**A**) and after (**B**) bilateral iliac stent implantation. Stents are implanted to achieve slight overstretching of the iliac arteries (B arrows).

facilitate interventional catheter placement. A single dose of heparin (100 U/ kg, iv) targeted to elevate activated clotting time (ACT) to greater than 250 s is administered prior to vascular injury and monitored using a Hemochron Whole Blood Coagulation System (Model 801). Additional heparin is administered if necessary to maintain anticoagulation. A 6F guide catheter (Cordis Corp.) is then passed antegrade under fluoroscopic guidance proximal to where the abdominal aorta bifurcates into the right and left iliac arteries. Radioopaque contrast media (Omnipaque, iohexol injection, Nycomed, Princeton, NJ, or equivalent) is used as necessary to facilitate visualization and placement of the guide catheter. If necessary, a radiopaque guide wire (0.0014-inch, Advanced Cardiovascular Systems, Inc., Temecula, CA) is used to help navigate the guide catheter into position.

Prior to angiography and vascular injury, nitroglycerine (50 µg, intraarterial) is administered through the guide catheter as a bolus injection. Quantitative angiograms are then performed for estimation of vessel size (luminal diameter of the targeted area for stenting), using the guide catheter as an internal reference (Fig. 1A). All angiograms used for quantitation are recorded on videotape for possible future evaluation. Once arteries have been sized, endothelial denudation is performed in the iliac arteries. A 3F Fogarty balloon embolectomy catheter (Baxter Healthcare Corp., Irvine, CA), is passed through the guide catheter into one of the iliac arteries to a level approx 4 cm distal to the bifurcation. The balloon is then inflated with 0.6 cc of air and withdrawn approx 3 cm with the feeling of resistance. This procedure is performed three times in the selected vessel and then duplicated in the contralateral iliac artery.

After performing denuding injury in the arteries, stents (i.e., Palmaz-Schatz balloon-expandable stents, Cordis/Johnson & Johnson, Miami, FL, or equivalent) are mounted on appropriately sized angioplasty balloons (2.5–3.5F, 15 mm Ninja, Cordis Corp., or equivalent) and prepared for deployment. Angioplasty catheters with stents are passed through the guide catheter under fluoroscopy and positioned into one of the iliac arteries to a level of the midpoint of endothelial denudation. Once properly positioned, stents are deployed by balloon inflation using an Indeflator Plus (Advanced Cardiovascular System, Inc.) to nominal balloon pressure (6–12 ATM), yielding a balloon/stent-to-artery ratio of 1.1–1.2:1.

After the second stent has been deployed and the angioplasty catheter has been withdrawn, nitroglycerine (50 μg, intraarterial) is injected via the guide catheter, and angiograms are obtained and recorded for quantification of midpoint in-stent luminal diameter (Fig. 1B). The guide catheter and arterial sheath are then removed, the carotid artery is ligated, the incision is closed, and animals are recovered from anesthesia and returned to their cages.

Treatment

In addition to the periprocedural heparin administered to prevent clotting during interventional procedures, animals were treated with oral aspirin (~10 mg/kg) starting 3 d before vascular injury and daily thereafter for the remainder of the study.

Follow-Up

If desired, prior to euthanasia, quantitative angiography of the midpoint in-stent luminal diameters may be determined after anesthesia and passage of a guide catheter via the left carotid artery. This measurement allows calculation of the degree of neointimal proliferation, or late luminal loss.

Necropsy

Upon completion of the 28-d in-life portion of the study, animals are anesthetized with pentobarbital and perfused prior to collecting vessels. Bromodeoxyuridine (BrDU, 50 mg/kg, Sigma) is administered 1 h before collection to allow for identification of proliferating cells. A thoracotomy is performed and cannula placed within the left ventricle directed up towards the aortic arch. A cut is made in the vena cava and the animal is perfused by gravity with 1 L of PBS followed by 1 L of 0.4% paraformaldehyde (PFA). The abdominal contents are removed and iliac arteries are carefully dissected both proximal and distal to the sites of injury and placed in PFA.

HISTOPATHOLOGY AND MORPHOMETRY

Specimens are embedded in methyl methacrylate mixed with *n*-butyl methacrylate (Sigma Chemical Co., St. Louis, MO) as previously described *(2)*. Five-

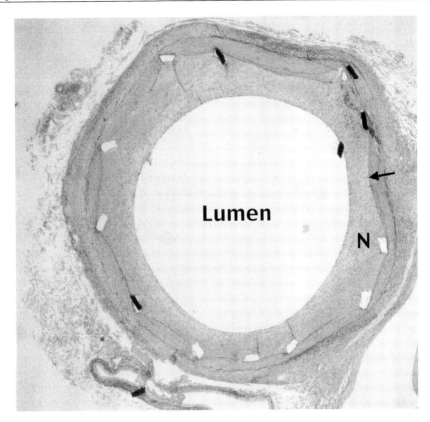

Fig. 2. Photomicrograph of monkey iliac artery 28 d after stent implantation (Verhoeff tissue elastin stain). A thick neointima **(N)** separates the internal elastic lamina (arrow) and stent struts from the lumen. (See color plate 2 appearing in the insert following p. 236).

μ sections are cut using a tungsten-carbide knife (Delaware Diamond Knives, Inc, Wilmington, DE). Tissue and cell structures as well as the depth of stent-related injury *(3)* are identified in histological sections by staining with Verhoeff's tissue elastin stain (Fig. 2) or hematoxylin and eosin. Neointimal, luminal, and medial cross-sectional areas are measured by computer-assisted digital planimetry. The luminal surface can be examined for adherent leukocytes.

Macrophages can be identified immunocytochemically with an antihuman macrophage antibody (HAM-56, DAKO Co, Carpenteria, CA). The number of proliferating cells can be quantified immunocytochemically on the basis of their incorporation of BrdU (anti-BrdU, DAKO Co., Carpenteria, CA), and smooth-muscle cells with anti-SMC actin (DAKO). Standard immunocytochemical protocols *(4)* are used in conjunction with heat-induced epitope retrieval. Sections are heated to 92°C in Target Retrieval Solution (DAKO Co, Carpenteria, CA), incubated with the primary antibody followed by a biotinylated sp-specific secondary antibody (Vector Laboratories Inc., Burlingame, CA), and stained with avidin-biotin peroxidase or avidin-biotin-alkaline phosphatase followed by 3,3–diaminobenzidine (Sigma Chemical Co, St. Louis, MO) or alkaline phosphatase (Vector Laboratories Inc., Burlingame, CA). Overall cell density was calculated by dividing the number of nuclei by the intimal area. The proportion of cells staining for HAM-56, SMC actin, or BrdU, in the intima or media, is calculated by dividing the number of positively stained cells by the total number of intimal or medial cells.

CONCLUSIONS

Nonhuman primates may offer advantages as experimental models in the study of vascular disease. Our examination of responses following endovascular stent placement in iliac arteries demonstrates brisk and concentric neointimal thickening comprising both smooth-muscle cells and cells of monocyte/macropahge origin. This finding has many parallels to responses in other species, and may be a central element in evaluating novel *biotherapeutics* intended for clinical use but with limited species cross-reactivity. It remains to be seen whether these models will also prove to be better predictors of human responses than nonprimate species have been.

ACKNOWLEDGMENT

This work was supported by grants from the National Institutes of Health (HL03104 to CR).

REFERENCES

1. Geary RL, Koyama N, Wang TW, Vergel S, Clowes AW. Failure of heparin to inhibit intimal hyperplasia in injured baboon arteries. Circulation 1995; 91:2972–2981.
2. Rogers C, Karnovsky MJ, Welt FGP, Edelman ER. Monocyte adhesion and neointimal hyperplasia in rabbits: coupled inhibitory effects of heparin. Arterioscler Thromb Vasc Biol 1996; 16:1312–1318.
3. Schwartz RS, Huber KC, Murphy JG, Edwards WD, Camrud AR, Vlietstra RE, et al. Restenosis and proportional neointimal response to coronary artery injury: results in a porcine model. J Am Coll Cardiol 1992; 19:267–274.
4. Rogers C, Edelman ER, Simon DI. A monoclonal antibody to Mac-1 (CD11b/CD18) blocks leukocyte recruitment and reduces intimal thickening after experimental angioplasty or stent implantation. Proc Natl Acad Sci 1998; 95:10,134–10,139.

5   Experimental Models of Arteriovenous Grafting

Afshin Ehsan, MD, Michael J. Mann, MD, and Victor J. Dzau, MD

INTRODUCTION

Venous tissue remains the most widely used arterial conduit for the treatment of occlusive coronary and peripheral vascular disease. However, neointima formation and the accelerated rate of atherosclerosis in these grafts leads to an unacceptably high failure rate, necessitating reoperation or revision in 50% of patients within 10 yr. Other conduit systems have proven to be less reliable because of limitations in availability or higher rates of thrombogenicity. Prosthetic arteriovenous (AV) conduits have become the predominant mode of long-term access for patients who require chronic hemodialysis. Expanded polytetrafluoroethylene (ePTFE) is the most commonly used prosthetic material in the construction of these grafts. The increased use of prosthetic conduits

From: *Contemporary Cardiology: Vascular Disease and Injury: Preclinical Research*
Edited by: D. I. Simon and C. Rogers © Humana Press Inc., Totowa, NJ

61

over the past 20 yr has accompanied an increase in the ages of patients on dialysis, and an increase both in the length of time patients are on dialysis and the severity of their vascular disease *(1)*. With the increased use of prosthetic conduits comes an increase in graft complications. Thrombosis of the graft, which is usually caused by venous outflow obstruction, is the most common complication, followed by infection and false aneurysm formation *(1,2)*. As a result, much emphasis has been placed on improving our understanding of the pathobiological effects of venous and prosthetic grafting, with the goal of improving long-term graft patency.

This challenge has led to the development of multiple animal models which can reproducibly create the pathobiology seen in both systems. More importantly, they allow us to gain insight into the dysfunctional mechanisms leading to failure, and the means to test novel therapeutic approaches for improving long-term graft patency. In this chapter we present an in-depth review of the variety of animal models available, with detailed information on the technical aspects of these models. We also provide guidelines for general pre- and postoperative care and available anesthetic and analgesic regimens required for successful implementation of these models. (In considering the appropriate anesthetic or analgesic regimens, please consult your facilities veterinarian for more detailed assistance). Finally, we discuss novel strategies for improving vein and AV graft patency through the prevention of neointimal hyperplasia, and the reduction of graft-wall thrombogenicity with the application of novel gene- and cell-based approaches to tissue bioengineering.

RODENT MODELS

Mouse Carotid Interposition Vein Graft

In choosing the strain of mice to be used, one must consider whether a particular strain is able to manifest certain background pathology which can influence vein graft biology, and which genetically altered strains are available and can provide relevant disease models. For studying vein graft disease, it may be important to work with models of experimental atherosclerosis, such as the apo E knockout mouse. Three-month-old mice, weighing 25–30 g should be used for vein grafting.

Mice are anesthetized with ip sodium pentobarbital (50 mg/kg body weight). Atropine sulfate (1.7 mg/kg body weight) is also administered in order to maintain the respiratory tract. The mouse is then secured to the bench in the supine position with the neck extended, and the skin is cleansed using 70% ethanol. Under a dissecting microscope, a midline incision is made on the ventral side of the neck from the lower aspect of the mandible to the sternum. The right cleidomastoid muscle is identified and resected. The right common carotid artery is mobilized from the level of the distal bifurcation, and the vessel is tied off in the middle segment, both proximally and distally, using 8-0 silk suture. The vessel is transected between the ties, and each end is passed through cuffs made of a polyethylene cannula with a 0.65-mm outer and 0.5-mm inner diameter (Portex LTD, London, United Kingdom). Each cuff is 1 mm in length, with a 1-mm handle or extension. The vessel along with the cuff handle is fixed by microhemostat clamps 4 mm in length (Martin, Tuttlingen, Germany). The sutures at both ends of the artery are removed, and a segment of the artery is carefully everted over the cuff with fine tweezers and fixed to the cuff with an 8-0 silk suture.

In this model, one can choose to use either the autologous external jugular vein, the isogenic jugular vein, or an isogenic vena cava such as the conduit. The right external jugular vein is exposed, and its branches are ligated using electrocautery. The proximal and distal ends are then tied off using 8-0 silk suture, and a 1-cm segment of the vessel is explanted. In order to harvest the vena cava, a midline abdominal incision is made in a donor mouse, and 0.5 mL of saline containing 100 U/mL of heparin is injected into the inferior vena cava. After approx 3 min, the anterior thoracic cage is opened from the level of the diaphragm and incised laterally to the internal mammary vessels. A 1-cm segment of the intrathoracic vena cava is dissected and removed. The grafts are then washed with saline containing 100 U/mL of heparin. Each end of the vein segment is sleeved over the artery cuffs and secured in place using 8-0 silk suture. The cuff handles are cut off when the anastomosis is complete, followed by removal of the vascular clamps. The skin is then closed with either a running or interrupted 6-0 silk suture (Fig. 1) *(42)*.

Rat Femoral Artery Interposition Vein Grafts

Male rats weighing between 325–400 g are anesthetized using either sodium pentobarbital (40 mg/kg) or ketamine (90 mg/kg) and xylazine (4 mg/kg) intraperitoneally. The animal is secured to the bench in the supine position and the skin is cleansed using 70% ethanol. Using a dissecting microscope, an incision is made in the right in the inguinal region, and the superficial epigastric vein and common femoral artery are dissected free from their surrounding tissue. The vein is tied off proximally and distally using 6-0 silk suture, and an 8-mm segment of the epigastric vein is excised and irrigated with heparinized saline. Hemostatic clamps are then placed proximally and distally on the artery, a 5-mm portion is excised, and the divided ends are flushed using heparinized saline. An end-to-end arteriovenous anastomosis is constructed using an interrupted 10-0 monofilament suture both proximally and distally. The clamps are removed to restore blood flow, and hemostasis is achieved. The wound is gently irrigated and closed using a running 5-0 silk suture (Fig. 2) *(3,4)*.

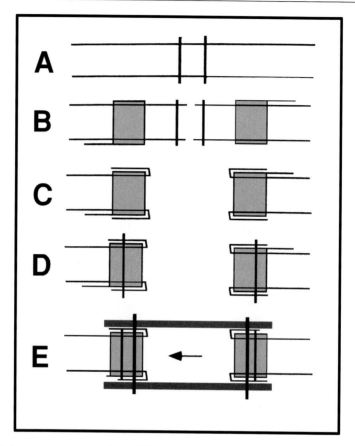

Fig. 1. Schematic representation of the murine vein graft model. The right common carotid artery is ligated with an 8-0 silk suture (**A**) and dissected between the middle ties
and passed through the cuffs, respectively (**B**). The vessel, together with the cuff handle,
is fixed with microhemostat clamps; the suture at the end of the artery is removed; and a
segment of the artery is turned inside out with a stent and fine tweezers to cover the cuff
body (**C**), which is fixed to the cuff with an 8-0 silk suture (**D**). A segment of the right
external jugular vein or vena cava (1 cm) is harvested and grafted between the two ends
of the carotid artery by sleeving the ends of the vein over the artery cuff and suturing them
together with an 8-0 ligature (**E**). The cuff handle is cut off, and the vascular clamps are
removed. Reproduced with permission from ref. *(42)*.

Rat Aortic Interposition Vein Graft

Male rats weighing between 250–350 g are anesthetized using ketamine (50
mg/kg) and xylazine (3 mg/kg) intramuscularly, supplemented with ip administration of ketamine for maintenance. The animal is secured to the bench in the
supine position, the skin is cleansed using 70% ethanol, and a midline neck
incision is made. Under a dissecting microscope, the jugular vein is isolated

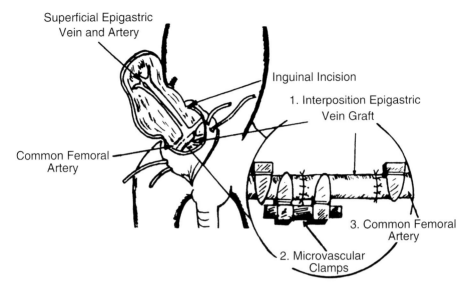

Superficial Epigastric
Vein and Artery

Inguinal Incision

1. Interposition Epigastric
Vein Graft

Common Femoral
Artery

3. Common Femoral
Artery

2. Microvascular
Clamps

Fig. 2. Schematic representation of the rat vein graft model. The inguinal fat pad is exposed and the superficial epigastric vein is dissected free from the surrounding tissue. Femoral vessels are isolated in preparation for grafting. Procedure is performed bilaterally in each rat. *Inset,* Superficial epigastric vein is interposition grafted to the femoral artery in an end-to-end fashion. Reproduced with permission from ref. *(3).*

and its branches are carefully ligated with a 5-0 silk suture. The vessel is then tied off proximally and distally, excised, and kept moist in a heparinized saline solution. The incision is closed using a running 5-0 silk suture, and using a midline abdominal incision, the abdominal aorta is identified and isolated. Hemostatic clamps are applied proximally and distally to the infrarenal portion of the aorta, and a 1-cm segment of the artery is excised. A 1-cm-segment vein is oriented in the reverse direction, and an end-to-end anastomosis is constructed using a running 10-0 monofilament suture. The clamps are removed to allow flow through the graft, and hemostasis is achieved. The wound is irrigated and the skin is closed using a running 5-0 silk suture *(5)*. Notably, Sterpetti et al. *(6)* has successfully implemented this model using the subdiaphragmatic vena cava from an isogenic rat to perform the bypass.

RABBIT MODELS

General Considerations for Rabbit Surgery

White New Zealand male rabbits weighing 3–3.5 kg should be used. Anesthesia is induced using either ketamine (2.5 mg/mL) and xylazine (0.09 mg/mL) intravenously (1-mL induction dose and 0.5-mL boluses as needed to maintain adequate anesthesia) or ketamine (22–50 mg/kg) and xylazine (2.5–10 mg/

kg) intramuscularly. For iv access, the marginal vein of the ear is cannulated with a 24-gauge angiocath. Intramuscular delivery of medications can be performed by injecting into either the anterior or posterior aspect of the thigh. Prophylactic antibiotics with coverage for gram-positive skin organisms are administered intramuscularly at the time of induction. Postoperatively, the animal can receive a number of opiate or nonsteroidal regimens delivered subcutaneously, intramuscularly, or intravenously for a period of time adequate to ensure comfort for the animal *(7)*.

Specific Models

CAROTID OR FEMORAL ARTERY INTERPOSITION VEIN GRAFT

The animal is placed in the supine position, and either the neck or the right inguinal region is prepped and draped in the usual sterile fashion. A dissecting microscope or loupe magnification is used. Under sterile conditions, a midline neck incision is made from the level of the larynx to the sternum or an oblique incision is made, and both the right femoral artery and vein are exposed. For the carotid model, a 3-cm segment of the right jugular vein is exposed proximal to its bifurcation. For the femoral model a 1.5–2-cm segment of the femoral vein is dissected. Branches are ligated using 4-0 silk suture, and the vessel is tied off proximally and distally and excised. Following excision, the vein is kept moist in a heparinized saline solution. Heparin, 1–200 U/kg, is administered intravenously and allowed to circulate for 1–2 min as either the right carotid or femoral artery is identified and dissected out. Hemostatic clamps are placed proximally and distally on the artery, and a 0.5-cm segment is excised. The vein is oriented in the reverse direction, and an end-to-end anastomosis is constructed using either an interrupted 7-0 or a running 10-0 monofilament suture. The clamps are then removed to allow flow through the graft, and hemostasis is achieved. The wound is irrigated, and the skin is closed using a running 4-0 monofilament suture *(8–11)*.

LARGE ANIMAL MODELS

General Considerations for Surgery on Large Animals

Animals are fasted for 12 h prior to surgery. Induction of anesthesia can be achieved by administration of a number of iv medications, and is followed by endotracheal intubation and maintenance of anesthesia using either halothane or isoflurane. Commonly used access sites are listed for each species in Table 1. To reduce rates of infection, the animals should receive prophylactic antibiotics with coverage for both gram-positive skin organisms and gram-negative organisms such as *E. coli*, approx 1 h before and 6 h after surgery. For long-term studies, the animals should also receive the same coverage for approx 5–7 d postoperatively. For effective management of postoperative pain, the animals

Table 1

Access Sites for Large Animals

Dogs	Sheep	Pigs	Baboons
Subcutaneous	Intravenous	Subcutaneous	Subcutaneous
Interscapular region	Jugular vein	Neck	Lateral thigh
Lateral thoracic region	Auricular v.	Flank	
Lumbar dorsal region	Cephalic v.		Intramuscular
	Saphenous v.	Intramuscular	Caudal thigh muscle
Intramuscular		Caudal thigh	
Caudal thigh		Semimembranous muscle	Intravenous
Semimembranosus muscle		Semitendinosus m.	Cephalic vein
Semitendinosus m.		Cranial thigh	Saphenous v.
		Gluteal m.	
Intravenous			
Saphenous vein		Intravenous	
Cephalic v.		Ear vein	
Jugular v.		Cephalic v.	
		Lateral saphenous v.	
		Median saphenous v.	

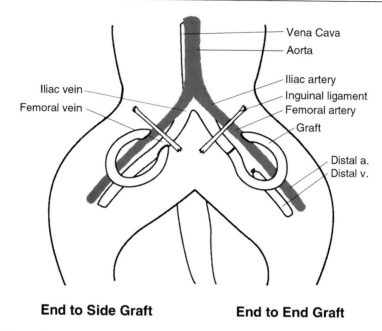

End to Side Graft   **End to End Graft**

Fig. 3. Schematic representation of the canine arteriovenous graft model. The graft is anastamosed to the femoral artery in an end-to-side fashion while the femoral venous anastamosis may be performed end-to-side or end-to-end. Reproduced with permission from ref. *(19)*.

can receive a number of opiate or nonsteroidal regimens delivered subcutaneously, intramuscularly, or intravenously for a period of time adequate to ensure comfort for the animal *(12–14,43)*. Finally, in an effort to further ensure proper wound healing or prevention of injury to chronic externalized grafts, the animals may wear a wide collar for 5–7 d, along with a protective jacket when necessary.

CANINE MODELS

Femoral Artery to Femoral Vein End-to-Side Loop Arteriovenous Graft

The most common model used in the study of pretreated or modified forms of ePTFE is the canine femoral artery to femoral vein end-to-side loop graft. Mongrel dogs (25–30 kg) are placed in the supine position. Under sterile conditions, using loupe magnification, the common femoral artery and vein are exposed bilaterally via a transverse incision 3 cm below the inguinal ligament. The animals are then systemically heparinized (100 U/kg), and the vessels are clamped proximally and distally. Using a 6-mm diameter and 25-mm ePTFE graft, an end-to-side anastomosis is made to both the artery and vein using a

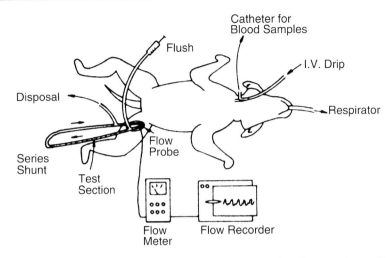

Fig. 4. Schematic of canine arteriovenous graft model showing shunt, catheter, flow measurement and recording instrumentation. Reproduced with permission from ref. *(20)*.

running 6-0 polypropylene suture. The arterial anastomosis is placed caudal to the venous anastomosis. The use of bilateral femoral vessels allows for internal controls, and therefore minimizes the number of animals needed for each study. The wounds are then closed in layers using a running 4-0 Vicryl suture *(15–18)* (Fig. 3). In a report by Fillinger, et al., it was determined that an end-to-end venous anastomosis does not significantly differ from an end-to-side venous anastomosis in terms of stability, turbulence, kinetic energy transfer, or magnitude of the hyperplastic response *(19)*.

Ex Vivo Arteriovenous Series Shunts

In order to assess the degree of thrombus deposition on various polymer surfaces, a canine ex vivo model for arteriovenous series shunt evaluation has been developed. This model allows for the testing of multiple polymeric surfaces in the same nonanticoagulated animal. For further details on the insertion of various polymers in series, please refer to the references cited *(20,21)*.

The model commonly used for acute ex vivo experiments requires exposure and ligation of the femoral artery and vein on one side under sterile conditions as previously described. The artery and vein are then cannulated with polyethylene tubing connected to the series shunt. The shunt section is initially filled with a degassed, divalent cation-free solution, such as Tyrode's solution, to prevent blood–air contact. A small branch artery, proximal to the shunt cannulation site, is cannulated with a polyethylene IV. 16-g catheter and connected to a syringe containing Tyrode's solution. The purpose of the branch cannulation is to enable the blood to be flushed out of the shunt following a predetermined interval of blood flow through the shunt. This method is necessary in order to detect the specific radiolabeled blood products deposited on the polymer surfaces. The flushing procedure consists of flushing 20 mL of Tyrode's solution through the shunt—thus returning the bulk of the blood in the shunt to the venous circulation— followed by flushing 35 mL of solution into the receptacle for disposal via a standard "T" on the venous end of the shunt (Fig. 4). This two-step procedure avoids dilution of the animal's blood with Tyrode's solution. Immediately after flushing, the joined test section is removed and fixed for further analysis. Another new set of test surfaces can be placed in series and tested at various time points as needed. Blood flow should be continuously monitored using a noninvasive electromagnetic flow transducer connected to a recorder. The animal is euthanized after the procedure *(20)*.

In an effort to assess long-term thrombus deposition on polymer surfaces, a model of chronically implanted iliac arteriovenous ex vivo shunt has been established. An abdominal incision is made under sterile conditions. The bowel and bladder are displaced, and the right common iliac vein and left external iliac artery are exposed. Approx 5 cm of the exposed vessel is isolated and ligated distally using 2-0 silk suture. Proximally, a ligature is temporarily placed under gentle tension to stop blood flow. An incision is made in the vessel wall and opened with forceps just large enough to insert the cannulating portion of the shunt a distance of 10 cm within the vessel. The shunt is sutured in place and positioned in a moderate curve along the floor of the abdominal cavity, using attachment points on the shunt at the junction of the vessel's distal ligature and the abdominal wall. It is then tunneled subcutaneously to the shoulder region of the animal, where it exits the body through a small incision with a Dacron cuff left just under the surface of the skin. The shunt is filled with sterile saline and clamped occlusively on the exteriorized ends. The abdominal incision is then closed in a layered fashion, and the exterior ends of the arterial and venous limbs are trimmed to the appropriate length, and connected in an abutted joint. Occluding clamps are removed and blood flow is established. Blood-flow rates are monitored with a Doppler ultrasonic blood-flow meter using an 8–MHz flat probe calibrated with the timed volumetric collection of blood *(21)* (Fig. 5).

Carotid or Femoral Artery Interposition Vein Graft

These model allows for the flexibility of using right and left arteries without significant morbidity. The neck or inguinal region is prepped and draped. Under sterile conditions, either a lateral neck incision or a longitudinal thigh incision is made. In the neck, a 4-cm segment of the external jugular vein is isolated distal to the internal and external maxillary veins and proximal to the brachiocephalic branch with careful ligation of all branches using a 4-0 silk suture. In the thigh, the femoral artery and vein are isolated, a 4-cm segment of the femo-

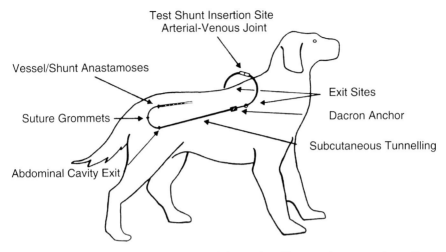

Test Shunt Insertion Site
Arterial-Venous Joint

Vessel/Shunt Anastamoses

Suture Grommets

Abdominal Cavity Exit

Exit Sites

Dacron Anchor

Subcutaneous Tunnelling

Fig. 5. Approximate anatomical position of the canine iliac arteriovenous shunt. Reproduced with permission from ref. *(21)*.

ral vein is dissected, and branches are ligated with 4-0 silk suture. The vein is tied off proximally and distally and excised, and is kept moist in a heparinized saline solution while either the carotid or femoral artery is dissected. In the neck, lateral incisions are closed using a running 4-0 Vicryl suture, and the carotid artery is isolated through a midline incision. The animal is heparinized (100 U/kg), the artery is clamped proximally and distally, and a 2-cm segment is excised. The vein is oriented in the reverse direction, and a spatulated end-to-end anastomosis is constructed using a running 7-0 monofilament suture. The clamps are removed to allow flow through the graft, and hemostasis is achieved. The wound is irrigated, and the skin is closed using a running 4-0 Vicryl suture *(22,23)*. In addition to the femoral and jugular veins, the cephalic vein is also an available conduit *(24)*.

SHEEP MODELS

Carotid Artery to Jugular Vein End-to-Side Loop Graft

Young adult sheep weighing approx 30–50 kg are placed in the supine position, and the neck is prepped and draped in the usual sterile manner. Under sterile conditions using loupe magnification, the right carotid artery and the left jugular vein are exposed through a single midline neck incision approx 10 cm in length. The animal is systemically heparinized (100 U/kg), and the vessels are clamped proximally and distally. Using a 6-mm diameter and an ePTFE graft 10–15 cm in length, an end-to-side anastomosis to both vessels is made with a running 7-0 monofilament suture. The graft should be laid across the neck in a superiorly arching loop configuration. The clamps are then removed to allow flow through the graft, and hemostasis is achieved. The wound is irrigated, and the skin is closed with a running 4-0 Vicryl suture *(25)*.

Femoral Artery Interposition Vein Graft

This model and the carotid artery interposition vein graft allow for the flexibility of using both femoral arteries for bypass reconstruction without significant morbidity to the animal. As mentioned previously, this can potentially reduce the number of animals needed because the contralateral reconstruction can act as an internal control. To begin, the animal is placed in the supine position and the inguinal region is prepped and draped in the usual sterile fashion. Under sterile conditions, a longitudinal thigh incision is made which extends to the level of the popliteal artery. Using loupe magnification, the femoral artery and vein are isolated. A segment of the femoral vein measuring approx 5–7 cm is dissected out, and using a 4-0 silk suture, its branches are ligated and the vessel is tied off proximally and distally and excised. Following excision, the vein is kept moist in a heparinized saline solution while the artery is dissected out. The animal is systemically heparinized (100 U/kg), and the femoral artery is clamped proximally and distally. With the vein oriented in the reverse direction, a spatulated end-to-side anastomosis is constructed from the proximal femoral artery to the above-knee popliteal artery, using a running 7-0 monofilament suture. The native femoral artery is then ligated between the proximal and distal anastomosis using a 4-0 silk suture. The clamps are removed to allow flow through the graft, and hemostasis is achieved. The wound is irrigated, and the skin is closed with a running 4-0 Vicryl suture *(26)*.

Carotid Artery Interposition Vein Graft

This model similarly allows for the flexibility of using both carotid arteries for bypass reconstruction without significant morbidity to the animal. The animal is placed in the supine position and the inguinal region is prepped and draped in the usual sterile fashion. Under sterile conditions, a longitudinal thigh incision is made, and using loupe magnification, one or both femoral veins are isolated. A segment measuring approx 4–5 cm of the vein is dissected out, and using a 4-0 silk suture, its branches are ligated, the vessel is tied off proximally and distally and excised. Following excision, the vein is kept moist in a heparinized saline solution while the incision is closed with a running 4-0 Vicryl suture. The neck is then prepped and draped, a midline incision is made, and one or both carotid arteries are isolated. The animal is systemically heparinized (100 U/kg), the carotid artery is clamped proximally and distally, and a 4–5-cm segment of the artery is excised. The vein is oriented in the reverse direction, and a spatulated end-to-end anastomosis is constructed using a running 7-0 monofilament suture. The clamps are removed to allow flow through the graft, and hemostasis is achieved. The wound is irrigated, and the skin is closed with a running 4-0 Vicryl suture *(27–29)*.

PORCINE MODEL
Carotid Interposition Vein Graft

Domestic crossbred pigs weighing approx 25–35 kg are placed in the supine position, and both thighs are prepped and draped in the usual sterile fashion. Under loupe magnification, bilateral long saphenous veins are isolated and their side branches are tied off with 3-0 silk suture. The vessel is tied off proximally and distally and excised. Following excision, the vein is kept moist in a heparinized saline solution while the incisions are closed with a running Vicryl suture. The neck is then prepped and draped, a midline incision is made, and one or both carotid arteries are isolated. The animal is systemically heparinized (150–300 U/kg), the carotid artery is clamped proximally and distally, and a 1–2-cm segment of the artery is excised. The vein is oriented in the reverse direction, and a spatulated end-to-end anastomosis is constructed using a running 8-0 monofilament suture. The clamps are removed to allow flow through the graft, and hemostasis is achieved. The wound is irrigated, and the skin is closed with a running 4-0 Vicryl suture *(30–32)*.

BABOON MODELS
Ex Vivo Chronic Arteriovenous Shunt

Nonhuman primate models offer a number of advantages for the study of potential human therapies to reduce arterial thrombosis. These advantages include:

1. Primate vascular anatomy;
2. Platelet structure, concentration, kinetics, and function similar to humans;
3. Coagulation, fibrinolytic, and inhibitor proteins in plasma similar to humans in concentration, kinetics, and function;
4. Proteins antigenically similar to humans permitting common use of immunologic probes and radioimmunoassays; and
5. Drug actions and pharmacokinetics similar to humans.

Male baboons (*papio* species) weighing between 10–15 kg are used after being dewormed and observed to be disease-free for at least 6 wk. Prior to placement of the chronic A-V cannula, the animals are acclimated to restraining chairs and contained in these chairs during the period of observation *(33)*. Silastic tubes are sterilized via autoclaving, and under sterile conditions, using the Seldinger technique, two 25-cm lengths of tubes, 3–4 mm in diameter (Dow

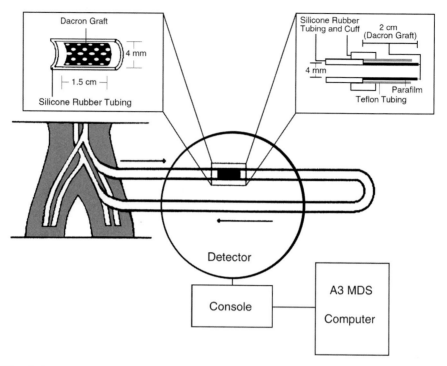

Fig. 6. Schematic representation of the experimental set-up to study platelet deposition. The enlarged device on the left was used for the long-term studies while the device on the right was used for the short-term studies. Reproduced with permission from ref. *(37)*.

Corning Corporation, Midland, MI), connected to 13–15-gauge vessel tips (Lifemed, Vernitron Corporation, Compton, CA) are inserted into the ipsilateral femoral artery and vein (Fig. 6). The two Silastic tubes can be secured using Dacron sewing cuffs at the exit skin sites and connected distally using a 1-cm (in length) and 3–4 cm (in diameter) blunt-edged Teflon connectors. Using this technique, one can generally perform up to four cannulations per femoral vessel in each baboon, thus permitting multiple reuse of each animal *(34–36)*. Cannula blood flow rate can be measured noninvasively with a Doppler ultrasonic flowmeter, using whole blood for calibration. The instrument can be equipped with an external "bobby pin"-type transducer probe that fits snugly around the Silastic tubing *(34,36)*.

Chronic Silastic A-V shunts in baboons can be rendered acutely thrombogenic under conditions of well-controlled flow and geometry by interposition of Dacron vascular grafts as extension segments of the A-V shunts *(34,37)*. Alternatively, irradiation of the Silastic tubing prior to insertion will also render the surface of the tubing acutely thrombogenic without total occlusion of the shunt *(36)*. As a result, these techniques are now among the most commonly used models for the study of a variety of antithrombotic therapies. The interposition of experimental luminal surfaces can also be employed as a means to evaluate the thrombogenicity of alternative graft materials *(35)*. Most importantly, these long-term Silastic shunts do not detectably shorten platelet survival or produce measurable platelet activation *(34,37)*. For details regarding construction of the Dacron interposition segments or means by which to quantify platelet deposition and thrombus formation, please refer to the references cited in this discussion.

FUTURE STRATEGIES FOR THE DEVELOPMENT OF ARTERIOVENOUS GRAFTS

As previously discussed, the most common cause of clinical graft failure is intimal hyperplasia at the venous anastomosis. The biology of this common phenomenon of vascular response to injury has attracted considerable attention in the hope of devising a means to treat or prevent vascular stenosis and occlusion. A central component of neointimal hyperplasia is the activation of medial vascular smooth muscle cells (VSMC) from their quiescent contractile state into a proliferative, secretory phenotype, and their subsequent migration across the internal elastic lamina and continued proliferation. Traditional pharmacotherapies have failed to ameliorate the course of neointimal hyperplasia in human clinical settings. Although numerous, redundant molecular factors are now known to stimulate VSMC proliferation in the injured vessel wall, the regulation of cell-cycle progression represents a final common pathway for intervention in the proliferative response. This regulation depends on the coordinated expression of multiple cell-cycle genes, and it has been demonstrated that blockade of a combination of these genes provides a more potent antiproliferative effect than inhibition of a single gene *(38)*. E2F—a transcription factor that is activated during cell-cycle progression—is responsible for the upregulated expression of up to a dozen cell cycle genes. A strategy for blocking neointimal hyperplasia and subsequent accelerated atherosclerosis in bypass vein grafts using intraoperative transfection of the vessel wall with decoy oligonucleotides that bear the consensus E2F binding site and block its transactivating activity is currently undergoing human clinical testing *(39,40)*. This approach can be modified for the intraoperative transfection of the arterial and venous vessels involved in A-V grafting for hemodialysis access. Such a treatment may reduce the development of perianastomotic intimal hyperplasia and subsequently prolong A-V graft patency.

Prosthetic materials such as PTFE or Dacron, which are often used in the construction of A-V grafts, have thrombogenic surfaces. A bioengineering, cell-based strategy for decreasing or eliminating this thrombogenicity may therefore yield a prosthetic graft capable of maintaining normal flow. Such a bioprosthesis may also be useful for delivering genetically engineered factors that could enhance graft function and survival or even provide an avenue for intravascular drug delivery. Isolation of autologous endothelial cells has been well-characterized, although clinically successful reduction of graft thrombogenicity via attempts at enhancing graft endothelialization with such cells has not yet been reported. It has been hypothesized that one can further enhance the function of these endothelial cells through the transfer of genes to autologous endothelial cells before seeding of the cells on the graft surface *(41)*. One such target gene is that which encodes vascular endothelial growth factor (VEGF), a potent endothelial cell mitogen. Secretion of this molecular agent from cells placed on the graft surface may promote endothelial survival and replication, and may yield improved and more rapid graft coverage with a nonthrombogenic endothelial layer.

CONCLUSION

It is important to consider the objectives of a study to determine the optimal animal model that can be used. The variety of existing animal models has provided researchers with the means to study the surgical aspects of arteriovenous grafting as well as its biologic ramifications. The use of these models also allows us now to further assess new and exciting methods to treat the processes of thrombogenesis and neointimal hyperplasia. In the long run, it is the translation of these novel therapeutic alternatives from bench to bedside that will lead to improvement in the care of human patients with occlusive vascular disease and chronic renal dysfunction.

REFERENCES

1. Zibari GB, Rohr MS, Landreneau MD, et al. Complications from permanent hemodialysis vascular access. Surgery 1988; 104:681–686.
2. Seshadri R. PTFE Grafts for Hemodialysis Access: techniques for insertion and management of complications. Ann Surg 1987; 206(5):666–673.
3. Faries PL, Marin ML, Veith FJ, et al. Immunolocalization and temporal distribution of cytokine expression during the development of vein graft intimal hyperplasia in an experimental model. J Vasc Surg 1996; 24:463–471.
4. Hoch JR, Stark VK, Turnispeed WD. The temporal relationship between the development of vein graft intimal hyperplasia and growth factor gene expression. J Vasc Surg 1995; 22:51–58.
5. Liu SQ. Prevention of focal intimal hyperplasia in rat vein grafts by using a tissue engineering approach. Atherosclerosis 1998; 140(2):365–377.
6. Sterpetti AV, Cucina A, Randone B, et al. Growth factor production by arterial and vein grafts: relevance to coronary artery bypass grafting. Surgery 1996; 120:460–467.
7. Lipman NS, Marini RP, Flecknell PA. Anesthesia and Analgesia in Rabbits. In: Kohn DF, Wixon SK, White WJ, Benson GJ, eds. Anesthesia and Analgesia in Laboratory Animals. Academic Press, 1997; 205–232.

8. Mann MJ, Gibbons GH, Kernoff RS, et al. Genetic engineering of vein grafts resistant to atherosclerosis. Proc Natl Acad Sci USA 1995; 92:4502–4506.

9. Zwolak RM, Adams MC, Clowes AW. Kinetics of vein graft hyperplasia: association with tangential stress. J Vasc Surg 1987; 5:126–136.

10. Davies MG, Klyachkin ML, Dalen H, et al. Regression of intimal hyperplasia with restoration of endothelium-dependent relaxing factor-mediated relaxation in experimental vein grafts. Surgery 1993; 114:258–271.

11. Yoshida K, Sugimoto K. Morphological and cytoskeletal changes in endothelial cells of vein grafts under arterial hemodynamic conditions in vivo. J Electron Microsc 1996; 45:428–435.

12. Harvey RC, Paddleford RP, Popilskis SJ, et al. Anesthesia and Analgesia in Dogs, Cats, and Ferrets. In: Kohn DF, Wixon SK, White WJ, Benson GJ, eds. Anesthesia and Analgesia in Laboratory Animals. Academic Press, 1997; 257–280.

13. Dunlop CI, Hoyt RF. Anesthesia and Analgesia in Ruminants. In: Kohn DF, Wixon SK, White WJ, Benson GJ, eds. Anesthesia and Analgesia in Laboratory Animals. Academic Press, 1997; 281–312.

14. Smith AC, Ehler WJ, Swindle MM. Anesthesia and Analgesia in Swine. In: Kohn DF, Wixon SK, White WJ, Benson GJ, eds. Anesthesia and Analgesia in Laboratory Animals. Academic Press, 1997; 313–336.

15. Lumsden AB, Chen C, Coyle KA, et al. Nonporous silicone polymer coating of expanded polytetrafluoroethylene grafts reduces graft neointimal hyperplasia in dog and baboon models. J Vasc Surg 1996; 24:825–833.

16. Drasler WJ, Wilson GJ, Stenoien MD, et al. A spun elastomeric graft for dialysis access. ASAIO Journal 1993; 39:114–119.

17. Trerotola SO, Fair JH, Davidson D, et al. Comparison of Gianturco Z stents and wallstents in hemodialysis access graft animal model. J Vasc Interv Rad 1995; 6:387–396.

18. Chen C, Ofenloch JC, Yiannakis YP, et al. Phosphorylcholine coating of ePTFE reduces platelet deposition and neointimal hyperplasia in arteriovenous grafts. J Surg Res 1998; 77:119–125.

19. Fillinger MF, Kerns DB, Bruch D, et al. Does the end-to-end anastomosis offer a functional advantage over the end-to-side venous anastomosis in high-output grafts? J Vasc Surg 1990; 12:676–690.

20. Lelah MD, Lambrecht LK, Cooper SL. A canine *ex vivo* series shunt for evaluating thrombus deposition on polymer surfaces. J Biomed Mat Res 1984; 18:475–496.

21. McCoy TJ, Wabers HD, Cooper SL. Series shunt evaluation of polyurethane vascular graft materials in chronically AV-shunted canines. J Biomed Mat Res 1990; 24:107–129.

22. Miller VM, Reigel MM, Hollier LH, et al. Endothelium-dependent responses in autogenous femoral veins grafted into the arterial circulation of the dog. J Clin 1987; 80:1350–1357.

23. Landymore RW, MacAulay MA, Fris J. Effect of aspirin on intimal hyperplasia and cholesterol uptake in experimental bypass grafts. Can J Cardiol 1991; 7(2):87–90.

24. Quist WC, LoGerfo FW. Prevention of smooth muscle cell phenotypic modulation in vein grafts: a histomorphometric study. J Vasc Surg 1992; 16:225–231.

25. Kenney DA, Tu R, Peterson RC, et al. Performance of a longitudinally compliant PTFE vascular prosthesis in an ovine A-V fistula model. ASAIO Trans 1990; 35:M761–M763.

26. Neville RF, Bartorelli AL, Sidway AN, et al. Vascular stent deployment in vein bypass grafts: observations in an animal model. Surgery 1994; 116:55–61.

27. Esquivel CO, Bjorck C-G, Bergentz S-E, et al. Reduced thrombogenic characteristics of expanded polytetrafluoroethylene and polyurethane arterial grafts after heparin bonding. Surgery 1984; 95:102–107.

28. Lannerstad O, Dougan P, Bergqvist D. Effects of different graft preparation techniques on the acute thrombogenicity of autologous vein grafts. An experimental study in sheep. Eur Surg Res 1987; 19:395–399.
29. Lannerstad O, Bjorck C-G, Dougan P, et al. The acute thrombogenicity of a compliant polyurethane arterial graft compared with autologous vein. An experimental study in sheep. Acta Chir Scand 1986; 152:187–190.
30. Angelini GD, Bryan AJ, Williams HMJ, et al. Distension promotes platelet and leukocyte adhesion and reduces short-term patency in pig arteriovenous bypass grafts. J Thorac Cardiovasc Surg 1990; 99:433–439.
31. Angelini GD, Izzat MB, Bryan AJ, et al. External stenting reduces early Cardiovgasc medial and neointimal thickening in a pig model of arteriovenous bypass grafting. J Thorac Cardiovasc Surg 1996; 112:79–84.
32. Mehta D, George SJ, Jeremy JY, et al. External stenting reduces long-term medial and neointimal thickening and platelet derived growth factor expression in a pig model of arteriovenous bypass grafting. Nat Med 1998; 4(2):235–239.
33. Young FA. Primate Control Systems. Proc Anim Care Panel 1957; 7:127–137.
34. Hanson SR, Kotze HF, Savage B, et al. Platelet interactions with dacron vascular grafts: a model of acute thrombosis in baboons. Arteriosclerosis 1985; 5:595–603.
35. Hanson SR, Harker LA, Ratner BD, et al. In vivo evaluation of artificial surfaces with a nonhuman primate model of arterial thrombosis. J Lab Clin Med 1980; 95:289–303.
36. Harker LA, Hanson SR, Kirkman TR. Experimental arterial thromboembolism in baboons: mechanisms, quantitation, and pharmacologic prevention. J Clin Invest 1979; 64:559–569.
37. Kotze HF, Lamprecht S, Badenhorst PN, et al. Transient interruption of arterial thrombosis by inhibition of factor Xa results in long-term antithrombotic effects in baboons. Thromb Haemostasis 1997; 77:1137–1142.
38. Morishita R, Gibbons GH, Ellison KE, et al. Single intraluminal delivery of antisense cdc2 kinase and proliferating-cell nuclear antigen oligonucleotides results in chronic inhibition of neointimal hyperplasia. Proc Natl Acad Sci USA 1993; 93:1458–1464.
39. Mann MJ, Kernoff R, Dzau VJ. Vein graft gene therapy using E2F decoy oligonucleotides: target gene inhibition in human veins and long term resistance to atherosclerosis in rabbits. Surgical Forum Volume, 1997; 48:242–244.
40. Mann MJ, Whittemore AD, Donaldson MC, et al. The PREVENT trial of vein graft genetic engineering: preliminary molecular and clinical findings. Circ 1998; 98:I321.
41. Wilson JM, Birinyi LK, Salomon RN, et al. Implantation of vascular grafts lined with genetically modified endothelial cells. Science 1989; 244:1344–1346.
42. Zou Y, Dietrich H, Hu Y, et al. Mouse model of venous bypass graft atherosclerosis. Amer J Path 1998; 153(4):1301–1310.
43. Popilskis SJ, Kohn DF. Anesthesia and Analgesia in Nonhuman Primates. In: Kohn DF, Wixon SK, White WJ, Benson GJ, Anesthesia and Analgesia in Laboratory Animals. Academic Press, 1997; 233–256.

6

Wire Denudation and Ligation Models of the Mouse Carotid Artery

Volkhard Lindner, MD, PhD

INTRODUCTION

Advances in genetic manipulation by gene targeting and introduction of transgenes have necessitated the development of arterial injury models for the mouse. Using genetically altered mice in these models would allow researchers to define the role of certain genes in the events associated with intimal lesion formation, remodeling, and endothelial cell growth. For the rat, the balloon catheter denudation model has become the most widely applied model for the study of these events. Adopting this balloon catheter injury model for the mouse carotid artery has presented a major technical challenge, largely because there is no commercially available catheter small enough to use with mice. In our search for other suitable devices that would achieve complete endothelial denudation, we developed the *guide wire denudation model (1)* and later, the technically less challenging *ligation model* that causes intimal hyperplasia in the absence of widespread endothelial denudation *(2)*. These two models are described in detail in this chapter.

MATERIALS AND EQUIPMENT

1. Ketamine (50 mg/mL).
2. Xylazine (20 mg/mL).
3. Insulin syringe (0.5 mL).
4. Ophthalmic ointment (Lacri-Lube, Allergan).

From: *Contemporary Cardiology: Vascular Disease and Injury: Preclinical Research*
Edited by: D. I. Simon and C. Rogers © Humana Press Inc., Totowa, NJ

5. Catheter (iv), 24-gauge, (Becton-Dickinson).
6. Tape
7. Surgery platform (e.g., 0.5-inch-thick Plexiglass, 13 cm x 15 cm, with stainless-steel screws to hold rubber bands for securing mouse).
8. Small rubber bands.
9. Dissecting microscope (e.g., Stemi 2000C, Zeiss, VWR Scientific Products).
10. Fiberoptic light source (e.g., ACE, EKE with dual gooseneck, Fostec, Auburn, NY).
11. Small hair clipper (inexpensive models can be obtained from Service Merchandise stores).
12. Betadine solution.
13. 2 × 2 inch gauze.
14. Cotton applicators.
15. Scalpel.
16. 6-0 silk surgical suture (e.g., Deknatel, Queens Village, NY).
17. Microdissecting forceps with curved tip (e.g., Aesculap, FD 281, Aesculap, San Francisco, CA).
18. Jeweler's forceps, straight, 4 3/4" (e.g., 160–55, George Tieman & Co., Hauppauge, NY).
19. Microforceps (e.g., Bracken, 10-1942, George Tieman & Co.).
20. Scissors, McPherson-Vannas, straight (e.g., 160–140, George Tieman & Co.).
21. Scissors, Stevens, straight blunt-tipped (e.g., 160–250, George Tieman & Co.).
22. Hemostat, 3 1/2", curved (e.g., 160–751, George Tieman & Co.).
23. Bulldog clamp, Johns Hopkins, 1 1/2," straight (e.g., 160–825, George Tieman & Co.).
24. Bulldog clamp, DeBakey, curved 5" (e.g., 70–551, George Tieman & Co.).
25. Michel wound clip applying forceps 5" (e.g., 160–912, George Tieman & Co.).
26. Michel wound clips, 7.5 mm (e.g., 160–898, George Tieman & Co.).
27. Guide wire from angioplasty catheter, 0.014".
28. Tubing, polyethylene (I.D. 0.023," O.D. 0.038," Becton Dickinson).
29. Epoxy glue.

PROCEDURES
Guide-Wire Denudation Model

The guide wire tip (approx 5 inches) is cut off from the remainder of the wire, and for better handling one end is inserted and glued into the tubing using epoxy glue. Used guide wires can usually be obtained from the cardiology department. It is important that the flexible guide-wire tip is curved, smooth, and undamaged (Fig. 1A, B). Introduction of the guide wire into the vessel can be facilitated with a trocar by inserting the wire into a 2.5-cm piece of polyethylene or thin-walled Teflon tubing with a bevel cut at the tip (Fig. 1A,B). The guide wire can be made smoother and stiffer by coating it with epoxy glue,

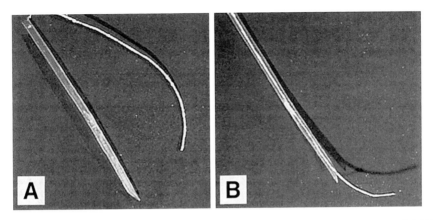

Fig. 1. Mouse guide-wire denudation model. (**A**) Trocar and curved guide-wire tip (0.014″) used for denudation of the common carotid artery. (**B**) Positioning of the trocar tip into the hole cut into the external carotid artery facilitates insertion of the wire.

which hardens quickly. Even spreading of the glue can be achieved by sliding the glue-coated wire through the tubing just before it hardens. This prevents the formation of glue droplets, which would make it impossible to insert the wire into the trocar.

ANIMALS AND ANESTHESIA

The initial studies used outbred female Swiss Webster mice (Simonsen Laboratories, Inc., Gilroy, CA) weighing 25–35 g. More recently, we have also applied the model to a number of different inbred strains. It should be emphasized that significant differences between the proliferative response of smooth-muscle cells (SMC) exist between strains. The animals were anesthetized by ip injection with a soln composed of ketamine (115 mg/kg body weight, Ketalar, Parke-Davis, Morris Plains, NJ) and xylazine (6.7 mg/kg, AnaSed, Lloyd Laboratories, Shenandoah, IA). The soln is prepared by injecting 1.7 mL of the xylazine stock (20 mg/mL) into a 10-mL vial of ketamine stock (50 mg/mL). Typically, a 0.5-mL insulin syringe is used for the ip injection of approx 50–70 µL of this soln for a mouse weighing 25 g.*

SURGICAL PROCEDURE

The mouse is placed with its back onto the Plexiglass platform with rubber bands attached to its hind legs. The rubber bands are attached to the screws protruding from the side of the platform, thereby stretching the legs. Another rubber band is used to hold down the head by the incisors. The front legs can be

---

* Note: Balb/C mice are very sensitive to this anesthetic combination, and require significantly lower doses (50–75% less).

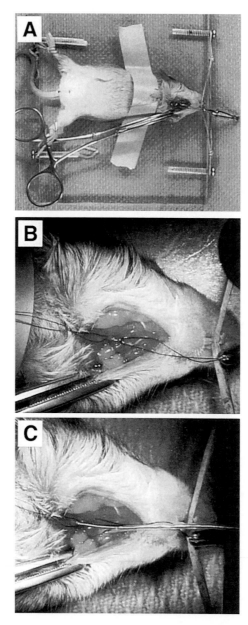

Fig. 2. Mouse guide-wire denudation model. (**A**) Positioning of the mouse with rubber bands and tape for dissection of the left external carotid artery. (**B**) Exposed external carotid artery with sutures in place. (**C**) Insertion of guide wire into the vessel.

kept away from the operating field with tape (Fig. 2A). Ointment is applied to the eyes to prevent drying of the cornea. The ventral part of the neck is shaved and the skin is disinfected with Betadine. A midline incision on the ventral side of the neck (1–1.5 cm) is made, and the salivary glands are moved laterally by blunt dissection. We usually perform the procedure on the left carotid artery because this vessel has no side branches (the right side has the subclavian artery), and endothelial regrowth can thus only occur from the carotid bifurcation and the aortic arch. For better access to the left carotid artery, the left salivary gland is held out of the way by the DeBakey clamp. The straight neck muscles are pushed medially while blunt dissection of the external carotid artery is performed with the microdissecting forceps with curved tips (Aesculap, FD 281). These forceps are highly suitable for separating the connective tissue from the vessel and placing the ligatures. The proximal ligature is placed around the external carotid artery just distal of the carotid bifurcation. The vessel is not tied off at this point. A small hemostat is attached to the ends of the ligature to apply tension caudally. This facilitates dissection of the more distal parts of the vessel, and the distal ligature should be placed as far distally around the external carotid artery as possible to isolate a relatively long segment of the vessel between ligatures. The distal ligature is tied into place, and tension is applied cranially by attaching the 1.5-inch bulldog clamp (Fig. 2B). A very small hole is cut into the vessel close to the distal ligature while blood flow is blocked with the proximal ligature. With the wire inside the trocar, the tip of the trocar is inserted into the hole with the bevel pointing down. The wire is advanced until it reaches the proximal ligature. The tension on the proximal ligature is relieved, and ligature is loosened around the vessel, thus allowing the wire to be advanced into the common carotid artery (Fig. 2C). Under rotation, the wire is moved back and forth along the entire length of the vessel (approx 2 cm from the hole in the external carotid) at least three times. The wire must move freely, and should not get caught at the hole in the vessel during the rotating motion. Advancing the wire too far in most cases will send it into the heart where it can cause serious damage, resulting in the death of the animal. After removal of the wire, to test whether clotting of the vessel occurred, the common carotid artery can be monitored for pulsation and color of the blood. If blood flows out of the hole briskly, clotting usually has not occurred. The proximal ligature on the external carotid is then tied, and the skin incision is closed using two wound clips.

HARVESTING OF VESSELS AND PERFUSION FIXATION

To assess the amount of endothelial regrowth from the carotid bifurcation and the aortic arch, Evans blue should be injected routinely a few minutes before euthanizing the animals. Evans blue (50 µL of a 5% soln in saline) is most conveniently injected into the renal vein via a 30-gauge needle after an abdominal incision is made in the anesthetized animal. If the injection is given via the tail vein, it is important that no air is injected and the hub of the needle is filled with soln. Injection of too much Evans blue will make the entire vasculature appear blue. The dye should be circulating for at least 2 min before perfusion fixation under physiological pressure with phosphate-buffered paraformalde-hyde (4%, 0.1M, pH 7.3) is carried out via a 24-gauge iv catheter placed into the left ventricle. Perfusion with 20 mL of fixative is usually sufficient, and can be followed by additional immersion fixation. The carotid arteries with the liga-ture in place are excised together with aortic arch, and endothelial regrowth occurring from the aortic arch and the carotid bifurcation is measured. The de-nuded (blue) segment of the carotid artery can be embedded in paraffin for analysis.

SMC PROLIFERATION AND ENDOTHELIAL-CELL REGROWTH

After complete endothelial denudation of the common carotid artery, the endothelium will grow back to completion within 3 wk. After 2 wk, the central portion of the vessel (2–3 mm) is still denuded, and this segment is suitable to study intimal lesion formation. If vessels show complete regrowth of endothe-lium much earlier than 2 wk, this is usually an indication that the denudation was incomplete. This is especially evident if patches of endothelium are present that are not connected to the endothelial outgrowth from the bifurcation and aortic arch. Thus, the pattern of endothelial regrowth can indicate whether en-dothelial denudation was complete. This is an important issue, because prolif-eration of SMC does usually not occur if an intact endothelium is present. Therefore, areas that were endothelialized earlier will show less intimal lesion development than areas that were endothelialized at later times. This problem can be resolved if only still-denuded areas are analyzed. If endothelial regrowth occurs before a neointima forms, increased numbers of medial SMC can often be observed (3).

The wire denudation causes damage to medial SMC, resulting in reduced medial SMC numbers 2 d after the procedure. SMC can be found in the intima at 8 d after denudation, and a small intimal lesion develops within 2 wk. This intimal lesion usually does not exceed 3–4 cell layers. A more extensive intimal lesion of a FVB mouse is shown in Fig. 3A.

CLINICAL RELEVANCE OF THE MODEL

Similar to the rat balloon injury model, this denudation model can be used to study factors that affect SMC and endothelial-cell proliferation and migration. Aspects of atherosclerosis can be addressed with the model when it is carried out in mice with mutations in genes involved in lipid metabolism. Achieving complete endothelial denudation in a reliable manner is technically challeng-ing, and there is definitely a learning curve with this model.

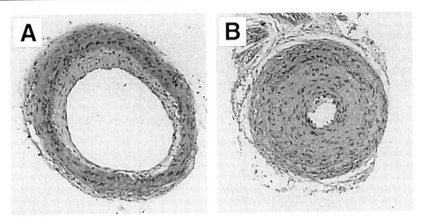

Fig. 3. Photomicrograph of cross-sectioned mouse carotid artery. (**A**) 2 wk after guidewire denudation. An intimal lesion has developed and there is also an increase in medial SMC number, indicating SMC proliferation. (**B**) 4 wk after ligation of the vessel at the bifurcation. An extensive SMC-rich intimal lesion has developed, and there is also considerable negative remodeling with shrinking of the vessel caused by the absence of net flow in the vessel. Hematoxylin-eosin stain, original magnification 125×.

Ligation Model

This model was described in detail in a recent publication *(2)*. The surgical procedure is very simple and requires very little time to perform. Yet the factors that cause intimal lesion formation and remodeling in this model are not completely understood.

SURGICAL PROCEDURE AND HARVESTING OF VESSELS

Dissection of the carotid bifurcation is essentially carried out as described in the previous section. The common carotid artery is then permanently tied off with a 6–0 silk ligature just proximal of the carotid bifurcation. The skin incision is closed as previously described. Just prior to perfusion fixation via the left ventricle, a small hole is cut proximal to the ligature to allow for good perfusion and draining of perfusate. Both common carotid arteries are excised, and for orientation, the ligature is left in place. The entire vessel is embedded, and 10 or more sections spanning the total length of the vessel are usually analyzed for morphometry. Sections are also routinely prepared from the contralateral nonligated vessel.

INTIMAL LESION FORMATION AND REMODELING

Clotting of the ligated vessel usually occurs only with a small segment next to the ligature. Oscillation of blood is apparent in the vessel, although there is no net flow. In FVB mice, this model is characterized by an initial loss of SMC with up to a 50% reduction in medial SMC at 2 d after the ligation. There is some loss and detachment of endothelium, but large-scale denudation is usually not observed. Infiltration with inflammatory cells is prominent in the adventitia and remodeling media. There is extensive SMC proliferation with neointima formation. Lesion development is typically more pronounced in more distal segments of the vessel. Within 4 wk, a thick neointima composed largely of SMC develops. The vessel also undergoes extensive negative remodeling with significant reductions in vessel diameter and lm area. Inflammatory cells appear to play a role in lesion formation as shown in a study of P-selectin-deficient mice exhibiting markedly reduced neointima formation and an absence of inflammatory cells *(4)*. The morphology of a typical lesion 4 wk after ligation is shown in Fig. 3B.

CLINICAL RELEVANCE OF THE MODEL

Remodeling and SMC proliferation are major events contributing to restenosis after angioplasty. The ligation model is well-suited to mimic these processes. Applying this model to gene-targeted mice will allow us to dissect the molecular mechanisms of the underlying cellular events.

REFERENCES

1. Lindner V, Fingerle J, Reidy MA. Mouse model of arterial injury. Circ Res 1993; 73:792–796
2. Kumar A, Lindner V. Remodeling with neointima formation in the mouse carotid artery after cessation of blood flow. Arterioscler Thromb Vasc Biol 1997; 17:2238–2244
3. Sullivan TR, Jr., Karas RH, Aronovitz M, Faller GT, Ziar JP, Smith JJ, et al. Estrogen inhibits the response-to-injury in a mouse carotid artery model. J Clin Invest 1995; 96:2482–2488.
4. Kumar A, Hoover JL, Simmons CA, Lindner V, Shebuski RJ. Remodeling and neointimal formation in the carotid artery of normal and P-selectin-deficient mice. Circulation 1997; 96:4333–4342.

7

Endothelial Denudation
and Arterial Dilation in the Mouse

Zhiping Chen, MD, Campbell Rogers, MD, and Daniel I. Simon, MD

INTRODUCTION

In order to define the role of specific genes in vascular injury and repair, investigators have pursued mouse models of arterial injury applied to transgenic and knockout strains. However, arterial lumen size (i.e., carotid- and femoral-artery diameter <0.5 mm) precludes endovascular balloon injury as typically performed in the rat and larger animals. We have recently developed a novel form of mechanical carotid-artery dilation and complete endothelial denudation based on the air-drying rat model of Fishman et al. (1) This mouse model shares much in common with widely studied and characterized experimental models of vascular injury, and takes advantage of the genetic diversity of the murine system.

MURINE MODEL FOR CAROTID-ARTERY DILATION AND ENDOTHELIAL DENUDATION

Male mice (8 wk old, weighing ~25 g) are anesthetized on day 0, using ketamine (80 mg/kg intraperitoneally; Fort Dodge Laboratories, Inc., Fort

From: *Contemporary Cardiology: Vascular Disease and Injury: Preclinical Research*
Edited by: D. I. Simon and C. Rogers © Humana Press Inc., Totowa, NJ

Table 1
Materials and Equipment

Anesthetics/analgesics
    Ketamine (100 mg/mL)
    Xylazine (20 mg/mL)
    Buprenex (0.3 mg/mL)
Angioplasty Inflation Device (Advanced Cardiovascular Systems/Guidant, Inc.,
    Santa Clara, CA)
Betadine solution
Cotton-tip applicators
Dissecting microscope (e.g., Nikon, SMZ-1B)
Forceps, curved (e.g., 11251–35, Fine Science Tools, Inc., Foster City, CA)
Forceps, straight (e.g., 10–2320, 10–1160, 10–1130, 10–1200, Biomedical Research
    Instruments, Inc., Rockville, MD)
Hemostatic Forceps (e.g., RS-7100, RS-7110, Roboz Surgical Instrument Co., Inc.,
    Rockville, MD)
Hair clipper
Microclips (RS-6500, Roboz)
Microclamps (e.g. 14–1000, Biomedical Research Instruments)
Needles, 30-gauge
Polyethylene tubing (PE-10, ID. 0.011", OD. 0.24", Becton Dickinson and Co.,
    Franklin Lakes NJ)
Scissors, straight (e.g., RS-5602, Roboz)
Scissors, curved (e.g., 11-2215, Biomedical Research Instruments)
Scalpel
Silk surgical suture, 5-0 and 6-0 (e.g., Deknatel, Fall River, MA)
Sponges
Sterile saline
Surgery platform
Syringes, 1 cc and 60 cc
Tape
Topical antibiotic ointment

Dodge, IA) and xylazine (5 mg/kg intraperitoneally). All surgery is performed using sterile techniques with the aid of a dissecting microscope. An equipment list is provided in Table 1. The mouse is placed in a supine position and secured by taping its feet to a platform. A 5–0 silk suture is attached to the incisor tooth, stretched, and taped on the platform to extend the neck. The ventral part of neck is prepared for surgery by clipping and disinfecting the skin surface with Betadine and 70% ethanol. A midline incision (~1.5 cm) is then made on the ventral side of the neck. In order to achieve complete endothelial denudation as well as controlled arterial stretching, we modified the air-drying model of

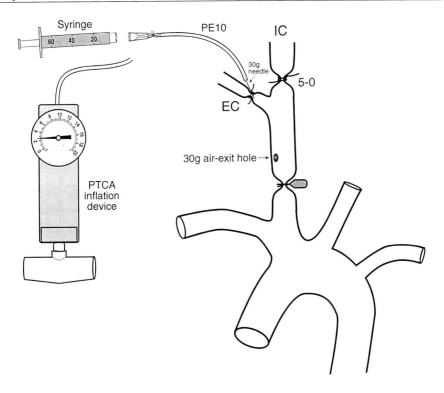

Fig. 1. Schematic illustration of mechanical carotid-artery dilation and complete endothelial denudation based on the air-drying rat model of Fishman et al. *(1)* Reproduced with permission from ref. *(2)*.

Fishman et al. (Fig. 1) *(1)*. The right carotid artery is surgically exposed and isolated from the surrounding tissues. The common carotid is isolated proximally as far as possible to obtain a relatively long segment of the common carotid artery. The proximal common carotid artery and internal carotid artery just beyond the internal–external carotid artery bifurcation are tied and looped with 5-0 silk sutures, respectively. Alternatively, the common and internal carotid arteries may be occluded with microvascular clamps. The external carotid artery is ligated with a 6-0 silk at the distal end. A transverse arteriotomy is made in the external carotid proximal to the ligature, introducing a 30-gauge needle that is advanced through the bifurcation and tied together with the common carotid by a 6-0 silk suture. Polyethylene tubing (PE-10, Becton Dickinson and Co., Franklin Lakes, NJ) is used to connect the needle to a saline-filled syringe, and luminal blood is removed by gently irrigating the isolated carotid segment. Thus, an isolated arterial segment is created (Fig. 1).

The syringe is replaced with an angioplasty inflation device (Advanced Cardiovascular Systems/Guidant, Inc., Santa Clara, CA) and the saline-filled isolated common carotid segment is dilated with 2.5 atm of pressure for 30 s. The inflation device is then replaced with an air-filled 60-mL syringe, and a 30-gauge air exit-hole is made at the proximal end of the common carotid. Endothelial denudation is performed by air-drying the carotid for 3 min (20 mL/min). After air-drying, the artery is refilled with saline to completely evacuate air, the needle is removed, and the external carotid is ligated proximal to the needle insertion site. Looped internal carotid sutures or microvascular clamps are removed to reestablish normal anterograde flow. A saline-damped cotton–tip applicator is applied to the air-exit hole in the common carotid to tamponade bleeding for about 2 min. Vigorous pulsation should be visible at this point. The wound is irrigated with saline, the incision is closed with running 5-0 silk suture, and topical antibiotic ointment is applied. Animals are allowed to awaken under a warming lamp. Total procedure time is approx 60 min. In our experience to date, all animals survive until the time of planned sacrifice without bleeding or infection.

TISSUE HARVEST AND PERFUSION FIXATION

After vascular injury, anesthesia is administered as described in the above section, the chest cavity opened, and the animals are sacrificed by right atrial exsanguination. A 22–gauge butterfly catheter is inserted into the left ventricle for in situ pressure perfusion at 100 mm Hg with 0.9% saline for 1 min, followed by fixation with 4% paraformaldehyde in $0.1M$ phosphate buffer, pH 7.3, for 10 min. The right and left common carotid arteries are excised and immersed in buffered paraformaldehyde. Spleen and small intestine from three Mac-1$^{+/+}$ and Mac-1$^{-/-}$ animals are harvested as control tissues for immunohistochemistry. All animals receive bromodeoxyuridine (BrdU), 50 mg/kg intraperitoneally, 18 h and 1 h before sacrifice.

Carotid arteries are embedded, and two cross-sections are cut 1 mm apart, and stained with hematoxylin, eosin, and Verhoeff's tissue-elastin stain. The lumen, intimal, and medial areas of each cross-sectional plane are measured using a microscope equipped with a CCD camera interfaced to a computer running NIH Image v1.60 software. Results for the two planes of each artery are averaged.

NEOINTIMAL FORMATION AND ARTERIAL REMODELING

We have recently characterized in detail the vascular repair response after mechanical carotid artery dilation and complete endothelial denudation in the C57BL/J6 strain *(2)*. Twenty-four h after injury, transmission electron micros-

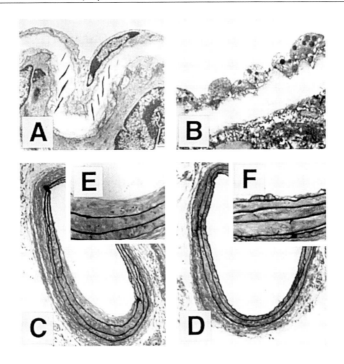

Fig. 2. Photomicrographs of mouse carotid arteries after arterial dilation and endothelial denudation. TEM from Mac-1$^{+/+}$ mice: (**A**) uninjured and (**B**) 24 h postinjury (original magnification: ×3000). VerHoeff elastin stain 28 d after vascular injury: (**C**) Mac-1$^{+/+}$ (×38); (**D**) Mac-1$^{-/-}$ (×38); (**E**) Mac-1$^{+/+}$ (×150); (**F**) Mac-1$^{-/-}$ (×150). Neointima separates the internal elastic lamina (arrows) from the lumen. Reproduced with permission from ref. *(2)* (See color plate 1 appearing in the insert following p. 236).

copy revealed that the injured arteries were completely denuded of endothelium and lined with a platelet monolayer (Fig. 2A,B). Arterial expansion at 2.5 atm leads to significant medial necrosis. Cellular and nuclear debris from smooth-muscle-cell (SMC) injury and death were visualized in the media. Intimal thickening began between 3 d and 7 d in this model and progressed significantly between 7 (mean–SEM: 0.0038–0.0012 mm^2) and 28 d (0.0112–0.0038 mm^2) (Fig. 2C,E). Significant medial thickening was also observed from 0 d (0.0133–0.0012 mm^2) to 28 d (0.0300–0.0028 mm^2) after injury. The intima:media area ratio (I:M) increased from 0.13–0.03 at 7 d to 0.34–0.13 at 28 d. Intimal and medial thickening were accompanied by progressive vessel enlargement or "positive remodeling" as determined by external elastic lamina (EEL) radius measurements in uninjured and 28 d postinjury vessels (0.104–0.015 mm to 0.204–0.006 mm).

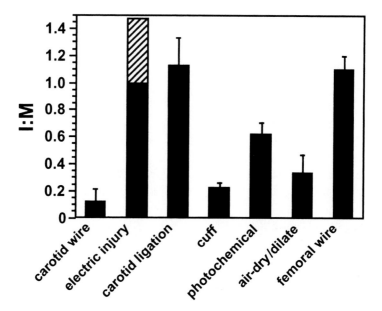

Fig. 3. Comparing mouse models of vascular injury. Ratio of intimal area to medial area (I:M, mean–SEM) is plotted for each published injury model as referenced in the text. In the case of electrical injury *(8)*, I:M is estimated due to total necrosis of the media and marked medial atrophy; neointimal is well-developed and is approx 12 cell layers thick.

Immunostaining for α-actin revealed that >80% of intimal cells were SMC (data not shown). We assessed cellular proliferation by using incorporation of BrdU at the time of sacrifice. Substantial proliferation was observed in this model at 7 d (18.6% of intimal cells) and fell significantly by 28 d (4.2% of intimal cells). In addition to SMC and platelets, leukocytes seem to play an important role in vascular repair in this model, since decreased accumulation of leukocytes in the vessel wall led to reduction in intimal proliferation and thickening in Mac-1 deficient mice in this model (Fig. 2) *(2)*.

MODEL OBSERVATIONS

This novel form of mechanical carotid artery dilation and complete endothelial denudation, based on the air-drying rat model of Fishman et al., *(1)* shares much in common with widely studied and characterized experimental models of vascular injury. It is fundamentally different from previously reported murine models of arterial injury in its ability to reliably achieve both endothelial and medial injury through an endovascular approach resulting in progressive intimal thickening over time. Prior murine models of neointimal thickening, including endovascular wire scraping, *(3–5)* perivascular cuffing *(6)*, ipsilateral carotid artery ligation, *(7)* and electrical- *(8)* or Rose Bengal/green light-induced injury, *(9)* are characterized by variable degrees of intimal and medial thickening, significant mural thrombus formation, or perivascular manipulation which may influence vessel-wall inflammation.

Intimal thickening after carotid-artery dilation and endothelial denudation is relatively modest, with I:M of 0.34–0.13 at 28 d. Significantly increased neointimal formation (I:M > 1.0) has been observed after carotid injury in LDL-receptor-deficient C57BL/J6 mice fed a high-fat diet (7.5% fat, 1.25% cholesterol) for 12 wk. We have also observed increased intimal thickening in mice housed in a nonisolator environment, suggesting that the biological response to vascular injury may be significantly modulated by local and systemic inflammatory factors.

Selecting an individual mouse model for vascular injury depends upon several factors, including ease of technique, method of injury (i.e., endovascular versus nonendovascular), and absence/presence of flow abnormalities or thrombus. Above all, many investigators desire a thick neointima. We have plotted the ratio of intima area to medial area for seven published models, including the recent report of femoral artery wire- and ligation-induced injury *(10)* (Fig. 3).

CONCLUSION

Restenosis is an orchestrated cellular response mediated by chemokines, cytokines, cell-adhesion molecules, extracellular matrix proteins, and proteases. Further studies of vascular repair after injury in mice genetically devoid of these components, perhaps coupled with murine models of atherosclerosis (i.e., apo E- and LDL receptor-deficient mice) using "double knockout" or bone marrow transplant approaches, will enable investigators to mechanistically explore vascular repair after mechanical injury in the setting of an atherosclerotic background, and to identify new targets for preventing clinical restenosis.

ACKNOWLEDGMENT

This work was supported by grants from the National Institute of Health (HL 57506 to Daniel I. Simon and HL 03104 to Campbell Rogers).

REFERENCES

1. Fishman JA, Ryan GB, Karnovsky MJ. Endothelial regeneration in the rat carotid artery and the significance of endothelial denudation in the pathogenesis of myointimal thickening. Lab Invest 1975; 32:339–351.
2. Simon DI, Chen Z, Seifert P, Edelman ER, Ballantyne CM, Rogers C. Decreased neointimal formation in Mac-1-/- mice reveals a role for inflammation in vascular repair after angioplasty. J Clin Invest 2000; 105:293–300.
3. Lindner V, Fingerle J, Reidy MA. Mouse model of arterial injury. Circ Res 1993; 73:792–796.

4. Sullivan TRJ, Karas RH, Aronovitz M, Faller GT, Ziar JP, Smith JJ, O'Donnell TFJ, Mendelsohn ME. Estrogen inhibits the response-to-injury in a mouse carotid artery model. J Clin Invest 1995; 96:2482–2488.

5. Akyurek LM, San H, Tashiro J, Nabel EG. A murine model of vascular injury and arterial gene transfer. Circulation 1999; 100:1–13.

6. Moroi M, Zhang L, Yasuda T, Virmani R, Gold HK, Fishman MC, et al. Interaction of genetic deficiency of endothelial nitric oxide, gender, and pregnancy in vascular response to injury in mice. J Clin Invest 1998; 101:1225–1232.

7. Kumar A, Lindner V. Remodeling with neointima formation in the mouse carotid artery after cessation of blood flow. Arterioscler Thromb Vasc Biol 1997; 17:2238–2244.

8. Carmeliet P, Moons L, Stassen JM, De Mol M, Bouche A, van den Oord JJ, et al. Vascular wound healing and neointima formation induced by perivascular electric injury in mice. Am J Pathol 1997; 150:761–776.

9. Kikuchi S, Umemura K, Kondo K, Saniabadi AR, Nakashima M. Photochemically induced endothelial injury in the mouse as a screening model for inhibitors of vascular intimal thickening. Arterioscler Thromb Vasc Bio 1998; 18:1069–1078.

10. Roque M, Fallon JT, Badimon JJ, Zhang WX, Taubman MB, Reis ED. Mouse model of femoral artery denudation injury associated with the rapid accumulation of adhesion molecules on the luminal surface and recruitment of neutrophils. Arterioscler Thromb Vasc Biol 2000; 20:335–342.

8 Vascular Photochemical Injury in the Mouse

Daniel T. Eitzman, MD and Randal J. Westrick, BS

CONTENTS

INTRODUCTION

The need for small animal models to study cardiovascular diseases has recently escalated with the advent of transgenic mouse technology. Advances in the transgenic mouse field have led to the production of numerous novel strains of mice with overexpression, targeted deletions, or replacement of selected genes of interest. The potential to uncover cause-and-effect relationships between the expression of virtually any gene in a whole animal and a measurable outcome is now a reality. Thus, mouse models designed to mimic the disease processes that occur in humans are extremely valuable. Because of the small size of the mouse cardiovascular system, downsizing of existing models or novel methods must be developed to study vascular disease in the mouse.

From: *Contemporary Cardiology: Vascular Disease and Injury: Preclinical Research*
Edited by: D. I. Simon and C. Rogers © Humana Press Inc., Totowa, NJ

In this chapter, we describe a relatively noninvasive method of inducing vascular injury and thrombosis in mice that is mediated by a reactive oxygen species also implicated in the development of human vascular diseases.

VASCULAR INJURY MODELS

Several vascular injury models have recenty been applied to the study of transgenic mice (1–5). Because of the relatively small size of the mouse, models that do not require extensive manipulation of the vasculature are especially useful. Ideally, the injury should target the endothelium, as this is the probable site of injury in most human vascular disease. The model also must be reproducible and easily standardized, with histological features similar to those occurring in human vasculopathy.

Photochemical-Induced Vascular Injury

Photochemical injury with tetrachlorotetraiodofluorescein, or rose bengal, is a relatively noninvasive method to elicit arterial injury, and is particularly useful for studying small animals such as mice. The injury is based on the photodynamic generation of singlet oxygen from systemically administered rose bengal after excitation with a green light (6) transmitted through the vessel wall. This model can be applied to vessels of virtually any size, has been used to elicit thrombosis in vessels as small as the rat retinal artery (7) and has recently been adapted for use in the mouse.

CAROTID ARTERIAL THROMBOSIS

To study the role of various murine genetic alterations on the development of arterial thrombus formation, we have focused on the carotid artery. This artery was chosen because of its accessibility and ease of monitoring flow. We have also performed experiments in the femoral artery, but have found that accurate flow monitoring is more difficult in this vessel because of its smaller size and the need to dissect free the adjacent femoral vein.

To access the carotid artery, the mouse is first anesthetized with sodium pentobarbital (70 mg/kg) (Butler, Columbus, OH), and the cervical area is swabbed with 70% ethanol. The mouse is positioned supine on a styrofoam platform with all four limbs extended laterally and taped to the surface. It is also very helpful to extend the neck by placing a loop of suture under the two front teeth of the mouse and fastening the superior aspect of the loop to a pin embedded in the styrofoam platform. After the mouse is appropriately positioned under a dissecting microscope (Nikon SMZ-2T, Mager Scientific, Inc., Dexter, MI), a midline cervical incision is made with a pair of scissors with the skin retracted upward to avoid injury to the trachea. Using blunt-tipped forceps, soft tissue to

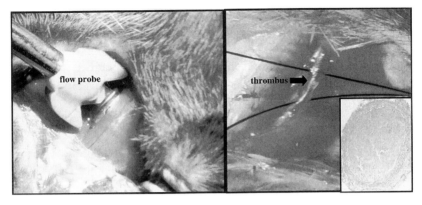

Fig. 1. Carotid arterial thrombosis following photochemical injury. Doppler flow-probe monitoring blood flow in carotid artery while artery is exposed to green light. (*left*) Gross appearance of clot in wild-type mouse, at which time no flow is apparent by Doppler. (*right*) Corresponding hematoxylin and eosin-stained section of occluded segment (*inset*).

the right of the trachea is dissected bluntly to expose the right carotid artery. Further blunt dissection on either side and under the carotid artery is necessary to allow placement of a flow probe. Retractors made from bent paper clips and rubber bands are used to retract the soft tissue on either side of the carotid artery.

For our thrombosis experiments, we use time to occlusive thrombosis as the primary endpoint. To document blood flow, we apply a model 0.5 VB ultrasonic flow-probe made by Transonics Systems (Ithaca, NY) connected to a Transonics T106 flow-meter with data acquisition software (WinDaq, DATAQ Instruments, Akron, OH). To facilitate placement of the flow-probe on the carotid artery, a piece of silk suture threaded under the carotid artery for intermittent gentle retraction is useful. The flow-probe is positioned under the carotid artery, and a few drops of warm saline are placed on the flow-probe to allow accurate flow detection. The probe is further manipulated to obtain a maximal flow signal (approx 0.7 mL/min). The probe position is maintained with alligator clips attached to a metal rod. With practice, the probe can be positioned without traction on the carotid artery while documenting excellent flow (Fig. 1).

Photochemical injury is initiated after the flow-probe is in place and is monitoring blood flow. First, a 1.5 mW green light (540 nm)-emitting laser (Melles Griot, Carlsbad, CA) is positioned 5 cm from the site of interest and held in place with clamps attached to a ring stand. This exposes approx 1 mm of the vessel to direct light. We prefer to have the light positioned and the flow-probe in place before the injection of rose bengal to precisely control for injury intensity and duration. Rose bengal (Fisher Scientific, Fair Lawn, NJ) is diluted to 10 mg/mL in phosphate-buffered saline and mixed well to dissolve all particulate matter. Fresh soln is prepared immediately before each group of experiments. To facilitate tail-vein injection, the tail is first swabbed with warm water to dilate the vein. The rose bengal is then injected at a concentration of 50 mg/kg (approx 0.10 mL) using a 27-gauge Precision Glide needle with a 1-mL latex-free syringe (Becton Dickinson and Co., Franklin Lakes, NJ). It is critical for reproducibility of this model that the tail-vein injections be performed by someone experienced in these techniques, as there is a learning curve for this method. Previous models using rose bengal in rodents to elicit vascular thrombosis have used lower concentrations of rose bengal to elicit thrombosis. However, the light source used in these models (Xenon lamps) is more intense (and more expensive) *(3,8)*.

The average time to occlusive thrombosis from the onset of injury under these conditions is approx 52 min in C57BL6/J mice *(9,10)*. This is associated with the gross appearance of a pearly white occlusive intraluminal filling defect (Fig. 1). It is important to note that we are measuring the time to vascular occlusion and not necessarily quantitating thrombus formation. It is apparent by flow reductions observed in the flow tracing, along with gross observations through the dissecting microscope, that a dynamic state of thrombus formation and lysis is occurring throughout the injury protocol prior to complete occlusion.

JUGULAR VEIN THROMBOSIS

We have also used this model to produce thrombosis in the mouse jugular vein. The jugular vein was also chosen because of its accessibility. The isolation procedure is identical to that of the carotid artery, although the dissection must be more delicate because of the fragile nature of the jugular vein. Positioning of the flow-probe is more difficult, as the vein collapses with minimal traction. However, an excellent flow signal can be obtained with flows of approx 0.6 mL/min. Rose bengal at a dose of 50 mg/kg produces occlusive thrombosis in approx 25 min. To increase the sensitivity of detecting changes between experimental groups, we have reduced the dose to 25 mg/kg, which increased the occlusion time to 40 min and appears to increase the sensitivity for detecting changes in fibrinolysis. As with the carotid artery, the occlusion is associated with an intraluminal filling defect observed through the dissecting microscope (Fig. 2).

STRAIN EFFECTS ON VASCULAR THROMBOSIS

The protocols described here apply to the C57BL6/J mouse strain. We have noted marked differences in the time to occlusive thrombosis in other mouse strains. For example, the 129Sv strain forms carotid arterial thrombosis in a significantly shorter period of time than the C57BL6/J strain. This is an important consideration when studying transgenic mouse strains, as most "knockout"

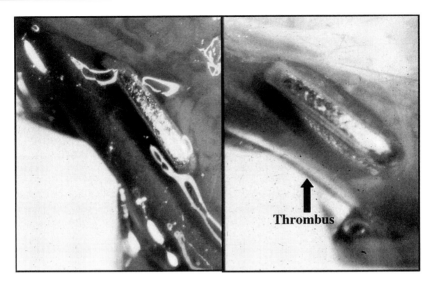

Fig. 2. Jugular Venous Thrombosis following photochemical injury. Jugular vein before injury (*left*). Thrombus in jugular vein following injury (*right*).

strains are a hybrid C57BL6/J–129Sv strain. Therefore we have routinely back-crossed the hybrid strain multiple generations to the C57BL6/J strain before formulating any conclusions regarding the effect of a genetic manipulation on vascular thrombosis.

INTIMAL HYPERPLASIA

Photochemical injury with rose bengal has recently been used to elicit intimal hyperplasia in the mouse femoral artery *(11)*. Although occlusive thrombosis occurs following injury, these investigators documented reestablishment of blood flow 24 h following injury. Histologically, at 24 h a rim of adherent platelets was observed, but otherwise the lm was not obstructed. Twenty-one d after injury, neointima that consisted almost entirely of smooth-muscle-cell (SMC) α-actin positive staining cells was observed *(11)*. We have also used this model to elicit neointima formation. In our model, persistent thrombus often occurs several days after injury to the femoral artery, which makes it difficult to distinguish neointima from organized thrombus (Fig. 3A). However, in the carotid artery, the lm is more likely to be free of residual thrombus 24 h after injury. Therefore, using the same conditions described for producing acute carotid arterial thrombosis, we have used this model to produce intimal hyperplasia in the carotid artery. The lesion formation is enhanced in the atherosclerotic-prone apo E-deficient mice, although a layer of lipid-laden foam cells is observed adjacent to the internal elastic lamina (Fig. 3B).

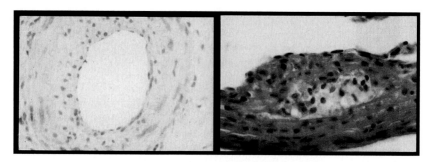

Fig. 3. Femoral and carotid neointima. Right femoral artery from 6-wk-wild-type C57Bl6/J mouse 3 wk after photochemical injury (*left*). Right carotid artery from 6-wk-old apo E-deficient C57Bl6/J mouse 3 wk after photochemical injury. Normal chow (*right*).

HISTOLOGICAL ANALYSIS

For analysis of injured arterial segments, mice are sedated with pentobarbital and then perfusion-fixed. A sternotomy is made, and 5 mL of a 4% phosphate-buffered paraformaldehyde solution is infused by left ventricular (LV) puncture with a 25-gauge needle. The right atrium is vented during this process by laceration with scissors. It is important for the infusing pressure of the fixative to be constant between experimental groups. This can be accomplished under the pressure of gravity with the infusate reservoir 3 ft above the animal connected to the needle by iv tubing. The injured arterial segment is then excised, placed in the fixative solution overnight, and transferred to 70% ethanol the following day. Tissues are embedded in paraffin and serial sections are made through the region of interest for hematoxyin and eosin staining or immunohistochemical analysis.

CONCLUSION

We believe that photochemical vascular injury in mice will be useful in the analysis of genetically modified mice to study factors involved in arterial and venous thrombosis as well as intimal hyperplasia. The ability of mouse models to predict outcomes in human disease states is uncertain, as even larger animal models have not been highly predictive. However, the advantages of transgenic technology currently available in mice models offer the potential for a highly informative resource.

ACKNOWLEDGMENTS

This work was supported by National Institute of Health grant HL03695-02.

REFERENCES

1. Carmeliet P, Moons L, Stassen J-M, De Mol M, Bouche A, van den Oord J, Kockx M, et al. Vascular wound healing and neointima formation induced by perivascular electric injury in mice. Am J Pathol 1997; 150:761–776.
2. Farrehi PM, Ozaki CK, Carmeliet P, Fay WP. Regulation of arterial thrombolysis by plasminogen activator inhibitor-1 in mice. Circulation 1998; 97:1002–1008.
3. Matsuno H, Uematsu T, Nagashima S, Nakashima M. Photochemically induced thrombosis model in rat femoral artery and evaluation of effects of Heparin and tissue-type plasminogen activator with use of this model. J Pharmacol Methods 1991; 25:303–318.
4. Harada K, Komuro I, Sugaya T, Murakami K, Yazaki Y. Vascular injury causes neointimal formation in angiotensin II type 1a receptor knockout mice. Circ Res 1999; 84:179–185.
5. Kumar A, Hoover JL, Simmons CA, Lindner V, Shebuski RJ. Remodeling and neointimal formation in the carotid artery of normal and P-selectin-deficient mice (see comments). Circulation 1996: 4333–4342.
6. Vandeplassche G, Bernier M, Kusama BM. Singlet oxygen and myocardial injury: ultrastructural, cytochemical and electrocardiographic consequences of photoactivation of rose bengal. J Mol Cell Cardiol 1990; 22:287–301.
7. Schmidt-Kastner R, Eysel UT. Ischemic damage visualized in flat mounts of rat retina after photochemically induced thrombosis. Brain Res Bull 1994; 34(5):487–491.
8. Takiguchi Y, Hirata Y, Wada K, Nakashima M. Arterial thrombosis model with photochemical reaction in guinea-pig and its property. Thromb Res 1992; 67:435–445.
9. Eitzman DT, Westrick RJ, Nabel EG, Ginsburg D. Plasminogen activator inhibitor-1 and vitronectin promote vascular thrombosis in mice. Blood 2000; 95(2): 577–580.
10. Eitzman DT, Westrick RJ, Xu Z, Tyson J, Ginsburg D. Hyperlipidemia promotes thrombosis following injury to atherosclerotic vessels. Atheroscler Thromb Vasc Biol. 2000; 20: 1831–1834.
11. Kikuchi S, Umemura K, Kondo K, Saniabadi AR, Nakashima M. Photochemically induced endothelial injury in the mouse as a screening model for inhibitors of vascular intimal thickening. Arterioscler Thromb Vasc Biol 1998; 18:1069–1078.

9 Mouse Model of Transluminal Femoral Artery Injury

Ernane D. Reis, MD, Susan S. Smyth, MD, PhD, and Barry S. Coller, MD

CONTENTS

INTRODUCTION

The growing use of percutaneous coronary interventions to treat vascular disease has reinforced the importance of understanding the molecular mechanisms involved in the arterial-wall response to injury. The difficulties in establishing robust animal models that simulate human disease have limited such studies *(1–3)*. Mouse models are particularly valuable because of the availability of mice with targeted gene disruptions. Such mice allow for the dissection of the molecular contributions to the vascular response and promise to help identify potential therapeutic targets *(4,5)*. A number of methods to produce external arterial injury in mice have been reported: ligation of the common carotid

From: *Contemporary Cardiology: Vascular Disease and Injury: Preclinical Research*
Edited by: D. I. Simon and C. Rogers © Humana Press Inc., Totowa, NJ

artery *(6)*, perivascular electrical injury of the carotid/femoral artery *(7)*, and placement of a polyethylene cuff *(8)*. The small size of mouse blood vessels has made it difficult to develop a reproducible model of endovascular injury. The reported endovascular methods rely on air *(9)* or wire *(10)* injury of the carotid artery. Since both vascular injury and arterial ligation have been independently demonstrated to induce intimal hyperplasia, we have developed a method that combines both endothelial denudation—induced by transluminal passage of a wire—and distal ligation of the mouse femoral artery. Our model is similar to models in larger animals, since platelet adhesion, recruitment of inflammatory cells, and neointimal formation follow the injury in a predictable manner *(11–13)*. We have found that the technical skills needed to perform the model can be acquired rapidly and that the results are highly reproducible. In this chapter, we present detailed methodology and characterize the response of the femoral arterial wall based on our experience with more than 1,000 procedures.

ANIMALS

Animal care and experimental procedures follow the recommendations of the Guide for the Care and Use of Laboratory Animals (Department of Health, Education, and Welfare, Publication No. NIH 85-23, 1996).

Generally, inbred mice are used; however, strain differences can be relevant and must be considered when interpreting results *(3)*. Most studies have used C57BL/6 mice. This strain is commonly used as the background for genetically modified mice, including hyperlipidemic mouse models such as the apolipoprotein-E (apo-E) knockout. C57BL/6 mice also have been preferred for gene-therapy studies using adenoviral vectors, because their immune system appears to allow longer expression of the transgene *(14)*. Consistent with previous findings *(8)*, we observed that C57BL/6 mice do not develop as much intimal hyperplasia as 129SV mice in our model (unpublished data). It is crucial, therefore, to have appropriate controls for these studies.

Male and female mice can be used for most studies. Although exogenous estrogen and oophorectomy have been reported to alter the arterial-wall response to injury in mice *(8,15)*, in experiments using wild-type, untreated adult mice, gender did not affect the response to femoral artery denudation *(11,12)*. Preliminary data using this model in hyperlipidemic mice also suggest that the response is independent of gender (unpublished data).

Adult mice (age >8 wk; weight ~20- to 30-g) are commonly used. Although successful arterial injury has been accomplished in 6-wk-old mice (~17 g), greater technical difficulty and sensitivity to anesthesia make such experiments more challenging.

Mice are fed either standard rodent chow (PMI Nutrition International, St. Louis, MO) or special diets (according to experimental design) and tap water *ad libitum*.

ANESTHESIA

Mice can be anesthetized by ip injection of pentobarbital (Nembutal®, Abbott Laboratories, North Chicago, IL) at 40–80 mg/kg body wt. At the lowest dosages, this drug usually induces general anesthesia in 10–15 min, and the anesthesia lasts 40–60 min. The ip route, however, results in variable responses, since some injections may be sc and others are intravisceral. Moreover, if reinjections are needed, the risks of complications such as ip bleeding and drug overdose increase. Pentobarbital anesthesia is also associated with cardiovascular depression caused by bradycardia.

We have found that general inhalational anesthesia is safer and easier to administer. To avoid the complications and difficulties of endotracheal intubation, the anesthetic may be given with spontaneous ventilation. To deliver inhalational anesthetics, we have developed a system that combines a vaporizer and a regulator. In the vaporizer, room air contacts filter paper soaked in isoflurane (Forane®, Baxter, Deerfield, IL). The isoflurane-saturated air is further mixed with room air and delivered to the mouse via a plastic nose cone. The regulator (Cole Palmer, Vernon Hills, IL) is used to titrate the content of isoflurane-saturated air (3.2–5.2 mL/min) and room air (100–130 mL/min).

SURGICAL TECHNIQUE

The animal is placed in the supine position with its paws fixed on the table and its lower extremities abducted and extended. The lower abdomen and both groins are depilated with an alkali cream (Nair®, Carter-Wallace, New York, NY) and cleansed with povidone-iodine 10% (Betadine®, Purdue Frederick, Norwalk, CT). The operation is performed with the assistance of a surgical microscope (Carl Zeiss, Thornwood, NY) under appropriate magnification (~×10 to ×20). A longitudinal groin incision is made, crossing the inguinal ligament. The femoral vessels are exposed at two sites: near the ligament and distal to the epigastric artery. Structures between these two sites—particularly the fat pad containing the epigastric vessels—are not dissected. Such limited dissection prevents unnecessary injury, and preserves collateral flow through the epigastric artery. For anatomy of mouse femoral vessels *see* Fig. 1 and Zhang et al. *(16)*. The segment of femoral artery between the take-offs of the epigastric and saphenous arteries is dissected free from the vein and nerve, and encircled with an 8-0 nylon suture (US Surgical, Norwalk, CT). The femoral artery and vein are then occluded temporarily using an atraumatic vascular mini-clamp (Accu-

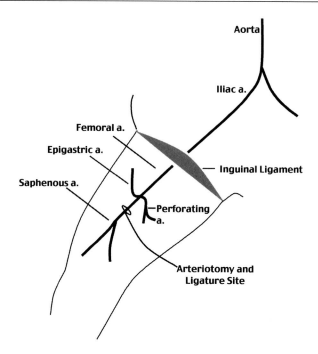

Fig. 1. Anatomy of the mouse femoral artery. The arteriotomy site for wire insertion is between the epigastric artery and the bifurcation of the femoral artery into the saphenous artery. The wire is advanced to the level of the aortic bifurcation.

rate Surgical and Scientific Instruments, Westbury, NY), placed just below the inguinal ligament. An arteriotomy is made approx 1 mm distal to the epigastric artery take-off. A 0.010" (0.25-mm) diameter angioplasty guide wire (ACS Hi-Torque APPROACH™, Advanced Cardiovascular Systems, Temecula, CA) is introduced into the arterial lumen, the clamp is removed, and then the wire is advanced ~1.5 cm, to the level of the aortic bifurcation. In our protocol the wire is advanced and pulled back three times, but this protocol can be modified for studies assessing different forms of vascular injury. The wire is then removed, and the arteriotomy site is ligated by tying the suture placed previously. The same procedure can be carried out on the contralateral side. Skin incisions are closed with continuous, 5-0 sutures of absorbable material (Vicryl®; Ethicon, Somerville, NJ). Bilateral arterial injury is usually completed in less than 30 min.

POSTOPERATIVE CARE

Postoperative analgesia can be provided with bupivacaine topical ointment, acetaminophen (Tylenol®) *per os*, or infiltration of the surgical site with 0.5%

lidocaine or bupivacaine. Mice are examined hourly until fully recovered from anesthesia and daily thereafter. Given the short procedure time and lack of exposure of the chest or abdominal cavities, postoperative warming is unnecessary. Mortality, mostly caused by anesthesia overdose, is less than 5%. Temporary paresis of the lower extremity is common, and may be caused by femoral-nerve contusion during dissection or clamping. Permanent motor deficit has not been noted. Foot necrosis occurs in less than 1% of limbs, and may be the result of arterial thrombosis.

HARVESTING AND PROCESSING OF SPECIMENS

To harvest the injured arteries, after deep anesthesia with pentobarbital or an inhalational agent, mice are perfused with 3–5 mL of phosphate-buffered saline (PBS, pH 7.4), followed by fresh 4% paraformaldehyde in PBS at 100 mmHg for 5 min. The perfusate is infused through a cannula (18–22 gauge; Angiocath®, Becton Dickinson, Sandy, UT) inserted into the chamber of the left ventricle and drained through an incision in the right atrium. After removal of the skin, abdominal wall, and viscera, the hindlimbs and pelvis are excised *en bloc*, fixed in 4% paraformaldehyde in PBS for 24 h, decalcified in 10% formic acid overnight, and reimmersed in paraformaldehyde solution for at least 1 h before cutting. The thighs, which contain the femoral vessels, are cut transversely from the inguinal ligament to the epigastric artery in 2-mm intervals, dividing the common femoral artery (~4-mm length) into two segments. These cuts undergo standard dehydration, paraffin-embedding, and sequential sectioning. Usually, multiple 5-μm cross-sections are obtained for immunohistochemistry or for staining with combined Masson-elastic (CME; to facilitate measurement of the arterial-wall layers) *(17)* or with hematoxylin-eosin (*see* Fig. 2).

HISTOMORPHOMETRY

Each cross-section is analyzed by two separate blinded investigators. For computerized morphometry, images are captured from a video camera attached to a light microscope and digitized. Lesions are quantified by computer-assisted planimetry (NIH Image 1.60 or ImagePro Plus® softwares). For each arterial segment, measurements are obtained of luminal area (LA); area bounded by internal elastic lamina (IEL; equivalent to the LA in the absence of intimal lesions); and area encircled by external elastic lamina (EEL; equivalent to overall vessel size). Derived calculations include medial area (EEL area minus IEL area), intimal area (IA; IEL area minus LA), and percentage of luminal narrowing ([IA/IA+LA]) × 100). The ratio IA/EEL can be used to assess remodeling *(18)*.

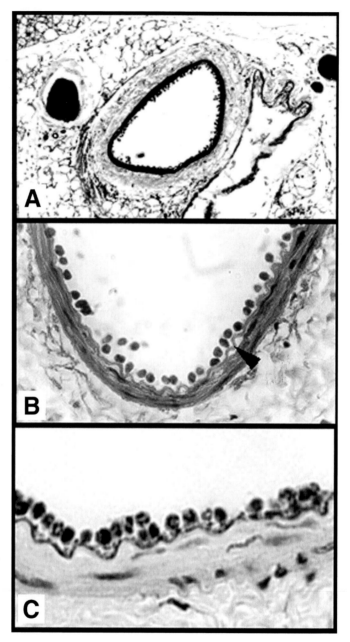

Fig. 2. Cross sections of mouse femoral arteries 1 h after transluminal wire injury. (**A**) Combined Masson elastic (CME) stain, showing the artery lying between the nerve (*left*) and vein (*right*). (**B**) Hematoxylin and eosin stain, showing arterial wall, with intact internal elastic lamina (arrowhead) and leukocyte accumulation on the injured luminal surface. (**C**) Immunohistochemisty using a rabbit polyclonal antimouse platelet antibody (Inner-Cell Technologies; Hopewel, NJ; brown-staining) showing platelet deposition along the injured wall and leukocytes attached to the platelets.

Endothelial-cell coverage can be assessed by identifying low-profile cells with central nuclei lining the luminal surface. Endothelial cells can be identified by immunohistochemical staining with, for example, antibodies to von Willebrand factor or PECAM-1 (CD31).

ACUTE RESPONSE TO INJURY

Immediately after injury, arteries display virtually complete endothelial denudation with minimal or no damage to the IEL. (In any given experimental group of mice, we observe disruption of less than 2% of the total length of IEL.) Platelets readily adhere to the denuded surface, with one to several layers of platelets present as early as 10–15 min after injury. Subsequently, from 30 min to 4 h, significant numbers of leukocytes attach directly to the platelets. Photomicrographs of arteries 1 h after injury illustrate the deposition of leukocytes (Fig. 2A–C) and platelets (Fig. 2C) on the vessel wall with excellent preservation of the IEL (Fig. 2B). Progressive endothelial regrowth occurs, and approx 90% of the luminal surface is re-endothelialized by 28 d (12).

NEOINTIMAL FORMATION

Intimal hyperplasia, defined as any proliferative lesion within the IEL circumference, is first detectable approx 7 d after vascular injury and increases thereafter. Average intima-to-media (I/M) ratios are approx 1/1 by 28 d in C57BL/6 mice (Fig. 3A). At 28 d, α-actin-expressing smooth muscle cells (SMCs) predominate within the neointima and substantial amounts of extracellular matrix are also present. Immunohistochemical studies demonstrate that the temporal sequence of expression of cell-cycle markers resembles the sequence found in studies of other animal models (19–21). ApoE knockout mice on a C57BL/6 background fed a Western diet can have more than 10-fold increases in their plasma lipid levels. Although these mice have no spontaneous lesions in the femoral artery at 8 wk of age (4), they develop exuberant, complex lesions 28 d after arterial injury. These lesions are rich in macrophages, foam cells, and deposits of extracellular cholesterol (Fig. 3B; Courtesy of Edward A. Fisher, MD, PhD, Mount Sinai School of Medicine, New York, NY).

LIMITATIONS OF THE MODEL

As with all other animal models of arterial injury, the degree of injury can vary in our model. Most variability is operator- or instrument-dependent, and can be reduced to a minimum by carefully designed and standardized procedures, including surgical technique and instrumentation. Appropriate controls are paramount. Since the temporary clamp used to prevent arterial blood flow has the potential to cause vascular injury, sham procedures were performed in

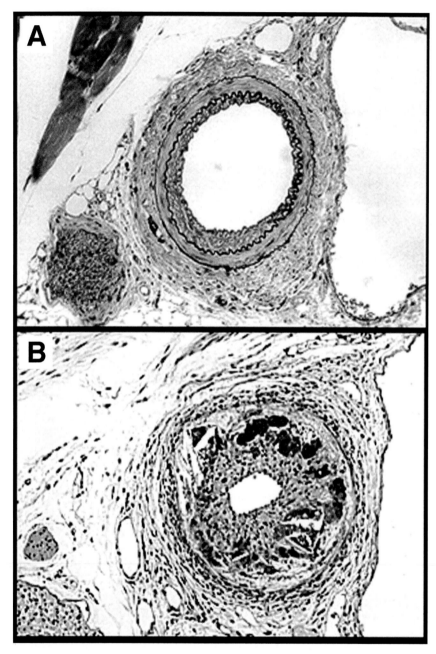

Fig. 3. Photomicrographs of mouse femoral artery cross-sections 4 wk after transluminal wire injury. (**A**) Wild-type C57BL/6 mouse; Combined Masson elastic staining. (**B**) Western-diet fed, apolipoprotein-E knockout mouse; immunostaining for macrophages (MOMA-2; rat antimouse macrophages-monocytes, 2 µg/mL; Serotec, Kidlington, UK).

which animals underwent all maneuvers (dissection, vascular clamping, arteriotomy, and ligation) except passage of the guide wire. No evidence of damage or vessel-wall reaction could be detected at 14 and 28 d postinjury in the area where the clamp was placed *(12)*.

In this model, the femoral artery is ligated distally; reduced blood flow may thus be a contributing factor to neointimal formation. As discussed above, in sham-operated mice, distal arterial ligation in the absence of endothelial denudation does not elicit intimal hyperplasia. Nonetheless, a reduction in blood flow caused by distal ligation of the artery may enhance the response to wire-denudation. The femoral artery has several small collaterals, and two prominent branches are consistently present: the superficial epigastric and perforating arteries (*see* Fig. 1). Although studies assessing blood-flow changes have not been conducted in this model, preserving these branches may be an important technical element to minimize the risk of thrombosis. In our model, femoral arteriotomy and ligature are done distal to these branches, and occlusive thrombus has been noted in only 10–15% of arteries *(12)*.

Adequate preparation of specimens is also important for consistent results. For example, poorly perfused arteries may appear collapsed on cross-sections, and thus morphometric analysis may be impaired. Lumen area is particularly influenced by vessel geometry, with a circular conformation resulting in maximal LA. Formulas based on length of IEL can be used to correct for distortion caused by eccentric sectioning because of either poor perfusion-fixation or angular cutting, but it is best to avoid distortions by adequate perfusion-fixation and perpendicular sectioning. Since perfusion-fixation is not performed when frozen sections are obtained, such specimens may not be adequate for complete morphometric analysis—for example, remodeling, cannot be evaluated.

CONCLUSION

Animal models of arterial injury are important for studying mechanisms of intimal hyperplasia and preclinical testing of new therapies *(1,2,5)*. The mouse is being used more frequently because genetically modified mice facilitate functional assessment of single or multiple genes in vivo. Although other techniques of injury have been described in mice, most of them use external approaches and thus, differ from the usual clinical scenarios in which injury occurs on the luminal surface—as in balloon angioplasty of coronary or peripheral arteries. One exception—wire denudation of the mouse carotid *(10)*—is considered technically difficult, and is prone to variability *(15)*. The air injury model *(9)* appears promising. Since in that model the endothelial damage is produced by desiccation rather than mechanical denudation, it may provide information that is complementary to that obtained in our model.

The technique of injury to the mouse femoral artery described here results in substantial amounts of intimal hyperplasia and is highly reproducible *(12,13,19)*. In this model, the endothelium is denuded by repeated passage of a standard angioplasty guide wire. The time course of neointimal formation is similar to that reported following balloon injury in rabbits *(22)*, pigs *(2)*, and baboons *(23)*. I/M ratios also are comparable to those obtained in larger animals *(12,24)*.

ACKNOWLEDGMENT

The authors wish to acknowledge the contributions of Dr. Heikke Vaananen, who devised the inhalatory anesthetic delivery system; Dr. John Fallon and Veronica Gulle for their expertise in performing/interpreting histomorphometry; and Drs. Merce Roque and Mark Taubman, whose input was essential in creating the model.

REFERENCES

1. Ferrell M, Fuster V, Gold HK, Chesebro JH. A dilemma for the 1990s. Choosing appropriate experimental animal models for the prevention of restenosis. Circulation 1992; 85:1630–1631.
2. Schwartz RS. Neointima and arterial injury: dogs, rats, pigs and more. Lab Invest 1994; 71:789-791 (editorial).
3. Carmeliet P, Moons L, Collen D. Mouse models of angiogenesis, arterial stenosis, atherosclerosis and hemostasis. Cardiovasc Res 1998; 39:8–33.
4. Breslow JL. Mouse models of atherosclerosis. Science 1996; 372:685–688.
5. Fuster V, Poon M, Willerson J. Learning from the transgenic mouse. Endothelium, adhesive molecules, and neointimal formation. Circulation 1998; 97:16–18.
6. Kumar A, Lindner V. Remodeling with neointima formation in the mouse carotid artery after cessation of blood flow. Arterioscler Thromb Vasc Biol 1997; 17:2238–2244.
7. Carmeliet P, Moons L, Stassen JM, De Mol M, Bouche A, van den Oord JJ, et al. Vascular wound healing and neointima formation induced by perivascular electric injury in mice. Am J Pathol 1997; 150:761–776.
8. Moroi M, Zhang L, Yasuda T, Virmani R, Gold HK, Fishman MC, et al. Interaction of genetic deficiency of endothelial nitric oxide, gender, and pregnancy in vascular response to injury in mice. J Clin Invest 1998; 101:1225–1232.
9. Simon DI, Chen Z, Seifert P, Edelman ER, Ballantyne CM, Rogers C. Decreased neointimal formation in Mac-1(-/-) mice reveals a role for inflammation in vascular repair after angioplasty. J Clin Invest 2000; 105:293–300.
10. Lindner V, Fingerle J, Reidy MA. Mouse model of arterial injury. Circ Res 1993; 73:792–796.
11. Reis ED, Roqué M, Zhang WX, Fallon JT, Weinberg H, Badimon JJ, et al. Neointimal hyperplasia after femoral artery transluminal injury in C57BL/6 and FVB mice. Surg Forum 1998; 49:303–305.
12. Roque M, Fallon JT, Badimon JJ, Zhang WX, Taubman MB, Reis ED. Mouse model of femoral artery denudation injury associated with the rapid accumulation of adhesion molecules on the luminal surface and recruitment of neutrophils. Arterioscler Thromb Vasc Biol 2000; 20:335–342.

13. Smyth SS, Reis ED, Zhang W, Fallon JT, Coller BS. β3-integrin-deficient mice are not protected from developing intimal hyperplasia after vascular injury. Blood 1999; 94 (Suppl. 1): 586a.

14. Rivard A, Silver M, Chen D, Kearney M, Magner M, Annex B, et al. Rescue of diabetes-related impairment of angiogenesis by intramuscular gene therapy with adeno-VEGF. Am J Pathol 1999; 154:355–363.

15. Iafrati MD, Karas RH, Aronovitz M, Kim S, Sullivan TR Jr, Lubahn DB, et al. Estrogen inhibits the vascular injury response in estrogen receptor alpha-deficient mice. Nat Med 1997; 3:545–548.

16. Zhang F, Shi DY, Kryger Z, Moon W, Lineaweaver WC, Buncke HJ. Development of a mouse limb transplantation model. Microsurgery 1999; 19:209–213.

17. Garvey W. Modified elastic tissue-Masson stain. Stain Technol 1984; 59:213–214.

18. Schwartz RS, Topol EJ, Serruys PW, Sangiorgi G, Holmes DR, Jr. Artery size, neointima, and remodeling: time for some standards. J Am Coll Cardiol 1998; 32:2087–2094.

19. Reis ED, Roqué M, Cordon-Cardo C, Fuster V, Badimon JJ. Time course of p27 expression after femoral arterial injury in the mouse. Surg Forum 1999; 50:482–483.

20. MacLellan WR, Majesky MW. Cell cycle regulators in vascular disease. Circulation 1997; 96:1717–1719.

21. Braun-Dullaeus RC, Mann MJ, Dzau VJ. Cell cycle progression. New therapeutic target for vascular proliferative disease. Circulation 1998; 98:82–89.

22. Doornekamp FNG, Borst C, Post MJ. Endothelial cell recoverage and intimal hyperplasia after endothelium removal with or without smooth muscle cell necrosis in the rabbit carotid artery. J Vasc Res 1996; 33:146–155.

23. Geary RL, Hohler TR, Vergel S, Kirkman TR, Clowes AW. Time course of flow-induced smooth muscle cell proliferation and intimal thickening in endothelialized baboon vascular grafts. Circ Res 1994; 74:14–23.

24. Clowes AW, Reidy MA, Clowes MM. Kinetics of cellular proliferation after arterial injury, III: endothelial and smooth muscle growth in chronically denuded vessels. Lab Invest 1986; 54:295–303.

II MODELS OF ARTERIAL THROMBOSIS

10 A Murine Model of Arterial Injury and Thrombosis

William P. Fay, MD, Andrew C. Parker, BS and Yanhong Zhu, MD

CONTENTS

INTRODUCTION

Mice are increasingly being used as models of human cardiovascular disease. (1) To a large extent, this has resulted from exciting advances in molecular genetics have enabled investigators to selectively modify the mouse genome to study the function of specific genes and proteins in vivo. In this chapter, we describe a method for studying arterial thrombosis in mice. This method exhibits several features observed in large animal thrombosis models. Therefore, it should prove useful to investigators examining the genetic determinants of thrombosis and thrombolysis at sites of arterial injury.

TARGET VESSELS AND METHODS FOR INDUCING THROMBOSIS

The carotid artery (diameter 0.6 mm), the femoral artery (diameter 0.4 mm), and the abdominal aorta (diameter 0.8 mm) are of sufficient size in adult mice

From: *Contemporary Cardiology: Vascular Disease and Injury: Preclinical Research*
Edited by: D. I. Simon and C. Rogers © Humana Press Inc., Totowa, NJ

to allow their use for thrombosis studies. We prefer the carotid artery for several reasons. It is accessible by simple dissection, and flow in the carotid can be measured with a miniature probe during short-term experiments. The carotid artery is also well-suited for chronic experiments, since the neck incision is easily closed with suture or staples and is not prone to infection. Complete occlusion of the carotid artery is well-tolerated by mice, and does not induce stroke because of collateral blood flow through the contralateral carotid artery. Several methods have been described for inducing thrombi in mouse arteries. These include electrical injury *(2)*, photochemical injury *(3)*, and chemical injury with ferric chloride *(4)*. However, electrical and photochemical injury have been characterized primarily in terms of their capacity to induce neointima formation. We have found ferric chloride injury to be a practical and reliable method for inducing acute, platelet-rich thrombi in mouse carotid arteries. The method, originally reported in rats *(5)*, is performed as follows:

1. Anesthetize mouse by ip injection of sodium pentobarbital 110 mg/kg. We usually study 6–8-wk-old mice (C57BL/6J) that weigh 20–25 g. Mice can be maintained under general anesthesia for >2 h without apparent adverse effects.
2. Secure mouse under dissecting microscope by taping limbs in extended position.
3. Make a midline incision in anterior neck and retract skin. Separate adipose and connective tissue by blunt dissection. The carotid arteries are located immediately lateral to the trachea (Fig.1). We prefer to use the left carotid artery. It is visible only after deeper dissection, and best found by its proximity to the vagus nerve.
4. Place a miniature flow-probe on the artery. We use a Model 0.5VB ultrasonic flow-probe (Transonic Systems, Ithaca, NY) that interfaces with an electronic flow-meter (Transonic Model T106). Several drops of saline are placed in the surgical wound to allow transmission of the ultrasound. Carotid artery blood flow in anesthetized mice ranges between 0.5 and 1.2 mL/min, with a mean of 0.7 mL/min. Permanent tracing of carotid artery blood flow can be recorded with a computerized data acquisition program (WinDaq, DATAQ Instruments, Akron, OH) or a strip chart recorder (Fig.2).
5. To induce thrombosis, place a 1×2-mm piece of filter paper (Whatman 1) saturated with 10% ferric chloride ($FeCl_3$) on the ventral surface of the carotid artery for 3.0 min. Saline must be aspirated from the wound before placing the filter paper on the artery. Therefore, blood flow cannot be monitored during the brief period of injury. After removing the ferric chloride-soaked filter paper from the arterial surface, saline is again placed in the wound, and carotid blood flow is recorded. We have found that 10% ferric chloride injury for 3 min usually induces occlusive thrombus formation in approx 20 min. Duration of injury and concentration of ferric chloride can be modified to achieve shorter or longer thrombosis times *(4,5)*.

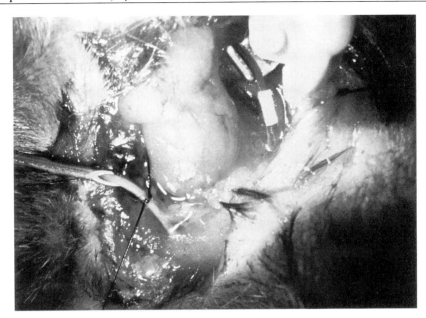

Fig. 1. Thrombosis protocol. The ventral neck of a mouse is viewed through a dissecting microscope during induction of carotid artery thrombosis (mouse head situated superiorly). A flow-probe is present on the left carotid artery. Filter paper saturated with 10% FeCl₃ is positioned on the artery proximal to the flow-probe. The right jugular vein is cannulated with 28G polypropylene tubing, which is sutured in place. Reprinted with permission from ref. *(6)*.

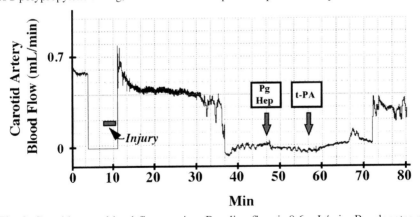

Fig. 2. Carotid artery blood-flow tracing. Baseline flow is 0.6 mL/min. Bar denotes period during which ferric chloride is applied to arterial surface. Artifactual reduction in flow during injury is caused by removal of saline from the surgical site to allow application of ferric chloride. Note cyclic flow variations prior to completely occlusive thrombus formation. Ten min after occlusion, heparin (200 U/kg bolus, 70 U/kg/h continuous infusion) and human plasminogen (50 mg/kg) were administered, and 10 min later, human t-PA 100 µg/kg/mL was infused. Flow was restored 14 min after initiation of t-PA infusion. Reprinted with permission from ref. *(6)*.

INTRAVENOUS INFUSIONS DURING OR AFTER ARTERIAL INJURY

For some experiments it is necessary to administer drugs, antibodies, or other reagents intravenously. Single bolus injections of ≤100μL can be administered via the lateral tail vein with an 27-gauge needle. If repeated or continuous infusions are necessary, the internal jugular vein (which is accessible via the same neck incision used to expose the carotid artery) can be cannulated with an L-Cath catheter placement set (Luther Medical Products, Tustin, CA) that contains 28G polyurethane tubing. After removing the introducer needle, the tubing remains in the lumen of the vein and is sutured in place (Fig.1). We have used this approach to infuse tissue-type plasminogen activator and heparin into mice at rates controlled by a Harvard infusion pump to study genetic factors that affect the response to thrombolytic agents (Fig.2) *(6)*.

HISTOLOGIC ANALYSIS OF INJURED CAROTID ARTERIES

Injured carotid artery segments can be retrieved for histologic analysis. We perfusion-fix the mouse arterial system according to the method of Carmeliet et al. *(2)*. After performing a midline sternotomy, the left ventricle is cannulated by direct cardiac puncture with an 25-gauge needle and an incision is made in the right atrial wall. Phosphate-buffered paraformaldehyde (4%) is infused into the left ventricle for 10 min from a reservoir situated 160 cm above the mouse. After excision, carotid artery segments are placed in 4% phosphate-buffered formaldehyde for 16 h, then transferred to 70% ethanol for storage until paraffin embedding. We have confirmed by light and electron microscopy that thrombi induced by ferric chloride are platelet-rich (Fig. 3).

IN VITRO ANALYSIS OF HEMOSTATIC FUNCTION IN MICE

It is often desirable to perform in vitro experiments in conjunction with in vivo studies. For example, in vitro platelet aggregation studies can be performed to determine if delayed vascular occlusion after injury is associated with reduced platelet function in vitro. Proper collection of blood is essential in performing in vitro clotting and platelet function assays. Although blood can be obtained from the retroorbital venous plexus of mice with a capillary tube, this method is not ideally suited for coagulation studies because it can cause tissue injury, thereby triggering tissue factor expression and thrombin formation. We prefer to collect blood by venipuncture of the surgically exposed inferior vena cava with an 25-gauge needle connected to a tuberculin syringe. With this approach, as much as 0.8 mL of blood can be collected into citrate or another appropriate anticoagulant. To process blood for in vitro platelet-function studies, place 1.0 mL samples of pooled, citrated whole blood in 1.5-mL polypro-

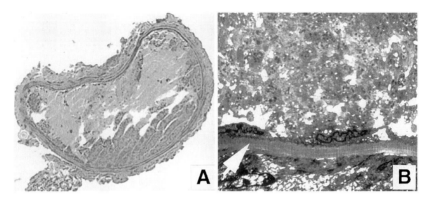

Fig. 3. Histologic analysis of murine carotid artery thrombi induced by ferric chloride. **(A)** Light microscopy, hematoxylin, and eosin staining (200× magnification). **(B)** Transmission electron microscopy showing that the thrombus is composed predominantly of platelets. Arrow indicates internal elastic lamina (3,400× magnification, lead citrate, and uranyl acetate stain).

pylene tubes. Centrifuge tubes (120g) for 8 min at room temperature in a swing-out rotor. After removing the platelet-rich plasma (PRP), the remaining blood can be centrifuged at 1200 g for 10 min to obtain platelet-poor plasma (PPP). The platelet count of PRP is measured, and PPP is used to adjust the platelet count of PRP to 2.5×10^8/mL. Using this approach, >1 mL of PRP suitable for aggregation studies can be obtained from three mice. Platelet aggregation in response to agonists such as ADP can be studied with 200-μL PRP samples in 7.25 x 55 mm siliconized, flat-bottom tubes by using a Model PAP-4 aggregometer (Bio/Data Corporation, Horsham, PA). Alternatively, aggregation of 100-μL PRP samples can be studied by using a previously described microtiter-plate aggregation assay *(7)*. Standard clotting assays (e.g., prothrombin time, activated partial thromboplastin time, thrombin time) can be performed on murine PPP using clinical reagents and machines used for human plasma.

PRECLINICAL APPLICATIONS OF THE MURINE FERRIC CHLORIDE MODEL

Much remains unknown regarding the in vivo function of the blood coagulation and fibrinolysis systems at sites of arterial injury. Identification and characterization of the molecular determinants of arterial thrombosis and thrombolysis will play a key role in enhancing our understanding of the pathogenesis of acute coronary-artery syndromes and stroke, and in designing strategies for improving treatment of these disorders. We consider ferric chloride injury of the mouse carotid-artery injury to be a useful and practical model for studying the regulation of thrombosis and thrombolysis within the complex environment of the intact artery. In recent experiments, we have used this model

Table 1
Genetic Modifications of the Murine Coagulation and Fibrinolysis Systems

Gene	Modification	Survival of homozygotes	References
Blood Coagulation System			
Fibrinogen	Knockout	Viable	13
Prothrombin	Knockout	Embryonic lethal	14
Factor V	Knockout	Embryonic lethal	15
	Knock-in (Leiden mutation)	Half die immediately after birth. Half normal.	16
Factor VII	Knockout	Embryonic lethal	17
Factor VIII	Knockout	Viable	18
Factor XI	Knockout	Viable	19
von Willebrand factor	Knockout	Viable	20
Thrombin receptor (PARI)	Knockout	Half die in utero. Half survive normally.	21
Protein C	Knockout	Embryonic lethal	22
Tissue factor	Knockout	Embryonic lethal	23,24
Tissue factor pathway inhibitor (TFPI)	Knockout	Embryonic lethal	25
Thrombomodulin	Knockout	Embryonic lethal	26
Blood Fibrinolytic System			
Plasminogen	Knockout	Viable	27,28
t-PA	Knockout	Viable	29
u-PA	Knockout	Viable	29
uPAR	Knockout	Viable	30,31
PAI-1	Knockout	Viable	11
	Transgenic	Viable	32,33
PAI-2	Knockout	Viable	34
Vitronectin	Knockout	Viable	35

to study the functions of vitronectin and plasminogen activator inhibitor-1 (PAI-1) in arterial thrombosis and thrombolysis, respectively *(4,6,8)*. The primary strength of the model is that it allows a uniform injury to be applied to a population of essentially genetically identical animals, or to groups of animals whose genetic differences are restricted to a single or a few genes. Therefore, it provides a powerful tool for studying molecular determinants of arterial thrombosis and thrombolysis. The major limitations of this model are the technical challenges posed by the small size of mice and the possibility that significant differences exist in the regulation of thrombosis and thrombolysis between mice and larger mammals, including humans. However, it is clear that high-quality, reproducible data can be obtained from mouse cardiovascular experiments *(9)*. Furthermore, comparisons of specific genetic mutations in mice and humans strongly suggest that mice can be used to model human disease processes *(10–12)*. Multiple components of the blood coagulation and fibrinolysis systems have been genetically modified in mice by gene targeting and transgenic strategies (*see* Table 1), and the list of targeted genes is growing rapidly. Therefore, we believe that this murine model will prove useful in studying the roles of a wide variety of genetic factors in thrombosis and thrombolysis within the distinct environment of the acutely injured artery.

ACKNOWLEDGMENT

This work was supported by National Institutes of Health grant HL57346.

REFERENCES

1. Doevendans PA, Hunter JJ, Lembo G, Wollert KC, Chien KR. Strategies for studying cardiovascular diseases in transgenic and gene-targeted mice In: Monastersky GM, Robi JM, eds: Strategies in Transgenic Animal Science. Washington, DC, American Society for Microbiology, 1995, pp. 107–144.

2. Carmeliet P, Moons L, Stassen J, De Mol M, Bouche A, van den Oord J, et al. Vascular wound healing and neointima formation induced by perivascular electric injury in mice. Am J Pathol 1997; 150:761–776.

3. Kikuchi S, Umemura K, Kondo K, Saniabadi AR, Nakashima M. Photochemically induced endothelial injury in the mouse as a screening model for inhibitors of vascular intimal thickening. Arterioscler Thromb Vasc Biol 1998; 18:1069–1078.

4. Farrehi PM, Ozaki CK, Carmeliet P, Fay WP. Regulation of arterial thrombolysis by plasminogen activator inhibitor-1 in mice. Circulation 1998; 97:1002–1008.

5. Kurz KD, Main BW, Sandusky GE. Rat model of arterial thrombosis induced by ferric chloride. Thromb Res 1990; 60:269–280.

6. Zhu Y, Carmeliet P, Fay WP. Plasminogen activator inhibitor-1 is a major determinant of arterial thrombolysis resistance Circulation 1999; 3050–3055.

7. Walkowiak B, Kesy A, Michalec L. Microplate reader—A convenient tool in studies of blood coagulation. Thromb Res 1997; 87:95–103.

8. Fay WP, Parker AC, Ansari MN, Zheng X, Ginsburg D. Vitronectin inhibits the thrombotic response to arterial injury in mice Blood 1999; 93:1825–1830.

9. Doevendans PA, Hunter JJ, Lembo G, Wollert KC, Chien KR. Strategies for studying cardiovascular diseases in transgenic and gene-targeted mice In: Monastersky GM, Robl JM, eds. Strategies in Transgenic Animal Science. Washington, DC, American Society for Microbiology, 1995, pp. 107–144.

10. Fay WP, Parker AC, Condrey LR, Shapiro AD. Human plasminogen activator inhibitor-1 (PAI-1) deficiency: characterization of a large kindred with a null mutation in the PAI-1 gene. Blood 1997; 90:204–208.

11. Carmeliet P, Stassen JM, Schoonjans L, Ream B, van den Oord JJ, De Mol M, et al. Plasminogen activator inhibitor-1 gene-deficient mice. II. Effects on hemostasis, thrombosis, and thrombolysis. J Clin Invest 1993; 92:2756–2760.

12. Carmeliet P, Mulligan RC, Collen D. Transgenic animals as tools for the study of fibrinolysis in vivo. J Int Med 1994; 236:455–459.

13. Suh TT, Holmback K, Jensen NJ, Daugherty CC, Small K, Simon DI, et al. Resolution of spontaneous bleeding events but failure of pregnancy in fibrinogen-deficient mice. Genes Dev 1995; 9:2020–2033.

14. Xue J, Wu Q, Westfield L, Tuley E, Lu D, Zhang Q, et al. Incomplete embryonic lethality and fatal neonatal hemorrhage caused by prothrombin deficiency in mice. Proc Natl Acad Sci USA 1998; 95:7603–7607.

15. Cui J, O'Shea KS, Purkayastha A, Saunders TL, Ginsburg D. Fatal perinatal haemorrhage and an incomplete block to embryonic development in mice lacking coagulation factor V. Nature 1996; 384:66–68.

16. Cui J, Purkayastha A, Yang A, Yang T, Gallagher K, Metz A, et al. Spontaneous thrombosis in mice carrying the APC resistance mutation (FV Leiden) introduced by gene targeting abstract. Blood 1996; 88 (Suppl 1):440a.

17. Rosen E, Chan J, Idusogie E, Clotman F, Vlasuk G, Luther T, et al. Mice lacking factor VII develop normally but suffer fatal perinatal bleeding. Nature 1997; 390(6657):290–294.

18. Bi L, Lawler A, Antonarakis S, High K, Gearhart J, Kazazian H. Targeted disruption of the mouse factor VIII gene produces a model of haemophilia A. Nat Genet 1995; 10:119–121.

19. Gailani D, Lasky N, Broze G. A murine model of factor XI deficiency. Blood Coagul Fibrinolysis 1997; 8:134–144.

20. Denis C, Methia N, Frenette P, Rayburn H, Ullman-Cullere M, Hynes R, et al. A mouse model of severe von Willebrand disease: defects in hemostasis and thrombosis. Proc Natl Acad Sci USA 1998; 95:9524–9529.

21. Connolly AJ, Ishihara H, Kahn ML, Farese RV, Jr, Coughlin SR. Role of the thrombin receptor in development and evidence for a second receptor. Nature 1996; 381:516–519.

22. Jalbert LR, Rosen ED, Moons L, Chan JC, Carmeliet P, Colleen D, et al. Inactivation of the gene for anticoagulant protein C causes lethal perinatal consumptive coagulopathy in mice. J Clin Invest 1998; 102: 1481–1488.

23. Toomey J, Kratzer K, Lasky N, Stanton J, Broze G. Targeted disruption of the murine tissue factor gene results in embryonic lethality. Blood 1996; 88(5):1583–1587.

24. Carmeliet P, Mackman N, Moons L, Luther T, Gressens P, Vlaederen I, et al. Role of tissue factor in embryonic blood vessel development. Nature 1996; 383(6595):73–75.

25. Huang Z, Higuchi D, Lasky N, Broze G. Tissue factor pathway inhibitor gene disruption produces intrauterine lethality in mice. Blood 1997; 90(3):944–951.

26. Rosenberg R. The absence of the blood clotting regulator thrombomodulin causes embryonic lethality in mice before development of a functional cardiovascular system. Thromb Haemostasis 1995; 74(1):52–57.

27. Bugge TH, Flick MJ, Daugherty CC, Degen JL. Plasminogen deficiency causes severe thrombosis but is compatible with development and reproduction. Genes Dev 1995; 9:794–807.

28. Ploplis V, Carmeliet P, Vazirzadeh S, Vlaenderen IV, Moons L, Plow E, et al. Effects of disruption of the plasminogen gene on thrombosis, growth, and health in mice. Circulation 1995; 92:2585–2593.

29. Carmeliet P, Schoonjans L, Kieckens L, Ream B, Degen J, Bronson R, et al. Physiological consequences of loss of plasminogen activator gene function in mice. Nature 1994; 368:419–424.

30. Bugge TH, Suh TT, Flick MJ, Daugherty CC, Romer J, Solberg H, et al. The receptor for urokinase-type plasminogen activator is not essential for mouse development or fertility. J Biol Chem 1995; 270:16,886–16,894.
31. Dewerchin M, Nuffelen AV, Wallays G, Bouche A, Moons L, Carmeliet P, et al. Generation and characterization of urokinase receptor-deficient mice. J Clin Invest 1996; 97:870–878.
32. Erickson LA, Fici GJ, Lund JE, Boyle TP, Polites HG, Marotti KR. Development of venous occlusions in mice transgenic for the plasminogen activator inhibitor-1 gene. Nature 1990; 346:74–76.
33. Eitzman DT, McCoy RD, Zheng X, Fay WP, Shen T, Ginsburg D, et al. Bleomycin-induced pulmonary fibrosis in transgenic mice that either lack or overexpress the murine plasminogen activator inhibitor-1 gene. J Clin Invest 1996; 97:232–237.
34. Dougherty K, Yang A, Harris J, Saunders T, Camper S, Ginsburg D. Targeted deletion of the murine plasminogen activator inhibitor-2 (PAI-2) gene by homologous recombination (Abstract). Blood 1995; 86 (Suppl 1):455a
35. Zheng X, Saunders TL, Camper SA, Samuelson LC, Ginsburg D. Vitronectin is not essential for normal mammalian development and fertility. Proc Natl Acad Sci USA 1995; 92:12,426–12,430.

11 Folts Cyclic Flow Animal Model for Studying In Vivo Platelet Activity and Platelet Interactions with Damaged Arterial Walls

John D. Folts, PhD, FACC

HISTORICAL BACKGROUND

Many attempts have been made to create partially obstructed coronary arteries in animals that can then be studied and manipulated to produce controlled decreases in coronary flow so that controlled increments of ischemia would be induced. Such a model would require the production of a fixed amount of stenosis, which would allow for essentially normal coronary flow with the animal at rest, but would cause ischemia and sudden death under many of the conditions known to increase the likelihood of sudden death in humans.

Over the years, many techniques have attempted to produce a stable discrete coronary lesion. Pneumatic occluders have had some success in temporary complete obstruction and in the production of graded increases in stenosis. Silk ligatures have been used to create very narrow and tight partial stenoses. Adjustable clamps, first used by Goldblatt on renal arteries, have been placed on coronary arteries to cause graded reductions in coronary flow. Micrometer-controlled snares placed around coronary arteries can also be used to effect graded decreases in coronary flow. All of these techniques produce narrow lesions 1–2 mm in length, which are difficult to control and which produce a very tight, uneven stenosis *(1)*. The coronary-artery lesions observed at autopsy in persons

From: *Contemporary Cardiology: Vascular Disease and Injury: Preclinical Research*
Edited by: D. I. Simon and C. Rogers © Humana Press Inc., Totowa, NJ

who died suddenly from coronary disease were usually 3–5 mm in length, and had a 50–80% reduction in lm diameter *(1)*.

Based on the preceding observations, the ideal requirements for an experimental model of coronary-artery stenosis with subsequent thrombosis are proposed as follows:

1. The technique should produce fixed amounts of coronary artery stenosis that can be increased or decreased under well-controlled conditions.
2. The technique should produce controlled degrees of intimal and medial damage, with exposure of subintimal structures such as collagen, elastin, and tissue factor.
3. The rate and size of a developing platelet thrombus should be detected by the changes in coronary flow measured with an electromagnetic or ultrasonic flowmeter placed on the stenosed coronary artery.
4. A means of collecting the platelet thrombus *in situ* in the narrowed coronary-artery segment for microscopic examination should be established.
5. The model should use a radiolucent device for producing stenosis so that coronary arteriography can be performed to confirm the degree of stenosis and to outline the thrombus in the narrowed lumen and detect any vasospasm. The model should be usable in surgically prepared anesthetized animals and in awake, chronically instrumented animals.

DESCRIPTION OF BASIC MODEL
Dogs

Dogs weighing between 12 and 30 kg of either sex may be utilized. They are premedicated with 3 mg/kg of morphine sulfate and are anesthetized 30 min later with 20 mg/kg of sodium pentobarbital given intravenously. The dogs are then intubated, and ventilation is maintained with 10 cc/kg of room air at 12–15 times/min using a Harvard® or Bird® respirator. Each dog is placed on its right side on a heating blanket. The blanket is adjusted to maintain the dog's core temperature at 38°C, which is the normal temperature for dogs. Arterial blood gases are determined every h and the tidal vol/respiratory rate adjusted accordingly to maintain the pH at approx 7.4, the P_{O2} at 75–85 mmHg, and the PCO_2 at approx 25 mmHg. Small increments of iv pentobarbital are given (30–60 mg) when needed to maintain general anesthesia. The three basic signs indicating that surgical anesthesia has been achieved are: (1) lack of a corneal reflex, (2) slack, relaxed jaw muscles, and (3) no movement or response to a painful stimulus such as pinching the tail.

The femoral artery and vein are surgically exposed, and isolated, and catheters are placed in them. The arterial catheter is attached to a pressure transducer which is connected to a strip chart recorder such as the Gould S 600. This provides a continuous measure of arterial blood pressure, and provides an arterial line for drawing blood samples for arterial blood-gas measurement.

A skin incision is made with the electrocautery, starting at the posterior border of the scapula to the sternum. The thoracic muscles are transected with the cautery from the posterior scapula to the costochondral junction. Care must be taken to avoid cutting through the parietal pleura, as the left lung will be just beneath the pleura. It is also important to look carefully for the internal mammary artery (internal thoracic artery in the dog) and vein which run parallel to and close to the sternum. If these are accidentally cut, they can be clamped and ligated with 2–0 silk suture. The chest is entered at the fifth intercostal space. The left lung is retracted dorsally with wet sponges. Then the pericardium is excised parallel to the phrenic nerve. Sutures (2-0 silk) are placed in the edge of the cut pericardium and retracted dorsally against the sponges covering the retracted left lung, forming a pericardial cradle. A 3-0 silk suture with an atraumatic curved needle is inserted into the epicardium in the lateral free wall of the left ventricle, avoiding any obvious epicardial branches. The suture is pulled toward the sternum (which also pulls the heart toward the sternum) to provide a better view of the main left coronary artery. The suture ends are clamped to the skin, and the left anterior coronary artery can now be easily visualized. To visualize the left circumflex coronary artery, the tip of the left atrial appendage is ligated with a 3-0 silk suture and then retracted dorsally. The left circumflex coronary artery is then visualized in the atrial/ventricular groove. To measure and record the electrocardiogram (ECG), a flexible wire is attached directly to the epicardial surface in the distribution of the coronary artery being studied—with care to avoid small epicardial branches—using a 5-0 prolene suture. This process provides a more sensitive ECG, and makes it possible to detect ST segment changes indicative of myocardial ischemia much sooner than if limb leads were used for recording the ECG. (Fig. 1,2) *(2)*. This is the active lead, comparable to a V_3 chest lead—with the other leads grounded to the animal. Either the left anterior descending coronary artery or the left circumflex coronary artery can be dissected out and utilized for the Folts cyclic flow model *(2)*. For some experiments, both arteries may be utilized.

One of the branches of the left coronary artery is carefully dissected free from the epicardial tissue at a length of 20–30 mm. When dissecting the left circumflex coronary artery (circ), great care must be taken to avoid the branches of the great cardiac vein which often overlay the circumflex coronary artery. When using the left anterior descending coronary artery (LAD), it is essential to avoid the venous branches which run very close and parallel to the LAD, and to look carefully for branches of the LAD which are on the underside of the LAD and perfuse the septum. If a branch of the circ or LAD is accidentally severed, it can be repaired with a double-armed 6-0 cardiovascular prolene su-

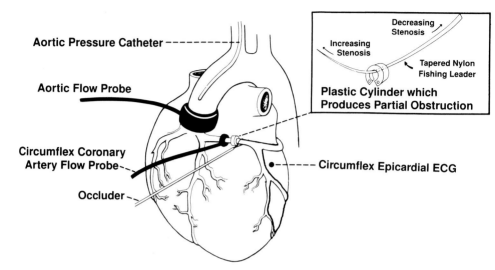

Fig. 1. Schematic of animal model for studying conditions similar to those of humans with coronary-artery disease. The figure shows the technique for producing fixed partial obstruction in a branch of the left circumflex coronary artery. A plastic cylinder 4–5 mm in length is placed to encircle and constrict the coronary artery, producing a 60–70% reduction in diameter. A smooth, tapered nylon fishline is placed between the inside wall of the plastic cylinder and the outside wall of the coronary artery. Fishline is then pulled in either direction to make slight increases or decreases in the amount of stenosis. LAD, left anterior descending coronary artery; ECG, electrocardiogram. (Reprinted with permission from Mehta J, ed., Platelets and Prostaglandins in Cardiovascular Disease. Mt. Kisco, NY, Futura, 1981).

ture. When the artery is isolated, either an electromagnetic flow-probe (Gould®), or a Doppler ultrasonic flow-probe (Transonic®) is placed on the artery proximal to where the stenosis will be placed to continuously measure coronary blood flow. When measuring coronary blood flow, without any stenosis, a temporary 20-s complete occlusion (using the occluder snare shown in Fig. 1) followed by release will produce a large increase in coronary blood flow called a reactive hyperemic response (RH) (shown at **A** in Fig. 2). Note that the electrocardiogram shown above **A** is normal.

Producing Intimal/Medial Damage and Stenosis

The plastic cylinders used to produce a 60–80% stenosis are made of Lexan®, a polycarbonate plastic, in a shape depicted in Fig. 1. They should be made with a range of internal diameters using metric drills. The most common sizes used are between 1.3 and 2.0 mm in 0.1-mm increments. The stenosing cylinders should be 4–5 mm in length *(2)*.

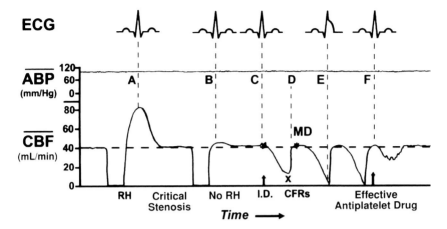

Fig. 2. Schematic diagram showing mean coronary blood flow (CBF) changes with no stenosis on the artery at (**A**). The electrocardiogram (ECG) at the top is normal, and when the coronary artery is totally occluded for only 20 s and then released, there is a large increase in flow called a reactive hyperemic response (RH). At (**B**), with critical stenosis (approx 70% diameter reduction) but no intimal damage (ID) when the artery is temporarily occluded for 20 s there is now no reactive hyperemia (RH). Flow is still steady and in the normal range, and the ECG is still normal. At (**C**) the ECG is still normal, but if intimal damage is produced in the area of stenosis, the coronary flow begins to decline. This is because of platelet aggregates collecting on the damaged walls in the narrowed lumen. With only intimal damage (ID), the growing platelet thrombus often breaks loose and embolizes distally (at X), and blood flow is restored. However, if the artery is clamped more forcefully at (**D**) to produce some medial damage (MD), the platelets adhere more vigorously in the stenosed lm. The platelet clot becomes larger, and is more adherent, and does not embolize, and the artery becomes totally occluded, (**E**) and now the occluded artery produces ECG signs of ischemia. At this point (**E**) the constricting cylinder must be gently shaken to dislodge the thrombus and restore coronary flow. If a potent, effective platelet inhibitor is given intravenously, (**F**), blood flow will be restored and the CFRs will be abolished, and the ECG will remain normal.

Fig. 3A–D show the steps involved in making the plastic cylinder, while Fig. 3E–G show how the cylinder is placed around an artery. The end product of each step is shown in the insert in the lower right-hand corner of each figure. The cylinder is made from round stock of Lexan® (Cadillac Plastics, Milwaukee, WI) with an approxmate diameter of 6 mm. Lexan® is a much better choice than lucite (Plexiglass), which cracks quite readily, or Teflon®, which is too slippery.

1. The Lexan® is secured in a vice clamp and a cylindrical section 4 mm in length is cut with a jeweler's saw, which has a relatively thin blade (Fig. 3A).

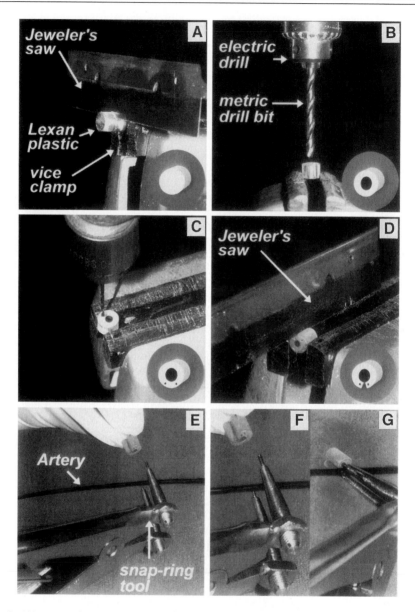

Fig. 3. (A) shows the various stages in constructing a plastic cylinder for placing around the coronary artery. It also shows how the Lexan® polycarbonate plastic is cut into a cylinder 4 mm in length with a jeweler's saw. (B) Demonstrates how the cylinder is held in a small vice clamp so that the metric drill bit can be used to produce the center hole where the artery will be placed. (C) Shows how the small metric drill is used to drill the two small holes which will be used to gently expand the cylinder for the artery to enter the lumen. (D) Shows how the "V" is cut into the cylinder, between the two small holes. The insert at the lower right of figures 3A–D shows the appearance of the cylinder at each stage

2. Next, the plastic cylinder is vertically secured in the vice clamp, and a center hole is made with a high-quality, sharp metric drill bit, moving slowly through the plastic. As the diameter of the drill producing the center hole must correspond to approx 70% of the diameter of the artery it will be placed around, cylinders with different center-hole diameters must be made to ensure a wide selection (Fig. 3B).
3. Two small holes ("guide holes") approx 1.3 mm in diameter are drilled as shown (Fig. 3C).
4. Finally, the "V" is cut into the cylinder with the jeweler's saw as shown. The space between the narrowest portion of the "V" should be kept to a minimum, so that the artery will not slip out. It is critically important to lightly sand the finished cylinder (No. 320 sandpaper) to ensure smooth surfaces free of burs that would otherwise damage the artery (Fig. 3D).
5. A pair of snap-ring pliers with tips that fit into the "guide holes" on the plastic cylinder is used to place the cylinder around the center. This tool can be purchased from most machine wholesale companies. Unlike most pliers, in which the tips move together when the handles are squeezed, these pliers are designed so that the tips move further apart when the handles are squeezed (Fig. 3E).
6. To place the cylinder on the exposed artery (shown as black tubing in the figures), the tips of the snap-ring tool are placed on either side of the artery. The tips are slipped into the two "guide holes" of the cylinder. Then, the handles of the snap ring tool are gently squeezed to open the "V" so that the artery can easily slip into the lm (center hole) of the cylinder. Pulling up gently with the tool facilitates the artery dropping through the "V" into the center hole. Once the artery is within the center hole, the snap-ring tool can be carefully released and slipped out of the guide holes (Fig. 3E–3G). The final appearance of the constricting cylinder in place on the coronary artery is shown in Fig. 1.

The artery diameter is measured with a caliper and one of the previously prepared cylinders chosen with an appropriate internal diameter which will narrow the artery by 60–80%. Small adjustments in the amount of stenosis can be made by placing a tapered nylon fishing leader between the outside of the coronary artery and inside the wall of the cylinder (Fig. 1). When the tapered line is pulled in one direction the amount of stenosis is increased, and when it is pulled in the other direction the amount of stenosis is decreased. When a critical stenosis—approx 70% (diameter reduction)—is produced, the mean coronary flow will still be in the normal range, but a temporary 20-s complete occlusion of the artery followed by release will not produce any reactive hyperemic (RH) re-

---

of construction. (E–G) show how the tips of the snap-ring pliers are placed on either side of the artery, which is shown in black. The tips of the snap-ring tool are placed in the two small holes of the plastic cylinder. This permits opening the "V" of the cylinder to let the artery slip into the larger center hole.

sponse (no RH as shown at **B** in Fig. 2). This method provides assurance that approx 70% stenosis has been achieved *(2,3)*. With a 70% stenosis—if no intimal damage has yet been produced—there will be essentially no change in coronary flow, and the electrocardiogram will be normal, as shown at **B** in Fig. 2. To produce moderate intimal damage of the arterial wall, the cylinder is moved 3–4 mm distally and the artery is clamped gently several times with a needle holder. The cylinder is then moved back on the artery to cover the area of intimal damage produced. When moderate intimal damage (ID) is produced, the flow will begin to decline, and then will be suddenly restored as shown at the X in the center of Fig. 2 at **C** and **D**. When more severe intimal and some medial damage (MD) is produced, the coronary flow will decline to zero, shown at **E** in Fig. 2. This decline in flow is caused by platelets adhering to the damaged, stenosed arterial wall. When the coronary flow reaches zero, there will be ECG ST segment changes indicative of ischemia as shown at **E** in Fig. 2 *(2)*. If the platelet-mediated thrombus does not break loose, restoring coronary flow, the plastic cylinder must be gently shaken. This process will embolize the thrombus, restoring coronary flow as shown at **E** in Fig. 2. Repeated cyclic flow reductions (CFRs) caused by acute platelet-mediated thrombus formation followed by distal embolization will occur for 4–6 h if no intervention is done. However, if an effective platelet inhibitor is given intravenously, the coronary flow will stabilize as shown at **F** on the right of Fig. 2 *(2,4–6)*. Using autologous Indium[M]-labeled platelets, we have shown that the rate of flow decline is directly related to the rate of platelet accumulation in the narrowed lm *(7)*. The CFRs are not caused by vasospasm in the narrowed lm *(8)*. This means that the frequency of CFRs per U of time is a direct on-line assay for in vivo platelet activity *(7,9)*. Thus, if something is done which increases in vivo platelet activity, the frequency of the CFRs will increase—such as when the dog is ventilated with cigarette smoke *(10)*. Conversely, if something is done which decreases in vivo platelet activity, the frequency of the CFRs with time will decrease or disappear. One example of this is giving aspirin, shown in Fig. 4.

Modification for Using Pigs

Because morphine produces excitement in pigs—which raises adrenaline levels and may also trigger malignant hyperthermia—pigs are premedicated with ketamine (Vetalar®) 20 mg/kg given intramuscularly. In addition, 0.4 mg of atropine is given intramuscularly to suppress excess salivation. A cut-down is made on the front foreleg and a catheter is placed in the vein. General anesthesia is then induced with 20 mg/kg of iv sodium pentobarbital. Supplemental anesthesia is given as needed.

Because the ribs are wide and flat in the pig, three or four ribs must be removed to provide adequate surgical exposure. Alternatively, a midsternotomy can be done with the pig on its back to provide exposure of the heart.

Aortic
Blood Pressure
(mmHg)

Circumflex
Coronary-Artery
Blood Flow
(mL/min)

Aortic
Blood Pressure
(mmHg)

Circumflex
Coronary-Artery
Blood Flow
(mL/min)

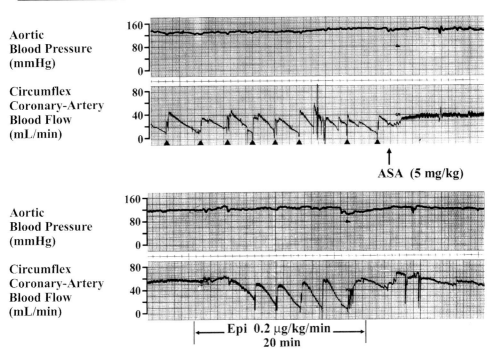

Fig. 4. This is an actual record of mean aortic blood pressure on the top and CFRs in the stenosed and damaged coronary artery. *(top)* On the right, aspirin (ASA) was given intravenously and within 3–4 min the CFRs were eliminated. At the bottom of the lower panel, the iv infusion of epinephrine (epi) causes the CFRs to return. When the epi infusion is stopped, the CFRs disappear again.

To Avoid Ischemia-Induced Ventricular Fibrillation

Experiments are usually conducted with a recording paper speed of 6 mm/ min; however, the ECG should be observed on a monitor at the usual speed of 25 or 50 mm/s. This allows continuous visualization of the changes in the ST segments of the ECG, and awareness of the onset of myocardial ischemia. This may occur during the dissection of the coronary artery or when the coronary blood flow has decreased to a low or zero value because of intraluminal occlusive thrombus. When ischemia occurs, the plastic cylinder is gently shaken to dislodge the platelet-mediated thrombus and restore blood flow, and the signs of ischemia—i.e., ST segment deviation from the isoelectric line—should disappear. If ventricular fibrillation occurs, it can be reversed with immediate cardioversion using internal paddles and 10–15 J of energy. It may be necessary to massage the heart to generate some aortic blood pressure, which produces some coronary flow. This flow will wash out some of the metabolic waste products and provide some myocardial oxygenation to facilitate cardioversion.

Cyclic Flow Reductions (CFRs)

Cyclic reductions in coronary flow will occur within 10 min after intimal and medial damage is produced, and a 60–80% stenosis is produced (Fig. 4). We and others have studied the cellular composition of the clot that gradually forms over 5–10 min and totally occludes the stenosed artery. The thrombus is intimally composed of aggregated platelets, damaged red cells, and very little fibrin. See these references for photomicrographs and electron micrographs of the thrombi in the narrowed lm (4,11,12).

In some instances, CFRs are not produced. Possible reasons are listed below:

1. Low platelet count <100,000/uL or hematocrit <30%;
2. Low body temperature <38°C;
3. Inadequate intimal and medial damage (see Fig. 2);
4. Not enough stenosis—i.e., less than 50% diameter reduction, with significant RH present (see Fig. 2);
5. Hypoxemia, acidemia—i.e., abnormal blood-gas values; or
6. Excess pentobarbital anesthesia (13) or use of halothane anesthesia (14). This occurs because excess pentobarbital or the normal concentration of halothane (0.5–1.0%) inhibits in vivo platelet activity (14).

Inhibition of CFRs with Aspirin, Restoration with IV Epinephrine

One of the first experiments done with the cyclic-flow model was to test the platelet-inhibitory effects of aspirin (15,16). CFRs were obtained as shown in Fig. 4. Five mg/kg of aspirin dissolved in saline (made basic, pH = 9 with a few drops of sodium hydroxide) was given intravenously. The CFRs were eliminated within 5 min (upper right of Fig. 4). Aspirin blocks the production of thromboxane A_2 by stimulated platelets, which is a potent recruiter of other platelets to collect in the narrowed lm and produce an occlusive thrombus. However, there are a variety of mediators in vivo besides thromboxane A_2, such as epinephrine that can activate platelets and help to produce a totally occlusive platelet-mediated clot in the stenosed lm despite pretreatment with aspirin (17). If epinephrine (0.1–0.2 µg/kg/min) is infused intravenously for 20–30 min, the platelet-inhibitory effect of aspirin can be overcome and the CFRs return. (shown in the bottom center of Fig. 4). The CFRs disappear when the epi infusion is stopped.

Since aspirin blocks only one of the many input stimuli, it is not surprising that epinephrine or other platelet stimuli can overcome the platelet-inhibitor effects of aspirin (see 18,19 for extensive review).

Effect of Increased Shear Stress on Platelet Activation

When platelets are inhibited by aspirin, they can also be reactivated by increased shear stress (18). Fig. 9 in Folts (41) shows a record from an experiment where platelet activity was decreased and the CFRs were eliminated with aspirin. However, when the amount of stenosis produced by the plastic cylinder was increased from 70% to 80% diameter reduction by pulling the tapered fish line (see Fig. 1) to produce increased stenosis and increased shear forces, the CFRs returned (Fig. 9 in 41). Thus, increased shear, through its action on the platelets produced by an increase in stenosis, can reactivate platelets despite pretreatment of platelets with aspirin (2,20). The model with increased stenosis and increased shear could be used to study the effects of drugs and other factors on shear-induced platelet activity.

DRUG STUDIES WITH THE CFR MODEL

The CFR animal model has been described as a good model for mimicking unstable angina as it occurs in patient with coronary-artery disease (21–23). A variety of platelet inhibitors have been tested in dogs using this model. Many of these drugs which eliminated the CFRs have gone on to successful clinical trials for treating unstable angina and acute coronary syndromes (see Folts for reviews) (18,19).

Study of Oral Agents in the CFR Model

To study an agent given orally to the anesthetized dog, the route of anesthesia is altered to produce less anesthetic depression of gastrointestinal function. The dog is given 3 mg/kg of morphine intramuscularly, followed by 5 mg/kg of ketamine (Vetalar®) intravenously to produce sedation. The skin and subcutaneous tissue overlying the brachial artery are infiltrated with local injections of 1% lidocaine. Then a cut-down is done on the right brachial artery and a catheter is advanced to the brachiocephalic artery under fluoroscopic guidance. With some practice this can be done blindly without fluoroscopy. This artery supplies three-fourths of the blood supply to the brain, as it supplies the right and left carotid artery and the right vertebral artery. Thus, only 5 mg/kg of pentobarbital can be given intraarterially instead of the 20 mg/kg that is normally needed when pentobarbital is given intravenously. If the catheter tip is properly placed in the brachiocephalic artery, the arterial blood pressure will show a transient decrease of 10–15 mmHg within 5–10 s, when 5 mg/kg of pentobarbital is given. All supplemental pentobarbital anesthesia is also given through this arterial line rather than intravenously (13,24). This mode of anesthesia provides a properly anesthetized brain which meets the criteria for surgical anesthesia mentioned earlier—but a more awake body. To avoid the need to wait for the stomach to empty in the anesthetized dog, the test substance may be given through a gastrostomy tube placed in the stomach wall with the tip in the duodenum (24). Red wine or purple grape juice was given intragastrically to anesthetized dogs displaying CFRs, and the CFRs were eliminated in two h (24,25). Capsules and powdered drugs can also be given via this route (24,26).

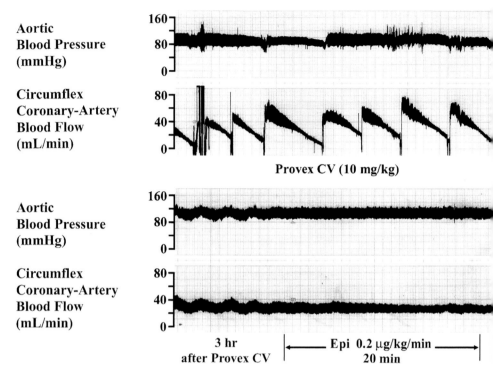

Fig. 5. This figure shows phasic aortic blood pressure, and coronary flow *(top)*. Note that CFRs are occurring at a regular rate. ProVex CV® (Melaleuca Inc., Idaho Falls, ID) is administered by stomach tube *(top, center)*. The record 3 h after the ProVex CV® was administered to the dog *(bottom)*. Note that the ProVex CV® has apparently been absorbed by the GI tract, entered the blood stream, inhibited the platelets, and eliminated the CFRs. Note that when epinephrine (epi) is infused intravenously, the CFRs do not return *(bottom right)*. This suggests the ProVex CV® has protected against the renewal of platelet activity by the epi.

Example: Testing an Orally Active Substance

PROVEX CV®

A commercial nutritional supplement called ProVex CV® (Melaleuca, Inc., Idaho Falls, ID) was studied in anesthetized dogs. The supplement contains polyphenolic compounds from grape-seed extract, grape-skin extract, ginkgo biloba, bilberry, and quercetin, a specific flavonoid. These substances are believed to have platelet-inhibitory as well as antioxidant properties. CFRs occurred on a regular basis, as shown at the top of Fig. 5. Three h after giving 15 mg/kg of ProVex CV® by stomach tube, the CFRs were gradually eliminated—indicating that the ProVex CV® was properly absorbed from the gut, reached the bloodstream, and achieved a blood concentration sufficiently high to significantly inhibit in vivo platelet activity, as shown at the bottom of Fig. 5. The CFRs are not renewed when epinephrine (epi) 0.2 &g/kg/min is infused as shown at the lower right in Fig. 5. This demonstrates that in the animal model, the ProVex CV® is a better platelet inhibitor than aspirin *(26)*. Ex vivo platelet aggregation studies in 14 human volunteers, taking ProVex CV® for 7 d also demonstrated significant antiplatelet properties *(26)*. This human study supports the platelet inhibition seen in the CFR model with ProVex CV® *(26)*.

Studies of the CFR Model in the Carotid Arteries of Rabbits or Monkeys

Dogs have become very expensive for research purposes. Thus, we have developed the use of rabbits, which are much less expensive, for thrombosis research *(2,27)*. Although rabbit hearts are too small to study the coronary arteries, the carotid arteries work well. Although primates would be very useful for thrombosis studies, they are very expensive. However, small primates such as cynomologous monkeys may be used—also by instrumenting the carotid arteries *(2,29)*.

Rabbits (3–4 kg) or cynomologous monkeys (3–5 kg) are anesthetized with 3 mg/kg of acepromazine intramuscularly followed by 30 mg/kg of ketamine (Vetalar®) intramuscularly. The femoral artery and vein are isolated and cannulated for blood-pressure measurement, and administration of fluids and sodium pentobarbital (15 mg) is given as needed to maintain anesthesia.

Through a midline incision in the neck, the trachea is isolated and cannulated with a curved 3–4 mm metal cannula to provide a tracheostomy, which facilitates breathing and prevents aspiration. Then the sternocleidomastoid muscle is transected on both sides of the neck with electrocautery, to allow exposure of both carotid arteries. Careful dissection is essential, because blood loss must be kept to a minimum in these small animals. A segment of the carotid artery is isolated, and either an electromagnetic or Doppler flow-probe is placed on it to continuously measure blood flow (Fig. 6). Distal to the flow-probe, the artery is clamped gently with rubber-covered forceps to produce intimal and medial damage (Fig. 6). The carotid arteries of rabbits or monkeys are more easily damaged than the coronary arteries of dogs, and thus must be handled very carefully. A 60–70% stenosis can be achieved by placing a plastic constrictor on the carotid artery that produces a 20% reduction in mean carotid blood flow. The tapered nylon fishing leader can be used to make small adjustments in carotid flow. The monkey's or rabbit's instrumented carotid artery will develop CFRs or cyclic-flow variations (CFVs), which are characterized by a sudden restoration of flow that occurs spontaneously or after gentle tapping of the cylinder *(2)*.

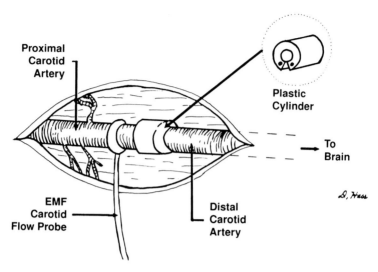

Fig. 6. This figure shows how the plastic cylinder (very similar to the one previously described) can be used to produce stenosis in a monkey or rabbit carotid artery. The electromagnetic flow (EMF) probe (or Doppler probe) should be placed on the surgically exposed carotid artery proximal to the stenosis. When necessary, the thrombus is dislodged by gently shaking the cylinder.

Potential Problems with Rabbit or Monkey Carotid Artery Model

CFRs may fail to occur for the same reasons provided for the dog. In addition, the blood flow may be too low in the carotid artery to produce the necessary turbulent flow in the area of stenosis. Turbulence is needed to bring the platelets into contact with the damaged arterial wall. In this case, occluding the contralateral carotid artery will often increase blood pressure, and the blood flow through the stenosed carotid artery and CFRs will begin.

In other cases, supplemental oxygen may be needed. This can be done by placement of a small tube which provides a flow of oxygen near the orifice of the tracheostomy tube. This will increase the oxygen content of the inspired air. The CFRs will continue for up to 3 h if no effective platelet inhibition is given. Several interesting studies have been done using rabbits and monkeys (30–32).

Studies in Chronic Awake Dogs

The dog may be prepared and instrumented as described earlier using the sterile surgical technique (3). The flow-probe cable and an arterial blood-pressure line can be tunneled under the skin to the withers area and exteriorized. The chest is then surgically closed in the usual fashion, and the dog is allowed to awaken. In the awake state, CFRs can still occur, and are measured with the flow-meter probe *(3,8,33)*. Dogs can be exercised on a treadmill, and the effects of exercise on in vivo platelet activity can be measured *(34)*. These studies are described in more detail in refs. *2,33–36*.

CFRs Recorded in Human Subjects with Arterial Stenosis Caused by Atherosclerosis

A range-gated ultrasound Doppler model flow-probe (Parks Electronic Lab, Beaverton, OR) can be placed on the skin over the popliteal artery in patients with peripheral vascular disease and stenosis in the large arteries in the leg. An acoustical gel is used to couple the sound from the ultrasonic crystals to the skin and to the artery beneath. Blood flow can be continuously monitored for hs. Patients with vascular disease in the legs may have intermittent claudication. These are periodic episodes of ischemic pain in the legs, even when at rest. This is believed to be the pathophysiologic equivalent of unstable angina in patients with coronary-artery disease. It is believed that some cases of periodic calf and ankle pain observed in patients with peripheral vascular disease may be caused by periodic platelet-mediated thrombus formation. Followed by embolization distally, this would produce CFRs in measured blood flow in the leg. These were observed in patients and were abolished temporarily with aspirin *(37)*.

Cyclic-flow reductions and CFVs have also been recorded in the coronary arteries of patients with coronary-artery narrowing caused by atherosclerotic plaque. Blood flow can be measured with a Doppler flow crystal placed on the end of a small (3F) catheter *(38)*. This flow measurement can be done in patients at the time of angioplasty by advancing the small Doppler catheter through the usual larger guide catheter into the coronary artery to be studied. Eichhorn et al. observed CFVs in the stenosed arteries of patients during coronary angioplasty *(38)*. The authors felt that these CFVs were caused by periodic formation of acute platelet-mediated thrombi followed by embolization distally—essentially the same as CFRs in the animal models *(38)*. It is important to note that these patients had CFVs despite pretreatment with Valium®, aspirin, and heparin. The CFVs may have occurred because the adrenalin levels were elevated in these patients, although the authors did not measure plasma adrenalin. Heparin and Valium® do not inhibit platelet activity. We have previously shown that heparin and aspirin do not protect against platelet-mediated cyclic flow reductions when adrenalin is elevated *(16,39)*.

A 0.18-inch guide wire has recently been developed with a Doppler crystal at the tip (Cardiometrics, Rancho Cordova, CA). This can be placed under fluoroscopic guidance through a guide catheter into one of the main diseased coronary branches of patients at the time of angioplasty. Monitoring blood flow continuously for 20 min also detected CFRs in these patients. These CFRs were seen in patients treated with aspirin, Valium, and heparin *(40)*. The CFRs were eliminated by giving 0.25 mg/kg of C7E3, a monoclonal antibody to the platelet GPIIb-IIIa fibrinogen receptor *(40)*. This antiplatelet agent was first tested in dogs and monkeys using the CFR models *(30)*.

Studies of Platelet Inhibitors in the CFR Model Leading to Clinical Trials

The following drugs/food substances have been shown to eliminate the CFRs, and to inhibit platelet activity in humans:

1. Aspirin *(16)*;
2. C7E3 (abciximab or ReoPro®) *(30)*;
3. Clopidogrel (Plavix) *(41)*;
4. Amlodipine *(42)*;
5. Nitroglycerin *(43)*;
6. Sodium nitroprusside *(44)*; and
7. Red wine and purple grape juice *(23)*.

Two drugs (prostacyclin PGI_2 and its analog Iloprost®) and dipyridamole (Persantine®) were unsuccessful in the dog CFR model and in clinical trials *(45–47)*. PGI_2 and Iloprost® produced unacceptable hypotension, and Persantine® was simply ineffective.

As new antiplatelet drugs are developed, they are likely to be tested in one of the CFR models. These models provide reliable indications of in vivo platelet activity over time. They also allow secondary thrombotic factors such as elevated catecholamines, increased medial damage, or increased shear forces to be tested. Animals can be studied in the awake or anesthetized state, and both oral and iv drugs can be tested.

REFERENCES

1. Folts JD. Experimental arterial platelet thrombosis, platelet inhibitors, and their possible clinical relevance. Cardiovasc Rev Rep 1982; 3:370–382.
2. Folts JD. An in vivo model of experimental arterial stenosis, intimal damage and periodic thrombosis. Circulation 1991; Suppl 4:IV3–14.
3. Folts JD, Gallagher K, Rowe GG. Hemodynamic effects of controlled degrees of coronary artery stenosis in short-term and long-term studies in dogs. J Thorac Cardiovasc Surg 1977; 73:722–727.
4. Folts JD. A model of experimental arterial platelet thrombosis, platelet inhibitors, and their possible clinical relevance: an update. Cardiovasc Rev Rep 1990; 11:10–26.
5. Ashton JH, Ogletree ML, Michel intramuscularly, Golino P, McNatt JM, Taylor AL, et al. Cooperative mediation by serotonin S_2 and thromboxane A_2/prostaglandin H_2 receptor activation of cyclic flow variations in dogs with severe coronary artery stenoses. Circulation 1987; 76:952–959.

6. Golino P, Ambrosio G, Ragni M, Pascucci I, Triggiani M, Oriente A, et al. Short-term and long-term role of platelet activating factor as a mediator of in vivo platelet aggregation. Circulation 1993; 88:1205–1214.
7. Maalej N, Holden JE, Folts JD. Effect of shear stress on acute platelet thrombus formation in canine stenosed carotid arteries: An in vivo quantitative study. Journal of Thrombosis and Thrombolysis 1998; 5:231–238.
8. Folts JD, Gallagher K, Rowe GG. Blood flow reductions in stenosed canine coronary arteries: vasospasm or platelet aggregation? Circulation 1982; 65:248–255.
9. Bush LR, Shebuski RJ. In vivo models of arterial thrombosis and thrombolysis. FASEB. J 1990; 4:3087–3098.
10. Gering SA, Folts JD. Exacerbation of acute platelet thrombus formation in stenosed dog coronary arteries with smoke from a non-tobacco-burning cigarette. J Lab Clin Med 1990; 116:728–736.
11. Bolli R, Ware A, Brandon TA, Weilbaecher DG, Mace ML. Platelet-mediated thrombosis in stenosed canine coronary arteries: inhibition by nicergoline, a platelet-active alpha-adrenergic antagonist. J Am Coll Cardiol 1984; 3:1417–1426.
12. Bush LR, Campbell WB, Buja M, Tilton G, Willerson JT. Effects of the selective thromboxane synthetase inhibitor dazoxiben on variations in cyclic blood flow in stenosed canine coronary arteries. Circulation 1984; 69:1161–1170.
13. O'Rourke ST, Folts JD, Albrecht RM. Inhibition of canine platelet aggregation by barbiturates. J Lab Clin Med 1986; 108:206–212.
14. Bertha BG, Folts JD, Nugent M, Rusy BF. Halothane, but not isoflurane or enflurane, protects against spontaneous and epinephrine-exacerbated acute thrombus formation in stenosed dog coronary arteries. Anesthesiology 1989; 71:96–102.
15. Folts JD, Crowell EB, Rowe GG. Platelet aggregation in partially obstructed coronary arteries and their inhibition with aspirin. Clin Res 1974; 22:595A.
16. Folts JD, Crowell EB, Rowe GG. Platelet aggregation in partially obstructed vessels and its elimination with aspirin. Circulation 1976; 54:365–370.
17. Rao GH, Escolar G, White JG. Epinephrine reverses the inhibitory influences of aspirin on platelet-vessel wall interactions. Thromb Res 1986; 44:65–74.
18. Folts JD. Drugs for the prevention of coronary thrombosis: from an animal model to clinical trials. Cardiovasc Drugs Ther 1995; 9:31–43.
19. Maalej N, Folts JD. Effect of shear stress on acute platelet thrombus formation in canine stenosed carotid arteries: An in vitro quantitative study.
20. Sherry S. Aspirin and antiplatelet drugs: the clinical approach. Cardiovasc Rev Rep 1984; 5:1208–1219.
21. Ikeda H, Koga Y, Kuwano K, Nakayama H, Ueno T, Yoshida N, et al. Cyclic flow variations in a conscious dog model of coronary artery stenosis and endothelial injury correlate with acute ischemic heart disease syndromes in humans. J Am Coll Cardiol 1993; 21:1008–1017.
22. Willerson JT, Golino P, Eidt J, Campbell WB, Buja LM. Specific platelet mediators and unstable coronary artery lesions. Experimental evidence and potential clinical implications. Circulation 1989; 80:198–205.
23. Demrow HS, Slane PR, Folts JD. Administration of wine and grape juice inhibits in vivo platelet activity and thrombosis in stenosed canine coronary arteries. Circulation 1995; 91:1182–1188.
24. Osman HE, Maalej N, Shanmuganayagam D. Grape juice but not orange or grapefruit juice inhibits platelet activity in dogs and monkeys. J Nutr 1998; 128:2307–2312.
25. Slane PR, Folts JD. Platelet inhibition in stenosed canine coronary arteries by quercetin and rutin, polyphenolic flavonoids found in red wine. Clin Res 1994; 42:162A.

26. Folts JD. Commercial mixture of flavonoids, ProVex CV, inhibits in vivo thrombosis and ex vivo platelet aggregation in dogs and humans. J Invest Med 1998; 46:199A.

27. Hill DS, Smith SR, Folts JD. The rabbit as a model for carotid artery stenosis, and periodic acute thrombosis. Fed Proc 1987; 46:421.

28. Folts JD, Mosher DF. Transient declines in stenosed monkey carotid artery blood flow due to acute platelet thrombus formation. Thromb Haemostasis 1983; 50:20.

29. Coller BS, Folts JD, Smith SR, Scudder LE, Jordan R. Abolition of in vivo platelet thrombus formation in primates with monoclonal antibodies to the platelet GPIIb/IIIa receptor. Correlation with bleeding time, platelet aggregation, and blockade of GPIIb/IIIa receptors. Circulation 1989; 80:1766–1774.

30. Schumacher WA, Goldenberg HJ, Harris DN, Ogletree ML. Effect of thromboxane receptor antagonists on renal artery thrombosis in the cynomologus monkey. J Pharmacol Exp Ther 1987; 243:460–466.

31. Pawashe AB, Golino P, Ambrosio G, Migliaccio F, Ragni M, Pascucci I, et al. A monoclonal antibody against rabbit tissue factor inhibits thrombus formation in stenotic injured rabbit carotid arteries. Circ Res 1994; 74:56–63.

32. Willerson JT, Yao SK, McNatt J, Benedict CR, Anderson HV, Golino P, et al. Frequency and severity of cyclic flow alternations and platelet aggregation predict the severity of neointimal proliferation following experimental coronary stenosis and endothelial injury. Proc Natl Acad Sci USA 1991; 88:10,624–10,628.

33. Eidt J, Ashton J, Golino P, McNatt J, Buja LM, Willerson JT. Treadmill exercise promotes cyclic alterations in coronary blood flow in dogs with coronary artery stenoses and endothelial injury. J Clin Invest 1989; 84:517–527.

34. Folts JD, Gering SA, Laibly SW, Bertha BG, Bonebrake FC, Keller JW. Effects of cigarette smoke and nicotine on platelets and experimental coronary artery thrombosis. Adv Exp Med Biol 1990; 273:339–58:339–358.

35. Folts JD, Bonebrake FC. The effects of cigarette smoke and nicotine on platelet thrombus formation in stenosed dog coronary arteries: inhibition with phentolamine. Circulation 1982; 65:465–470.

36. Eichhorn EJ, Grayburn PA, Willard JE, Anderson HV, Bedotto JB, Carry M, et al. Spontaneous alterations in coronary blood flow velocity before and after coronary angioplasty in patients with severe angina. J Am Coll Cardiol 1991; 17:43–52.

37. Folts JD. Cigarette smoking and thrombus formation. Am Heart J 1988; 116:1657–1658.

38. Anderson HV, Kirkeeide RL, Krishnaswami A, Weigelt LA, Revana M, Weisman HF, et al. Cyclic flow variations after coronary angiogplasty in humans: clinical and angiographic characteristics and elimination with 7E3 monoclonal antiplatelet antibody. J Am Coll Cardiol 1994; 23:1031–1037.

39. Yao SK, McNatt J, Cui K, Anderson HV, Maffrand JP, Buja LM, et al. Combined ADP and thromboxane A2 antagonism prevents cyclic flow variations in stenosed and endothelium-injured arteries in nonhuman primates. Circulation 1993; 88:2888–2893.

40. Folts JD. Inhibition of platelet activity in vivo by amlodipine alone and combined with aspirin. Int J Cardiol 1997; 62:S111–S117.

41. Folts JD, Stamler J, Loscalzo J. Intravenous nitroglycerin infusion inhibits cyclic blood flow responses caused by periodic platelet thrombus formation in stenosed canine coronary arteries. Circulation 1991; 83:2122–2127.

42. Rovin JD, Stamler JS, Loscalzo J, Folts JD. Sodium nitroprusside, an endothelium-derived relaxing factor congener, increases platelet cyclic GMP levels and inhibits epinephrine-exacerbated in vivo platelet thrombus formation in stenosed canine coronary arteries. J Cardiovasc Pharmacol 1993; 22:626–631.

43. Folts JD, Rowe GG. Dipyridamole does not inhibit thrombus formation in stenosed canine coronary arteries nor does it augment the inhibitory effect of low dose aspirin. Journal of Vascular Medicine and Biology 1989; 1:255–261.
44. Schafer AI. Antiplatelet therapy. Am J Med 1996; 101:199–209X.
45. Fitzgerald GA. Dipyridamole. N Engl J Med 1987; 316:1247–1257.

III CHRONIC ATHEROSCLEROTIC MODELS

12 Mouse Models of Atherosclerosis

Wulf Palinski, MD, Claudio Napoli, MD, and Peter D. Reaven, MD

CONTENTS

INTRODUCTION

Mice are rapidly becoming the preferred model for studies of the pathogenesis of atherosclerosis *(1–10)*. Although wild-type mice are inherently resistant to hypercholesterolemia and atherogenesis, identification of genes determining the susceptibility of mice to atherosclerosis and advances in gene knockout and transgene techniques have led to the generation of murine models that develop extensive atherosclerosis. These models offer new insights into atherogenic mechanisms of apolipoproteins, enzymes, and receptors involved in lipid metabolism, lipoprotein oxidation and glycation, adhesion molecules and cytokines, and the humoral and cellular immune system, as well as gene regulation in vascular cells. The use of murine models for studies testing the antiatherogenic efficacy of drugs, gene transfer, or immune modulation is made

From: *Contemporary Cardiology: Vascular Disease and Injury: Preclinical Research*
Edited by: D. I. Simon and C. Rogers © Humana Press Inc., Totowa, NJ

possible by the availability of morphometric techniques that allow quantification of the size of atherosclerotic lesions throughout the mouse aorta, irrespec-
tive of the degree of hypercholesterolemia and atherogenesis achieved. This
chapter reviews murine models of atherosclerosis and provides a detailed overview of the distribution and composition of atherosclerotic lesions in these mice
and the preparative techniques and computer-assisted image analysis methods
used to quantify lesion size. This is followed by a review of some of the principal research applications of murine models.

MURINE MODELS OF HYPERCHOLESTEROLEMIA AND ATHEROSCLEROSIS

Mice Developing Mild to Moderate Atherosclerosis

The lipoprotein profile of wild-type mice differs significantly from that of
humans and primates. Total plasma cholesterol levels in mice are very low, and
most of their cholesterol is carried in high density lipoproteins (HDL). Mice
also lack cholesteryl ester transfer protein (CETP), which mediates the ex-
change of HDL cholesterol esters with VLDL triglycerides. Even when fed
high-fat diets, wild-type mice do not develop significant atherosclerosis. In contrast, in C57BL/6 mice, an inbred strain with a genetic susceptibility to hypercholesterolemia, high-fat diets induce a two- to threefold increase in TC levels
and a relative shift of cholesterol from HDL towards atherogenic lipoprotein
fractions (11–15). By itself, this degree of hypercholesterolemia is insufficient
to induce atherogenesis. However, when combined with cholic acid, which
seems to enhance inflammation (16), prolonged exposure to high-fat diets leads
to the accumulation of macrophages in the aortic intima. These are not generally accepted as true early stages of atherosclerosis for the followiong reasons:
they are mostly limited to the aortic root (under the leaflets of the aortic valve)
where turbulent flow conditions prevail; their formation depends on cholic acid;
and, most importantly, they do not progress toward more advanced atherosclerotic lesions.

Nevertheless, the C57BL/6 strain has been essential to enhance the susceptibility to atherosclerosis of other murine strains in which specific genes have
been knocked out or overexpressed, such as the 129 strain. After repeated cross-
breeding into the C57BL/6 background, such models have been extensively
used to study the consequences of overexpression of murine or human
apoproteins—particularly apolipoprotein (apo) A-I and A-II (17–19). These
studies have shown that high plasma levels of apo A-I strongly reduce lesion
formation (consistent with the inverse correlation between HDL levels and heart
disease in humans), whereas overexpression of apo A-II enhances lesion size.
This suggests that, in addition to the plasma level of HDL, its apoprotein composition is an important determinant of atherogenesis. Results obtained with a

model combining overexpression of human apo B and knockout of apo A-I suggested that HDL deficiency requires elevated LDL levels in order to be atherogenic, whereas in the absence of hypercholesterolemia, HDL deficiency does not increase lesion formation (20). Overexpression of apo A-IV also reduces atherogenesis (21). Other studies have investigated the atherogenic effects of overexpression of human apo(a) alone (22,23) or in combination with apo B, (24–26) as well as that of apo B100 and apo B48 (27–29). A murine model of abetalipoproteinemia has also been generated in mice. However, only heterozygotes proved to be viable (30).

Mice Developing Extensive Atherosclerosis

The theoretical objections regarding the nature of "atherosclerosis" in many of the models discussed here have recently been overcome by the development of two models in which extensive hypercholesterolemia and advanced atherosclerotic lesions occur spontaneously or in response to high-fat diets.

The first of these is the apoE-deficient (apoE$^{-/-}$) mouse, developed independently by the groups of Breslow and Maeda (31,32). These knockout mice are unable to generate apoE, and consequently show marked elevation of plasma levels of apoproteins which are normally cleared by receptors binding to apoE, mainly chylomicrons and VLDL. Intermediate density lipoprotein (IDL) and LDL levels are raised to a lesser extent. Even on a regular chow, these mice usually develop plasma cholesterol levels of 600 mg/dL or more. Further increases to more than 1,200 mg/dL are achieved by cholate-free diets with increased cholesterol content (0.15%), termed "Western diets" by Breslow and colleagues. As described here, these mice develop advanced lesions throughout the aorta (33–35).

The second model is the LDL receptor-deficient (LDLR$^{-/-}$) mouse (36). Although these mice have the same genetic defect as humans with familial hypercholesterolemia and LDL receptor-deficient (WHHL) rabbits, LDLR$^{-/-}$ mice develop only "moderately" elevated plasma cholesterol levels (250–300 mg/dL) when fed regular mouse chow. However, levels of about 1,200 mg/dL are easily achieved by high-fat, high cholesterol diets. In analogy to the apoE$^{-/-}$ model, these extreme cholesterol levels induce extensive atherosclerosis throughout the aorta (37–39). In contrast to the apoE$^{-/-}$ mouse, in LDLR$^{-/-}$ mice most of the cholesterol is carried in the IDL/LDL fraction.

To obtain a more homogeneous genetic background and to remove as much as possible athero-resistance traits derived from the 129 strain, apoE$^{-/-}$ and LDLR$^{-/-}$, mice have been back-crossed with C57BL/6 mice for 10 generations (Jackson Laboratories). Both models have been extensively used for studies of atherogenic mechanisms, for intervention studies with drugs, and to investigate the role of the immune system in atherosclerosis. In addition, murine models of human familial combined hyperlipoproteinemia (40) and models of genetic

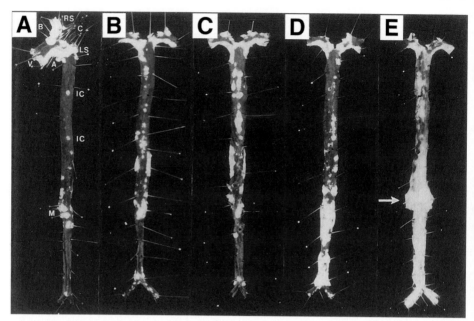

Fig. 1. *En face* preparations of unstained aortas from homozygous apoE[-/-] and LDLR[-/-] mice fed different atherogenic diets for up to 6 mo. (**A**) Anatomically correct preparations. Predilection sites of atherosclerotic lesions are the small curvature of the arch (A) and the branch sites of the brachiocephalic (**B**), the right subclavian (RS), the left common carotid (**C**) and subclavian (LS), some intercostal arteries (IC), the mesenteric and renal arteries (M), and the iliac bifurcation. "V" indicates the position of the aortic valve. Scale = mm. (**B–E**) Representative aortas showing typical progression of atherosclerosis. In these preparations, the aortic arch was split and one half was folded over to the right side to obtain a flat surface for image analysis. (**B,C**) Initially, lesions at the predilection sites described above undergo significant thickening and also begin to expand laterally. (**D,E**) Further atherogenesis occurs mostly in the abdominal aorta, whereas complete coverage of the thoracic aorta is seldom seen. Panel E also shows a gross dilatation of the abdominal aorta (arrow) indicative of an aneurysm. (Composite panel using arteries from experiments described in refs. *35,38,39,70*)

defects that affect receptor-mediated plasma clearance of lipoproteins, such as apo E3–Leiden *(41,42)*, have been developed.

PREDILECTION SITES AND COMPOSITION OF MURINE ATHEROSCLEROTIC LESIONS

The following section describes distribution and characteristics of atherosclerotic lesions observed in apoE[-/-] and LDLR[-/-] mice, but the findings may also apply in part to double apoE and LDL receptor knockout mice *(43)* and other murine models in which high cholesterol levels have been sustained for prolonged periods. In both apoE[-/-] and LDLR[-/-] mice, the earliest lesions appear in the vicinity of the aortic valve (Figs. 1A, 2A). This is eventually followed by a more or less simultaneous appearance of lesions at typical predilection sites in the aorta: the small curvature of the arch; the orifices of the brachiocephalic, left subclavian, and common carotid artery; the branch sites of the mesenteric and renal arteries; and the iliac bifurcation (Fig. 1A). Contrary to rabbit models, lesion formation at branch sites of the intercostal arteries is highly unpredictable in mice. Lesions formed at the above-described predilection sites then grow towards the lumen and begin to expand laterally (Fig. 1B,C). Upon very prolonged exposure to extreme hypercholesterolemia, additional atherogenesis occurs mainly in the abdominal aorta, whereas the thoracic aorta is seldom completely covered by lesions (Fig. 1D,E). In advanced lesions, erosion of the intimal surface and medial involvement is frequently seen and sometimes leads to formation of aneurysms. The gross dilatation of the abdominal aorta, shown in Fig. 1E, suggests that mice often survive such aneurysms for prolonged periods. However, cardiovascular mortality is increased in mice with advanced atherosclerosis, in contrast to WHHL rabbits which have normal lifespans.

Lesions in apoE$^{-/-}$ and LDLR$^{-/-}$ mice have been extensively characterized *(33–35,38)* and have been shown to share many of the features found in human atherosclerosis. Representative examples are shown in Fig. 2. The earliest lesions in the vicinity of the aortic valve (Fig. 2A,B) and other predilection sites throughout the aorta consist mostly of macrophage/foam cells. Lesions shown in these figures are similar to those found in the aortic root of C57BL/6 mice not subjected to additional genetic alteration. In apoE$^{-/-}$ and LDLR$^{-/-}$ mice, lesions in both the aorta and the aortic root begin to form fibrous caps (Fig. 2C). These transitional lesions may progress toward classical atheromas with a single large necrotic core (Fig. 2D). However, other advanced lesions show multiple and sometimes overlapping necrotic cores and fibrous caps.

After prolonged exposure to high cholesterol levels, very large lesions are often found in the aortic origin. These lesions spread towards the leaflets and often cause considerable stenosis (Fig. 2E). Lesions causing extensive stenosis can also be seen in some coronary arteries (Fig. 2F). A recent paper reporting hypoxia-induced electrocardiographic changes and other indicators of prolonged myocardial ischemia in LDLR$^{-/-}$ mice *(44)* and the observation of spontaneous thrombosis in murine aortas (Calara, Napoli and Palinski, unpublished data) suggest that coronary atherosclerosis in mice may result in clinical sequelae. In addition to macrophages (Fig. 2B) *(33–35)* and some T-cells *(45)*, early and advanced lesions contain modified lipoproteins. Immunocytochemistry shows both "oxidation-specific" epitopes—i.e., epitopes generated during the oxidation of LDL and other lipoproteins *(35,46,47)*—and epitopes of advanced glycation endproducts (AGE) (Fig. 2G) *(48)*. Murine lesions are also rich in immunoglobulins G and M (Fig. 2H) *(9,35,38)*. These immunoglobulins

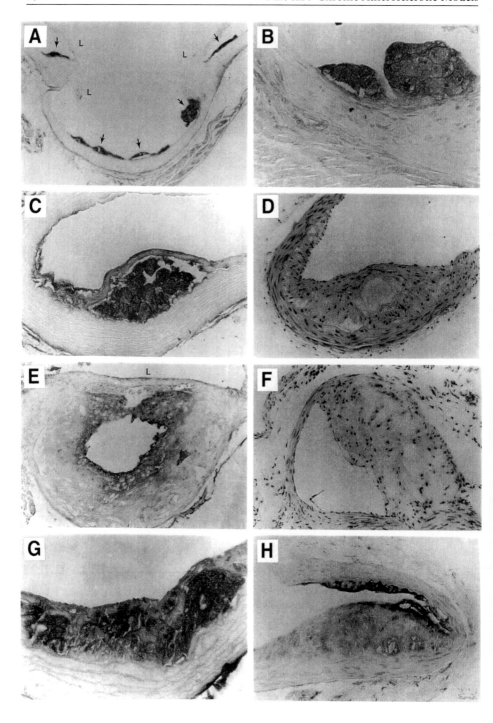

are likely to include autoantibodies to oxidized LDL, *(9,35,38,49)* and are frequently found in the same intimal areas as macrophages and "oxidation-specific" epitopes *(35)*. T-cells are prevalent in murine lesions *(45,50)* and a recent paper also reported the presence of B-cells, which were generally though to be absent from atherosclerotic lesions *(51)*.

Murine atherosclerosis is frequently associated with disruption of the media and large aneurysms have been observed (Fig. 1E) *(33–35,39)*. Medial atrophy often occurs in areas of acute inflammation, and recent evidence shows that metalloproteinases play an important role in medial remodeling and cardiac rupture in mice *(52,53)*. Murine models have been extensively used to study thrombosis and hemostasis (reviewed in 7), but induction of thrombosis in these models has usually been dependent on exogenous vascular injury. However, deep erosion or rupture of murine atherosclerotic lesions in the aorta, and in coronary arteries, may occur spontaneously in mice with extensive atherosclerosis, in particular older apoE$^{-/-}$ mice, and give rise to thrombus formation (Calara, Napoli and Palinski, unpublished data). The incidence of spontaneous plaque erosion/rupture and thrombosis appears to be much lower than in humans, and the lack of a single well-defined fibrous cap (similar to that seen in the classical human atheroma) in many large lipid-rich murine lesions makes it difficult to differentiate between plaque fissure and deep erosion in mice.

Very advanced atherosclerotic lesions of apoE$^{-/-}$ mice also contain *vasa vasorum* in the deep subintimal areas and vicinity of the internal elastic lamina *(54)*. Inhibition of capillary growth by angiogenesis inhibitors significantly inhibited atherogenesis *(54)*. As a result, ApoE$^{-/-}$ mice may be useful to test antiatherogenic interventions targeting factors involved in neovascularization.

Fig. 2. Representative photomicrographs of different stages of atherosclerotic lesions in apoE$^{-/-}$ and LDLR$^{-/-}$ mice. (**A,B**) Sections through the aortic origin showing parts of the valve leaflets (L) and the sinus of Valsalva. Immunostaining with an antibody to murine macrophages highlights several small lesions (arrows). Higher magnification (**B**) shows that these early lesions consist mostly of macrophage/foam cells. (**C**) Transitional lesion in the aorta of an apoE$^{-/-}$ mouse with a distinct fibrous cap. (**D**) Atheroma with a well established necrotic core in the aortic origin of an apoE$^{-/-}$ mouse stained with hematoxylin/eosin. (**E**) Very extensive lesion in the aortic origin of an LDLR$^{-/-}$ mouse. Note that the lesion has grown towards the valve leaflet (L) and caused severe stenosis. (**F**) High magnification of a coronary artery of an LDLR$^{-/-}$ mouse partially occluded by a lesion. (**G**) In addition to macrophages and some T-cells, *(36)* lesions are rich in immunoglobulins. Dark areas indicate presence of IgG or IgM (double immunostaining). Immunoglobulins are frequently found in the same intimal areas as macrophages and "oxidation-specific" epitopes *(35,38)*. (**H**) Advanced aortic lesion immunostained with an antibody against advanced glycation endproducts (AGE). AGE epitopes are present even in euglycemic mice and often co-localize with oxidation-specific epitopes. Reprinted with permission from refs. *35* (A,B), *38* (E), and *48* (H).

QUANTITATIVE DETERMINATION
OF ATHEROSCLEROSIS IN MICE

Preparative Methods

Two basic approaches can be used to quantify atherosclerosis in mice. The first and more widely used was introduced by Paigen et al., and measures lesion areas in cross-sections through the aortic root *(55)*. The second was developed by Palinski and colleagues, and determines atherosclerosis in the entire aorta, expressing results as the percent of surface area covered by lesions *(35,39)*. The initial tissue preparation is similar for both methods. Mice are anesthetized with ether or metafane. The thorax is opened and the systemic circulation is perfused for 15–20 min with phosphate-buffered saline (PBS) containing 20 μM BHT and 2 μM EDTA, pH 7.4, via a 21G cannula inserted into the left ventricle. Physiological pressure is achieved by suspending the buffer reservoir 80–100 cm above the heart and allowing free outflow of the perfusate from an incision into the right atrium. For most purposes, this is sufficient to remove the blood. However, to further reduce cell adhesion to the arterial wall, the lungs may be tied off prior to perfusion. The aortic tree is then perfused for 15 min with a fixative, such as formal-sucrose (4% paraformaldehyde, 5% sucrose, 20 μM EDTA, pH 7.4).

Preparation of the Aortic Tree

Although the diameter of the mouse aorta is very small, a method to obtain e*n-face* preparations of the murine aorta similar to those of larger animal models and humans has been developed *(35)*. The aorta is exposed from the heart to the iliac bifurcation and carefully dissected from the surrounding tissue. Suitable instruments are available from several manufacturers and include extra-delicate Mini-Vanna spring scissors, straight, sharp, #15000–00, 7.5 cm; *idem* 10 cm, #15024–00; extra fine Graefe forceps #11150–10, 10 cm; Dumont #5 beveled forceps, fine shanks, #11251–30, 11 cm; Dumont forceps #7b, curved shanks with serrated tips, #11271–30, 11 cm; cover glass forceps, smooth tips, straight, #11074–02, 10.5 cm (all from Fine Science Tools, Foster City, CA). Minor branching arteries—e.g., the intercostal arteries, are cut off and the adventitia is removed *in situ*, as much as possible. The aorta is then opened longitudinally while still attached to (and held in place by) the heart and the major branching arteries. The tip of a small (eye surgical) scissors is inserted through a partial transverse incision into one femoral artery and slid forward. After longitudinally opening one femoral artery, the procedure is repeated for the second femoral artery and the aorta. The primary incision follows the ventral side of the aorta and the inner curvature of the arch. To obtain a flat preparation of the arch for imaging, a second incision is made along the major curvature of the arch and through the orifices of the brachiocephalic trunc and the left common carotid and subclavian arteries. The remaining branches of the major arteries are then cut off. The aorta is removed from the heart to approx 3 mm distal to the iliac bifurcation and pinned out on a black wax surface in a dissecting pan (Fisher Scientific, #09–002–20), using 0.2-mm-diameter stainless-steel pins (Fine Science Tools, #26002–20). Each pin is placed either well within a lesion or well away from lesions, so that the image of the pin can be edited out in the electronic image without arbitrary editing of lesion edges. The aortas are then subjected to an additional fixation with formal-sucrose for 12 h, and stained with Sudan IV.

Staining of the Aorta

5 g Sudan IV are added to 500 mL 70% ethanol and 500 mL 100% acetone; mixed thoroughly in a biosafety cabinet and filter (Whatman #4.) The stained can be stored and reused, but should be filtered prior to each use. Staining procedure: arteries are rinsed for 5 min in 70% ethanol, Sudan-stained for 6 min, de-stained with 80% ethanol for approx 3 min or until nonlesioned areas of the aorta are free of staining, and rinsed with buffer.

Preparation of the Heart

After dissection, the upper half of the heart containing the aortic origin is gently dissected with a fresh razor blade (the cutting plane should be parallel to the aortic valve) (55). Further preparation of the heart may follow several approaches. The original Paigen method uses oil-red O staining to visualize lipids in the sections. This requires frozen sections, as the ethanol gradients used for paraffin embedding dissolve most of the free lipids from tissues. Although lipid staining greatly facilitates the detection of lesion boundaries, freezing damages cell membranes. Preparation of cryosections is slower, and more sections are lost than during sectioning using paraffin-embedded tissues. Note that perfusion-fixation is not needed to prepare frozen tissues. Embedding of the heart in OTC medium, freezing in liquid nitrogen, and cryo-sectioning are performed by standard procedures. An alternative approach is to continue fixation of the heart overnight, followed by paraffin embedding.

Sequential 7–10-μm thick sections are cut from the apex towards the base of the heart until the aortic valve leaflets appear. From this point, serial sections are collected for morphometry of atherosclerotic lesions. The number of sections needed is discussed in the following sections. To facilitate morphometry, paraffin-embedded sections can be stained by conventional histological techniques—i.e. with hematoxylin and eosin or with stains that particularly enhance the contrast between the lesion and the surrounding normal tissue, particularly the internal elastic lamina (elastic fiber stains).

Quantitation of Atherosclerosis by Computer-Assisted Image Analysis

The first step in analysis consists of capturing electronic images *(39)*. In principle, three approaches can be used. Images of the Sudan-stained aorta (or segments thereof) can be captured with a color (RGB) video camera or a high-resolution digital camera. Alternatively, the aorta can be conventionally photographed and the photographic slide (or print) can be scanned. Resolution of RGB cameras is limited, as they conform to the NTSC (i.e., television) standard. Some digital cameras offer considerably higher resolution, but do not read that of fine-grain film. Thus, the best images should be obtained by using photographic images and a high-resolution scanner (e.g., 2000 dots per inch). However, the resulting electronic image files will be exceedingly large, slowing down image analysis and potentially exceeding the capacity of the imaging (video) board. When setting up an imaging facility, it should be kept in mind that the accuracy of the image analysis will be determined to a far greater extent by the preparative skills and by the time and effort of the investigator performing the analysis than by the hardware. We routinely determine atherosclerosis in murine aortas on three separate 24-bit color images of the aorta (arch and upper thoracic aorta, lower thoracic and upper abdominal aorta, and lower abdominal aorta) captured with a Sony DXC-960MD three-chip color video camera *(39)*. The use of several higher magnification images partially compensates for the low resolution of the video camera.

The extent of atherosclerosis in the entire aorta is then quantitated by computer-assisted image analysis. Various software packages are available for this purpose. Although the features and sequence of steps vary between these programs, the basic approach is similar. Here we describe the procedure for Bioscan Optimas software (Bioscan, Seattle, WA) in an IBM-based system *(39)*. The first step consists of the retouching of the needle holes in the captured image (Fig. 3, *top*). The edge of the segment is traced using an automated feature of the software (Fig. 3, *middle*). The extent of atherosclerosis is then determined using a selection of threshold ranges in the three basic colors (Fig. 3, *bottom*). The total aortic surface area and the lesion area are then calculated by the program. If desired, the total surface area can be corrected by subtracting the area of the orifices of branching arteries, determined by a different threshold. The extent of atherosclerosis is then expressed as the percent of surface area of the entire aorta covered by Sudan-positive atherosclerotic lesions.

The threshold ranges are initially determined on a few randomly selected arteries. The operator defines several atherosclerotic areas. The lowest and highest threshold values for these areas determined by the software are then used as the default threshold. Even though the default threshold should be accurate for most images of arteries stained and captured under identical conditions, during

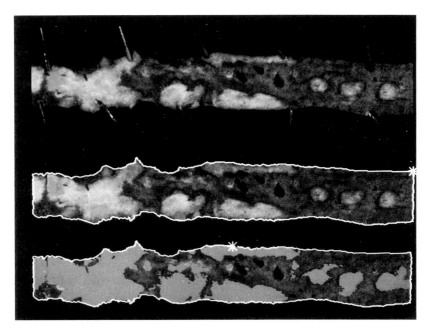

Fig. 3. Stages of the image analysis process: Raw digital image of a Sudan-stained segment of a mouse aorta (*top*). After editing out the needles, the segment is outlined by the edge-detection feature of the software (*middle*). The area corresponding to the selected threshold is highlighted (*bottom*) and the shape and size of lesions is compared to that of the actual lesions. The software then determines the total surface area of the vascular segment and the threshold (lesion) area. Reprinted with permission from ref. *(39)*.

image analysis the threshold must be verified for each aortic segment to ensure that it is accurate. This is done by comparing the shape and size of individual lesions in the highlighted threshold image (Fig. 3, *bottom*) to that of the actual lesions in the artery viewed through a stereo microscope, and adjusting the threshold range until the two match. In some instances when many very small lesions occur next to advanced atheromas, parts of the image must be analyzed separately, as no single threshold can be found that accurately reflects all lesions.

Determination of the extent of atherosclerosis in cross-sections of the aortic origin can be performed with the same software or by "low-tech" methods (e.g., counting squares under the microscope). Three images are captured of each cross-section through the aortic origin, each roughly comprising the area under one valve leaflet, using a microscope-mounted RGB video camera. The luminal lesion edge can be easily traced automatically, but the intima-media border is usually traced manually. Even if an elastin stain is used, automatic tracing of the abluminal edge of the lesions requires frequent operator intervention, because advanced murine atherosclerosis often disrupts the internal elastic lamina and involves the media. Lesion areas from the three images are then added to obtain the lesion area for the entire cross-section, and results are reported as the average of all sections analyzed.

Comparison of Morphometric Techniques

Both of the techniques discussed in the previous section have inherent advantages and disadvantages. Clearly, for most murine models that do not develop extensive hypercholesterolemia, lesion formation is essentially limited to the aortic origin, and the Paigen method is therefore the only choice. In models with more extensive atherogenesis, both methods can be used. Once atherosclerosis covers more than 3–5% of the aortic tree, lesion sizes measured by both techniques correlate reasonably well *(39)*. Obviously, once lesions in the aortic origin have reached a stage where further growth is no longer possible, such correlation can no longer be assumed. Furthermore, several preliminary reports suggest that differences in atherogenic mechanisms may exist between the aortic origin and the rest of the aorta. In this context, it is noteworthy that male LDLR$^{-/-}$ and apoE$^{-/-}$ mice have substantially more atherosclerosis in the entire aorta than females, *(39,56)* whereas the opposite is generally true for the aortic origin of murine models.

The advantage of the Paigen method is that it provides a measure of luminal growth of lesions, and allows for the calculation of lesion volumes from serial sections, whereas the measurement of the surface area provides a two-dimensional parameter that cannot differentiate between early and advanced lesions. On the other hand, the *en face* preparation of the aorta by the Palinski method can be completed in about 1–1.5 h by a skilled investigator or technician, and morphometry is equally fast. When performed on a sufficiently large number of sections, the determination of atherosclerosis in the aortic origin is far more labor-intensive. No consensus exists as to how many sections are needed for an accurate assessment of atherosclerosis. Paigen and colleagues used all or intermittent sections through the sinus of Valsalva from the first appearance of a valve leaflet until the aorta assumed a round shape (near the branch sites of the coronaries) for quantification of lesions. This is equivalent to about 0.25 mm of the aortic origin. Veniant et al. quantified 60 sections obtained at 20-μm intervals, representing 1.2 mm of the aorta *(29)*, while others feel that only 5 sections are sufficient. Apart from the fact that measurement of a larger segment of the aortic origin is inherently less susceptible to random variability in lesion distribution in the aortic origin, the size of the lesions also determines the number of sections required. Clearly, the area of large lesions is less likely to change dramatically, from section to section, whereas small lesions can be easily missed when only a few sections are analyzed. Thus, the choice of method largely depends on the goals and experimental conditions of each study. If results are to be compared to those of human, primate, or rabbit studies which use *en face* determinations of atherosclerosis, the Palinski method is more appropriate. A recent report also suggests that more consistent results are obtained by surface measurements of the entire aorta *(29)*. Other investigators have used combinations of the two methods, or new variations—e.g., cross-sections through the aortic root combined with longitudinal cross-sections through the arch *(57)*. However, the most important issue is not which method is preferable, but that accurate determinations of the extent of atherosclerosis in murine models are possible independent of the extent of lesions achieved. Both surface and cross-sectional lesion area correlate reasonably well with the aortic weight *(58)*. In mice with extensive atherosclerosis, most of the total weight actually represents the atherosclerotic intima, and aortic weight is therefore a simple, cumulative measure of atherosclerosis, especially when combined with additional parameters, such as the lesion content in oxidized lipoproteins *(58)* or cholesterol.

STUDIES USING APOE$^{-/-}$ AND LDLR$^{-/-}$ MICE

Although the lipoprotein profiles of apoE$^{-/-}$ and LDLR$^{-/-}$ mice are very different, as we have seen, extensive atherosclerosis can be induced in both models. However, it is important to keep in mind that the atherogenic mechanisms may be somewhat different. In addition to hypercholesterolemia, atherogenesis in apoE$^{-/-}$ mice may also be influenced by the inability of macrophages in atherosclerotic lesions to generate apoE, which may interfere with reverse cholesterol transport. Effects of apoE on the immune system have also been reported *(59)*. Another difference is the spontaneous development of hypercholesterolemia in apoE$^{-/-}$ mice. In our experience, LDLR$^{-/-}$ mice show less variability in plasma cholesterol levels. LDLR$^{-/-}$ mice are also particularly attractive for many intervention studies that affect the cholesterol level, because cholesterol levels in different experimental groups can more easily be matched by modulating the fat and cholesterol content of their diets. In general, the extent of atherosclerosis correlates with cholesterol levels when mice with a broad range of hypercholesterolemia are analyzed together. Within the narrow range of a typical experiment, such correlation often cannot be established.

ApoE$^{-/-}$ mice have been used to demonstrate that apo A-I has a powerful antiatherogenic effect, even under conditions of extreme hypercholesterolemia *(60,61)*. A number of elegant studies showed that macrophage-specific expression of human apoE or bone-marrow transplantation of apoE-positive macrophages reduces atherogenesis in apoE$^{-/-}$ mice *(8,62–64)*. Conversely, when irradiated normal mice were reconstituted with apoE$^{-/-}$ macrophages, atherosclerosis was increased *(65)*. The finding that macrophage-specific expression of apoE reduced atherogenesis independently of reducing plasma cholesterol levels also provides strong evidence for the importance of apoE generated by macrophages in atherosclerotic lesions for reverse cholesterol transport *(59)*. Oxidation of LDL and other lipoproteins is considered to be an important contributor to atherogenesis *(10,47,66)*. Oxidized LDL has chemotactic and cytotoxic properties and is eagerly taken up by scavenger receptors of intimal macrophages, greatly enhancing foam-cell formation. More recently, it has also been recognized that oxidative processes may affect the regulation of gene expression by vascular cells and modulate expression of a number of adhesion molecules and cytokines that influence atherogenesis. For example, intracellular signaling via the nuclear factor kappa B (NFκB) is oxidation sensitive *(66)*. OxLDL may also downregulate proinflammatory genes by promoting expression of the peroxysome proliferator-activated receptor gamma (PPARγ) *(67)*. Even mildly oxidized LDL activates multiple apoptotic signaling pathways *(68)*. Finally, OxLDL interferes with vascular relaxation in response to nitric oxide, which in turn may modulate lesion formation *(69)*.

Because extensive lipid peroxidation occurs in apoE$^{-/-}$ and LDLR$^{-/-}$ mice *(35,38,49)*, both models have been used to test the antiatherogenic efficacy of interventions with natural and synthetic antioxidants *(70–78)*. Reduced lesion formation in mice overexpressing paraoxonase also supports the atherogenicity of lipoprotein oxidation *(79)*.

USE OF MURINE MODELS TO INVESTIGATE THE ROLE OF THE IMMUNE SYSTEM IN ATHEROGENESIS

The involvement of the immune system in atherogenesis has long been hypothesized *(4,80)*. As described in the previous section, atherosclerotic lesions contain immunoglobulins and immuno-competent cells, such as macrophages and several subclasses of T-lymphocytes, and several markers of their activation (IL-2 receptors on T-lymphocytes, class II histocompatibility antigens, interferon γ, and C5b-9 complement complexes) *(80)*. However, it is not known whether the involvement of the immune system enhances or protects against atherosclerosis, and by what mechanisms *(9)*. Immune responses clearly play a major role in transplant atherosclerosis *(81)*. Yet a protective role is suggested by the observation of increased atherosclerosis in immune-compromised animals.

Murine models may be particularly valuable to investigate the role of the immune system in atherogenesis because a number of murine strains with well-characterized deficiencies of the humoral and cellular immune system are available that can be crossed with strains which develop extensive atherosclerosis. Murine studies which support a protective role of the immune system include the demonstration that MHC class I-deficient C57BL/6 mice (which lack cy-tolytic T-cells and have impaired natural killer-cell activity) developed a three-fold increase in lesions in the aortic valve region when fed a high-fat diet (82). Cyclosporine treatment of hypercholesterolemic mice, which suppresses T-cells also accelerated atherosclerosis (83). Finally, a protective role of the anti-in-flammatory interleukin IL-10 has recently been reported (84). In contrast, apoE$^{-/-}$ mice crossed with Rag-1 knockout mice (combined cellular and hu-moral immune deficiency) showed a 42% decrease in atherosclerosis when fed a regular diet, compared to apoE$^{-/-}$ mice. However, the same immune-deficient apoE$^{-/-}$ mice showed no significant decrease in atherosclerosis when fed a high-fat diet which resulted in plasma cholesterol levels of approx 1800 mg/dL (85,86). Other evidence for a proatherogenic role of specific factors involved in immune reactions includes the fact that mice lacking INFγ or the INFγ receptor (50,87), the IL-8 receptor (88), or the p55 component of the TNF receptor (89) showed decreased atherogenesis. A strong proatherogenic effect of IL-1 has also been reported (90). Antibody blocking of the CD40 ligand (CD40L, also known as CD154) markedly reduced early atherogenesis in LDLR$^{-/-}$ mice (57). Another study also provided evidence for the atherogenic role of CD40 signal-ing, but suggested an atherogenic role of this pathway mostly in advanced stages of atherosclerosis (91).

Apo E$^{-/-}$ and LDLR$^{-/-}$ mice have proven invaluable in the study of the immu-nological consequences of LDL oxidation (review in ref. 9). During the oxida-tion of LDL, reactive aldehydes are generated that form adducts with lysine and histidine residues of apo B and other proteins, giving rise to a large number of immunogenic neoepitopes (35,38,46). Oxidized LDL (OxLDL) formed in ath-erosclerotic lesions or elsewhere triggers a complex humoral immune response in vivo and autoantibodies binding to various epitopes of OxLDL have been described in humans and animal models of atherosclerosis (46). Atheroscle-rotic apoE$^{-/-}$ and LDLR$^{-/-}$ mice have high titers of such autoantibodies (35,38) and monoclonal antibodies recognizing a very broad spectrum of oxidized pro-teins, apoproteins, phospholipids, and adducts thereof have been cloned from non-immunized atherosclerotic apoE$^{-/-}$ mice (49,92,93). Extensive evidence suggests that the titers of such antibodies may be of diagnostic and/or prognos-tic value in humans (9,94) and a direct correlation between the extent of athero-sclerosis and the antibody titer has been established in LDLR$^{-/-}$ mice (38). Very recently, we have demonstrated that continued immunization of LDLR$^{-/-}$ mice with malondialdehyde (MDA)-modified LDL—a model of OxLDL—yielded a highly significant reduction of atherosclerosis in the aortic origin (95), con-firming the results of a similar intervention in WHHL rabbits (96). A protective effect of immunization with MDA-LDL was also reported in apoE$^{-/-}$ mice (97). However, in our study (95) the protective effect of immunization with MDA-LDL did not appear to be primarily due to the induction of very high titers of autoantibodies against oxidation-specific epitopes, as immunization with normal LDL preparations—which was oxidized far less extensively and did not result in dramatic rises in autoantibody titers, also significantly reduced atherogenesis in LDLR$^{-/-}$ mice. A more likely explanation would be, the beneficial effect of immunization stems from the modulation of cellular immune responses. The group of Dr. Hansson recently reported that during the progression of atherosclerosis, shifts from one T-cell subset to another occur (98). Decreasing T-cell numbers in more advanced lesions have also been reported (99). Shifts in T-cell populations may influence the balance of pro—and antiatherogenic factors secreted in lesions. For example, TH1 cells secrete INFγ, which exert proatherogenic effects in early lesions (50)—even in the absence of leukocytes (100). Thus, a decrease of Th1 cells in response to immunization with oxidized LDL could reduce atherogenesis via a decrease of atherogenic cytokines and interleukins. However, immunization with other antigens, e.g., heat shock proteins (thought to be part of a defensive mechanism of cells stressed by chemical or physical injury) or with beta2 glycoprotein I enhanced atherogenesis in mice (101,102). Passive transfer of immunoglobulins (which results in down-regulation of the recipient's humoral and cellular immune system) also reduced atherogenesis (103). Thus, it is evident that different components of the immune system activated by different immuno-modulation may exert pro- or antiatherogenic effects.

Murine models are also increasingly used to study the role of macrophages in atherosclerosis, particularly their recruitment into the intima (104–111), the role of different scavenger receptors (112,113), and macrophage gene regulation (114). The "op" mouse, which lacks macrophage colony-stimulating factor (MCSF) and therefore has greatly reduced macrophage numbers, has been crossed with the apoE$^{-/-}$ mouse to test whether macrophages enhance atherogenesis (115). Although confounding systemic consequences of impaired macrophage numbers were obvious in op mouse, the size of their lesions was markedly reduced (115). Additional support for a detrimental role of macrophages was provided by reduced atherogenesis in mice lacking CCR2, the receptor for MCP-1 (104,105). Notably, INFγ was also decreased in lesions of crosses between CCR2$^{-/-}$ and apoE$^{-/-}$ mice (105).

The recruitment of circulating monocytes and T-cells has been the focus of particularly intense investigation. For example, it has been shown that VCAM-1 and ICAM-1 are upregulated at predilection sites of atherosclerosis (106,107). An involvement of VCAM-1 and P-selectin for mononuclear rolling has been shown by intravital microscopy (108), and a contribution of these molecules to lesion growth demonstrated in apoE$^{-/-}$ mice (109). Crosses of double knockout mice lacking P- and E-selectin with LDLR$^{-/-}$ mice also developed significantly less atherosclerosis (110). Inhibition of alpha 4 integrin and ICAM-1 in apoE$^{-/-}$ mice had similar effects (111).

MURINE MODELS OF DIABETES AND ATHEROSCLEROSIS

A relatively new but very promising use of murine models is the investigation of potential atherogenic mechanisms of diabetes. Although other animal models of congenic or streptozotocin-induced diabetes exist—and insulin resistance can be achieved in rats by a diet rich in fructose—rats do not develop significant atherosclerosis, even when given high-fat diets. To generate a murine model of diabetes with extensive atherosclerosis, apoE$^{-/-}$ or LDLR$^{-/-}$ mice can be crossed with mice with an inherited diabetic condition *(116)*. Alternatively, diabetes may be achieved by streptozotocin in an atherosclerosis-susceptible murine model *(117)*.

Again, the LDLR$^{-/-}$ mouse is a particularly attractive model, because it allows one to match the cholesterol levels of experimental groups and thus to determine potential atherogenic effects of diabetes independent of the modulation of cholesterol levels. In studies by Reaven and colleagues, extensive hyperglycemia was achieved in LDLR$^{-/-}$ mice by ip injection of streptozotocin, but the plasma glucose could be moderated by providing small amounts of slow-release insulin. This also prevented the extreme hypertriglyceridemia and excess mortality frequently seen in other models. Lipid profiles of diabetic mice were similar to those of poorly controlled diabetic patients, with increased VLDL levels and slightly reduced HDL levels. However, despite the presence of hyperglycemia, diabetic dyslipidemia, and enhanced formation of AGE in the vessel wall, diabetic mice did not show enhanced aortic atherosclerosis. Although these results suggest a very limited role of hyperglycemia and AGE formation in atherogenesis, it remains to be determined whether diabetes does not have the same atherogenic effect in LDLR$^{-/-}$ mice as in humans, or whether the results in mice were overshadowed by the marked hypercholesterolemia in this experiment (1000 mg/dL). Another study obtained similar results in C57BL/6 mice, in which plasma cholesterol levels were only modestly elevated (290 mg/dL), but increased lesion formation was observed in the aortic origin in diabetic BALB/c mice *(118)*. This raises the possibility that there may be differences in the susceptibility to proatherogenic effects of diabetes between murine strains. Interestingly, infusion of AGE in mice has been reported to increase expression of VCAM-1 *(119)*, one of the mechanisms by which diabetes may enhance atherogenesis.

Very recently, attempts have been made to generate a model of insulin resistance (IR) in LDLR$^{-/-}$ mice *(120)*. A fructose-rich diet resulted in marked hypercholesterolemia, but failed to induce marked IR in LDLR$^{-/-}$ mice. Surprisingly, the fructose diet also enhanced atherosclerosis, compared to mice in which similar cholesterol levels had been induced by a Western diet. More importantly, the same study showed that the Western diet not only induced hypercholesterolemia, but also a marked hyperinsulinemia and IR in mice *(120)*.

Previous studies had suggested that high-fat diets may lead to IR *(121,122)*. Nevertheless, the observation of IR in LDLR$^{-/-}$ mice given standard Western diets may complicate the interpretation of many atherosclerosis studies using similar diets. To avoid the overriding effects of marked hypercholesterolemia, future studies on the role of IR in atherogenesis should be carried out at lower cholesterol levels. A potential approach would be to induce IR in LDLR$^{-/-}$ mice by a diet with a more moderate fat content and to compare atherosclerosis to that of a control group receiving the same diet but supplemented with an insulin-sensitizing agent *(120)*.

Finally, both LDLR$^{-/-}$ and apoE$^{-/-}$ mice have been being used to determine the effects of PPARγ ligands, such as rosiglitazone, troglitazone and analogues, on atherogenesis *(123)*.

CONCLUSION

As outlined above, murine models are eminently suitable to study the atherogenic role of apoproteins, enzymes, and receptors involved in lipid metabolism, vascular cells and their secretory products, immune responses, lipid oxidation and glycation, and insulin resistance. Nevertheless, some differences remain that limit the validity of results obtained in mice for humans. For example, the murine lipid metabolism is quite different because mice lack CETP, which may have both pro- and antiatherogenic consequences *(124,125)*. The normal lipoprotein profile of mice is also quite different from that of humans, in particular in regard to HDL. Physiological consequences of the much smaller size of mice must also be considered. For example, early fatty streaks consisting of a few layers of foam cells may significantly restrict the lumen *(126)* and cause hemodynamic changes in the mouse, whereas similar lesions are negligible in human arteries, except perhaps in the aorta of human fetuses of hypercholesterolemic mothers, where fatty streaks are already formed *(10,127)*. Finally, phenomena influenced by physical distances, such as diffusion of oxygen and plasma proteins, are likely to be different in murine lesions. However, the low cost and relative ease of genetic manipulation make murine models of atherosclerosis a very valuable research tool.

ACKNOWLEDGMENT

The present review was supported by NHLBI grant HL56989 (La Jolla Specialized Center of Research in Molecular Medicine and Atherosclerosis).

REFERENCES

1. Rubin EM, Smith DJ. Atherosclerosis in mice: getting to the heart of a polygenic disorder. Trends Genet 1994; 10:199–203.

2. Shih DM, Welch C, and Lusis AJ. New insights into atherosclerosis from studies with mouse models. Molec Med Today 1995; 1:364–372.

3. Breslow JL. Mouse models of atherosclerosis. Science 1996; 272: 685–688.

4. Lichtman AH, Cybulsky M, and Luscinskas FW. Immunology of atherosclerosis: the promise of mouse models. Am J Pathol 1996; 149:351–357.

5. Chien KR, and Grace AA. Principles of cardiovascular molecular and cellular biology. In: Braunwald E, ed. Heart Disease, 5th ed., WB Saunders, Philadelphia, 1997; 1626–1649.

6. Fuster V, Poon M, and Willerson JT. Learning from the transgenic mouse: endothelium, adhesive molecules, and neointimal formation. Circulation 1998; 97:16–18.

7. Carmeliet P, Moons L, and Collen D. Mouse models of angiogenesis, arterial stenosis, atherosclerosis and hemostasis. Cardiovasc Res 1998; 39:8–33.

8. Linton MF, and Fazio S. Macrophages, lipoprotein metabolism, and atherosclerosis: insights from murine bone marrow transplantation studies. Curr Opin Lipidol 1999; 10:97–105.

9. Palinski W and Witztum JL. Immune responses to oxidative neoepitopes on LDL and phospholipids modulate the development of atherosclerosis. J Intern Med 2000; 247:371–380.

10. Palinski W and Napoli C. Pathophysiological events during pregnancy influence the development of atherosclerosis. Trends Cardiovasc Med 1999; 9:205–214.

11. Paigen B, Mitchell D, Reue K, Morrow A, Lusis AJ, and LeBoef RC. Ath-1, a gene determining atherosclerosis susceptibility and high density lipoprotein levels in mice. Proc Natl Acad Sci USA 1987; 84:3763–3767.

12. Paigen B, Nesbitt MN, Mitchell D, Albee D, and LeBoeuf RC. Ath-2, a second gene determining atherosclerosis susceptibility and high density lipoprotein levels in mice. Genetics 1989; 122:163–168.

13. LeBoeuf RC, Doolittle MH, Montcalm A, Martin DC, Reue K, and Lusis AJ. Phenotypic characterization of the Ath-1 gene controlling high density lipoprotein levels and susceptibility to atherosclerosis. J Lipid Res 1990; 31:91–101.

14. Paigen B, Ishida BY, Verstuyft J, Winters RB, and Albee D. Atherosclerosis susceptibility differences among progenitors of recombinant inbred strains of mice. Arteriosclerosis 1990; 10:316–323.

15. Hyman RW, Frank S, Warden CH, Daluiski A, Heller R, and Lusis AJ. Quantitative trait locus analysis of susceptibility to diet-induced atherosclerosis in recombinant inbred mice. Biochem Genetics 1994; 32:397–407.

15. Liao F, Andalibi A, deBeer FC, Fogelman AM, and Lusis AJ. Genetic control of inflammatory gene induction and NF-kappa B-like transcription factor activation in response to an atherogenic diet in mice. J Clin Invest 1993; 91:2572–2579.

17. Rubin EM, Krauss RM, Spangler EA, Versuyft JG, and Clift SM. Inhibition of early atherogenesis in transgenic mice by human apolipoprotein A-I. Nature 1991; 353:265–267.

18. Schulz JR, Versuyft JG, Gong EL, Nichols AV, and Rubin EM. Protein composition determines the anti-atherogenic properties of HDL in transgenic mice. Nature 1993; 365:762–765.

19. Warden CH, Hedrick CC, Qiao JH, Castellani LW, and Lusis AJ. Atherosclerosis in transgenic mice overexpressing apolipoprotein A-II. Science 1993; 261:469–72.

20. Hughes, SD, Verstuyft J, and Rubin EM. HDL deficiency in genetically engineered mice requires elevated LDL to accelerate atherogenesis. Arterioscler Thromb Vasc Biol 1997; 17:1725–1729.

21. Duverger N, Tremp G, Caillaud JM, Emmanuel F, Castro G, Fruchart JC, Steinmetz A, and Denefle P. Protection against atherogenesis in mice mediated by human apolipoprotein A-IV. Science 1996; 273:966–968.

22. Lawn RM, Wade DP, Hammer RE, Chiesa G, Verstuyft JG, and Rubin EM. Atherogenesis in transgenic mice expressing human apolipoprotein(a). Nature 1992; 360:670–672.

23. Hughes SD, Lou XJ, Ighani S, Verstuyft J, Grainger DJ, Lawn RM, and Rubin EM. Lipoprotein(a) vascular accumulation in mice. In vivo analysis of the role of lysine binding sites using recombinant adenovirus. J Clin Invest 1997; 100:1493–1500.
24. Linton MRF, Farese RV Jr, Chiesa G, Grass DS, Chin P, Hammer RE, Hobbs HH, and Young SG. Transgenic mice expressing high plasma concentrations of human apolipoprotein B100 and lipoprotein(a). J Clin Invest 1993; 92:3029–3037.
25. Callow MJ, Verstuyft J, Tangirala R, Palinski W, and Rubin EM. Atherogenesis in transgenic mice with human apolipoprotein B and lipoprotein(a). J Clin Invest 1995; 96:1639–1646.
26. Mancini FP, Newland DL, Mooser V, Murata J, Marcovina S, Young SG, Hammer RE, Sanan DA, and Hobbs HH. Relative contributions of apolipoprotein(a) and apolipoprotein B to the development of fatty lesions in the proximal aorta of mice. Arterioscler Thromb Vasc Biol 1995; 15:1911–1916.
27. Young SG, Farese RV Jr, Pierotti V, Taylor S, Grass DS, and Linton MF. Transgenic mice expressing human apo B100 and apo B48. Curr Opin Lipidol 1994; 5:94–101.
28. Purcell-Huynh DA, Farese RV, Johnson DF, Flynn LM, Pierotti V, Newland DL, Linton MF, Sanan DA, and Young SG. Transgenic mice expressing high levels of human apolipoprotein B develop severe atherosclerotic lesions in response to a high-fat diet. J Clin Invest 1995; 95:2246–2257.
29. Veniant MM, Pierotti V, Newland D, Cham CM, Sanan DA, Walzem RL, and Young SG. Susceptibility to atherosclerosis in mice expressing exclusively apolipoprotein B48 or apolipoprotein B100. J Clin Invest 1997; 100:180–188.
30. Raabe M, Flynn LM, Zlot CH, Wong JS, Veniant MM, Hamilton RL, and Young SG. Knockout of the abetalipoproteinemia gene in mice: reduced lipoprotein secretion in heterozygotes and embryonic lethality in homozygotes. Proc Natl Acad Sci USA 1998; 95:8686–8691.
31. Plump AS, Smith JD, Hayek T, Aalto-Setala K, Walsh A, Verstuyft JG, Rubin EM, and Breslow JL. Severe hypercholesterolemia and atherosclerosis in apolipoprotein E-deficient mice created by homologous recombination in ES cells. Cell 1992; 71:343–353.
32. Zhang SH, Reddick RL, Piedrahita JA, and Maeda N. Spontaneous hypercholesterolemia and arterial lesions in mice lacking apolipoprotein E. Science 1992; 258:468–471.
33. Reddick RL, Zhang SH, and Maeda N. Atherosclerosis in mice lacking apoE. Evaluation of lesional development and progression. Arterioscler Thromb 1994; 14:141–147.
34. Nakashima Y, Plump AS, Raines EW, Breslow JL, and Ross R. ApoE-deficient mice develop lesions of all phases of atherosclerosis throughout the aortic tree. Arterioscler Thromb 1994; 14:133–140.
35. Palinski W, Ord V, Plump AS, Breslow JL, Steinberg D, and Witztum JL. ApoE-deficient mice are a model of lipoprotein oxidation in atherogenesis: demonstration of oxidation-specific epitopes in lesions and high titers of autoantibodies to malondialdehyde-lysine in serum. Arterioscler Thromb 1994; 14:605–616.
36. Ishibashi S, Brown MS, Goldstein JL, Gerard RD, Hammer RE, and Herz J. Hypercholesterolemia in low density lipoprotein receptor knockout mice and its reversal by adenovirus-mediated gene delivery. J Clin Invest 1993; 92:883–893.
37. Ishibashi S, Goldstein JL, Brown MS, Herz J, and Burns DK. Massive xanthomatosis and atherosclerosis in cholesterol-fed LDL receptor-negative mice. J Clin Invest 1994; 93:1885–1893.
38. Palinski W, Tangirala RK, Miller E, Young SG, and Witztum JL. Increased autoantibody titers against epitopes of oxidized LDL in LDL receptor-deficient mice with increased atherosclerosis. Arterioscler Thromb Vasc Biol 1995; 15:1569–1576.
39. Tangirala RK, Rubin EM, and Palinski W. Quantitation of atherosclerosis in murine models: correlation between lesions in the aortic origin and in the entire aorta, and differences in the

extent of lesions between sexes in LDL receptor-deficient and apoprotein E-deficient mice. J Lipid Res 1995; 36:2320–2328.

40. Masucci-Magoulas L, Goldberg IJ, Bisgaier CL, Serajuddin H, Francone OL, Breslow JL, and Tall AR. A mouse model with features of familial combined hyperlipidemia. Science 1997; 275:391–394.

41. van Vlijmen BJ, van den Maagdenberg AM, Gijbels MJ, van der Boom H, HogenEsch H, Frants RR, Hofker MH, and Havekes LM. Diet-induced hyperlipoproteinemia and athero-sclerosis in apolipoprotein E3–Leiden transgenic mice. J Clin Invest 1994; 93:1403–1410.

42. Lutgens E, Daemen M, Kockx M, Doevendans P, Hofker M, Havekes L, Wellens H, and de Muinck ED. Atherosclerosis in APOE3–Leiden transgenic mice: from proliferative to athero-matous stage. Circulation 1999; 99:276–283.

43. Ishibashi S, Herz J, Maeda N, Goldstein JL, and Brown MS. The two-receptor model of lipoprotein clearance: tests of the hypothesis in "knockout" mice lacking the low density lipoprotein receptor, apolipoprotein E, or both proteins. Proc Natl Acad Sci USA 1994; 91:4431–4435.

44. Caligiuri G, Levy B, Pernow J, Thorén P, and Hansson GK. Myocardial infarction mediated by endothelin receptor signaling in hypercholesterolemic mice. Proc Natl Acad Sci USA 1999; 96:6920–6924.

45. Zhou X, Stemme S, and Hansson GK. Evidence for a local immune response in atheroscle-rosis. CD4+ cells infiltrate lesions of apolipoprotein-E-deficient mice. Am J Pathol 1996; 149:359–366.

46. Palinski W, Rosenfeld ME, Ylä-Herttuala S, Gurtner GC, Socher SA, Butler S, Parthasarathy S, Carew TE, Steinberg D, and Witztum JL. Low density lipoprotein undergoes oxidative modification in vivo. Proc Natl Acad Sci USA 1989; 86:1372–1376.

47. Steinberg D. Low density lipoprotein oxidation and its pathobiological significance. J Biol Chem 1997; 272:20963–20966.

48. Reaven P, Merat S, Casanada F, Sutphin M, and Palinski W. Effect of streptozotocin induced hyperglycemia on lipid profiles, formation of advanced glycation endproducts in lesions and extent of atherosclerosis in LDL receptor deficient mice. Arterioscler Thromb Vasc Biol 1997; 17:2250–2256.

49. Palinski W, Hörkkö S, Miller E, Steinbrecher UP, Powell HC, Curtiss LK, and Witztum JL. Cloning of monoclonal autoantibodies to epitopes of oxidized lipoproteins from apoE-defi-cient mice. Demonstration of epitopes of oxidized low density lipoprotein in human plasma. J Clin Invest 1996; 98:800–814.

50. Gupta S, Pablo AM, Jiang X, Wang N, Tall AR, and Schindler C. IFN-gamma potentiates atherosclerosis in ApoE knock-out mice. J Clin Invest 1997; 99:2752–2761.

51. Zhou X, and Hansson GK. Detection of B cells and proinflammatory cytokines in atheroscle-rotic plaques of hypercholesterolaemic apolipoprotein E knockout mice. Scand J Immunol 1999; 50:25–30.

52. Carmeliet P, Moons L, Lijnen R, Baes M, Lemaître V, Tipping P, et al. Urokinase-generated plasmin activates matrix metalloproteinases during aneurysm formation. Nat Genet 1997; 17:439–444.

53. Heymans S, Luttun A, Nuyens D, Theilmeier G, Creemers E, Moons L, et al. Inhibition of plasminogen activators or matrix metalloproteinases prevents cardiac rupture but impairs therapeutic angiogenesis and causes cardiac failure. Nat Med 1999; 5:1135–1142.

54. Moulton KS, Heller E, Konerding MA, Flynn E, Palinski W, and Folkman J. Angiogenesis inhibitors endostatin or TNP-470 reduce intimal neovascularization and plaque growth in apolipoprotein E-deficient mice. Circulation 1999; 99:1726–1732.

55. Paigen B, Morrow PA, Holmes D, Mitchell D, and Williams RA. Quantitative assessment of atherosclerotic lesions in mice. Atherosclerosis 1987; 68:231–240.

56. Marsh MM, Walker VR, Curtiss LK, and Banka CL. Protection against atherosclerosis by estrogen is independent of plasma cholesterol levels in LDL receptor-deficient mice. J Lipid Res 1999; 40:893–900.
57. Mach F, Schönbeck U, Sukhova GK, Atkinson E, and Libby P. Reduction of atherosclerosis in mice by inhibition of CD40 signalling. Nature 1998; 394:200–203.
58. Tsimikas S, Shortal BP, Witztum JL, and Palinski W. In vivo uptake of radiolabeled MDA2, an oxidation-specific monoclonal antibody, provides an accurate measure of atherosclerotic lesions rich in oxidized LDL and is highly sensitive to their regression. Arterioscler Thromb Vasc Biol 2000; 20:689–697.
59. Mahley RW. Apolipoprotein E. Cholesterol transport proteins with expanding role in cell biology. Science 1988; 240:622–630.
60. Plump AS, Scott CJ, and Breslow JL. Human apolipoprotein A-I gene expression increases high density lipoprotein and suppresses atherosclerosis in the apolipoprotein E-deficient mouse. Proc Natl Acad Sci USA 1994; 91:9607–9611.
61. Paszty C, Maeda N, Verstuyft J, and Rubin EM. Apolipoprotein AI transgene corrects apolipoprotein E deficiency-induced atherosclerosis in mice. J Clin Invest 1994; 94:899–903.
62. Bellosta S, Mahley RW, Sanan DA, Murata J, Newland DL, Taylor JM, and Pitas RE. Macrophage-specific expression of human apolipoprotein E reduces atherosclerosis in hypercholesterolemic apolipoprotein E-null mice. J Clin Invest 1995; 96:2170–2179.
63. Linton MF, Atkinson JB, and Fazio S. Prevention of atherosclerosis in apolipoprotein E-deficient mice by bone marrow transplantation. Science 1995; 267:1034–1037.
64. Boisvert WA, Spangenberg J, and Curtiss LK. Treatment of severe hypercholesterolemia in apolipoprotein E-deficient mice by bone marrow transplantation. J Clin Invest 1995; 96:1118–1124.
65. Fazio S, Babaev VR, Murray AB, Hasty AH, Carter KJ, Gleaves LA, Atkinson JB, and Linton MF. Increased atherosclerosis in mice reconstituted with apolipoprotein E null macrophages. Proc Natl Acad Sci USA 1997; 94:4647–4652.
66. Berliner JA, Navab M, Fogelman AM, Frank JS, Demer LL, Edwards PA, Watson AD, and Lusis AJ. Atherosclerosis: Basic mechanisms. Oxidation, inflammation, and genetics. Circulation 1995; 91:2488–2496.
67. Ricote M, Huang J, Fajas L, Li A, Welch J, Najib J, Witztum JL, Auwerx J, Palinski W, and Glass CK. Expression of the peroxisome proliferator-activated receptor γ in human atherosclerosis and regulation in macrophages by colony stimulating factors and oxidized low density lipoprotein. Proc Natl Acad Sci USA 1998; 95:7614–7619.
68. Napoli C, Quehenberger O, de Nigris F, Abete P, Glass CK, and Palinski W. Apoptosis induced by mildly oxidized LDL involves multiple apoptotic signaling pathways in human coronary cells. FASEB J 2000; 15: in press.
69. Bonthu S, Heistad DD, Chappell DA, Lamping KG, and Faraci FM. Atherosclerosis, vascular remodeling, and impairment of endothelium-dependent relaxation in genetically altered hyperlipidemic mice. Arterioscler Thromb Vasc Biol 1997; 17:2333–2340.
70. Tangirala RK, Casanada F, Witztum JL, Steinberg D, and Palinski W. Effect of the antioxidant N,N'-diphenyl 1,4–phenylenediamine (DPPD) on atherogenesis in apoE-deficient mice. Arterioscler Thromb Vasc Biol 1995; 15:1625–1630.
71. Zhang SH, Reddick RL, Avdievich E, Surles LK, Jones RG, Reynolds JB, Quarfordt SH, and Maeda N. Paradoxical enhancement of atherosclerosis by probucol treatment in apolipoprotein E-deficient mice. J Clin Invest 1997; 99:2858–2866.
72. Bird DA, Tangirala RK, Fruebis J, Steinberg D, Witztum JL, and Palinski W. Effect of probucol on LDL oxidation and atherosclerosis in LDL receptor-deficient mice. J Lipid Res 1998; 39:1079–1090.

73. Hayek, T, Attias J, Smith J, Breslow JL, and Keidar S. Antiatherosclerotic and antioxidative effects of captopril in apolipoprotein E-deficient mice. J Cardiovasc Pharmacol 1998; 31:540–544.

74. Praticò D, Tangirala RK, Rader DJ, Rokach J, and FitzGerald GA. Vitamin E suppresses isoprostane generation in vivo and reduces atherosclerosis in apoE-deficient mice. Nature Med 1998; 4:1189–1192.

75. Crawford RS, Kirk EA, Rosenfeld ME, LeBoeuf RC, and Chait A. Dietary antioxidants inhibit development of fatty streak lesions in the LDL receptor-deficient mouse. Arterioscler Thromb Vasc Biol 1998; 18:1506–1513.

76. Cynshi O, Kawabe Y, Suzuki T, Takashima Y, Kaise H, Nakamura M, et al. Antiatherogenic effects of the antioxidant BO-653 in three different animal models. Proc Natl Acad Sci USA 1998; 95:10123–10128.

77. Moghadasian MH, McManus BM, Godin DV, Rodrigues B, and Frohlich JJ. Proatherogenic and antiatherogenic effects of probucol and phytosterols in a apolipoprotein E-deficient mice: possible mechanisms of action. Circulation 1999; 99:1733–1739.

78. Witting PK, Pettersson K, Ostlund-Lindqvist AM, Westerlund C, Eriksson AW, and Stocker R. Inhibition by a coantioxidant of aortic lipoprotein lipid peroxidation and atherosclerosis in apolipoprotein E and low density lipoprotein receptor gene double knockout mice. FASEB J 1999; 13:667–675.

79. Shih DM, Gu L, Hama S, Xia YR, Navab M, Fogelman AM, and Lusis AJ. Genetic-dietary regulation of serum paraoxonase expression and its role in atherogenesis in a mouse model. J Clin Invest 1996; 97:1630–1639.

80. Libby P, and Hansson GK. Involvement of the immune system in human atherogenesis. Current knowledge and unanswered questions. Lab Invest 1991; 64:5–15.

81. Shi C, Lee WS, He Q, Zhang D, Fletcher DL, Newell JB, and Haber E. Immunologic basis of transplant-associated arteriosclerosis. Proc Natl Acad Sci USA 1996; 93:4051–4056.

82. Fyfe AI, Qiao JH, and Lusis AJ. Immune deficient mice develop typical atherosclerotic fatty streaks when fed an atherogenic diet. J Clin Invest 1994; 94:2516–2520.

83. Emeson EE, Shen ML, Bell CG, and Qureshi A. Inhibition of atherosclerosis in CD4 T-cell-ablated and nude (nu/nu) C57BL/6 hyperlipidemic mice. Am J Pathol 1996; 149:675–685.

84. Mallat, Z, Besnard S, Duriez M, Deleuze V, Emmanuel F, Bureau MF, et al. Protective role of interleukin-10 in atherosclerosis. Circ Res 1999; 85:17–24.

85. Dansky HM, Charlton SA, Harper MM, and Smith JD. T and B lymphocytes play a minor role in atherosclerotic plaque formation in the apolipoprotein E-deficient mouse. Proc Natl Acad Sci USA 1997; 94:4642–4646.

86. Daugherty A, Pure E, Delfel-Butteiger D, Chen S, Leferovich J, Roselaar SE, and Rader DJ. The effects of total lymphocyte deficiency on the extent of atherosclerosis in apolipoprotein E-/- mice. J Clin Invest 1997; 100:1575–1580.

87. Nagano H, Mitchell RN, Taylor MK, Hasegawa S, Tilney NL, and Libby P. Interferon-gamma deficiency prevents coronary arteriosclerosis but not myocardial rejection in transplanted mouse hearts. J Clin Invest 1997; 100:550–557.

88. Boisvert WA, Santiago R, Curtiss LK, and Terkeltaub RA. A leukocyte homologue of the IL-8 receptor CXCR-2 mediates the accumulation of macrophages in atherosclerotic lesions of LDL receptor-deficient mice. J Clin Invest 1998; 101:353–363.

89. Schreyer SA, Peschon JJ, and LeBoeuf RC. Accelerated atherosclerosis in mice lacking tumor necrosis factor receptor p55. J Biol Chem 1996; 271:26174–26178.

90. Elhage R, Maret A, Pieraggi MT, Thiers JC, Arnal JF, and Bayard F. Differential effects of interleukin-1 receptor antagonist and tumor necrosis factor binding protein on fatty-streak formation in apolipoprotein E-deficient mice. Circulation 1998; 97:242–244.

172 Part III / Chronic Atherosclerotic Models

91. Lutgens E, Gorelik L, Daemen MJ, de Muinck ED, Grewal IS, Koteliansky VE, and Flavell RA. Requirement for CD154 in the progression of atherosclerosis. Nat Med 1999; 5:1313–1316.
92. Hörkkö S, Miller E, Dudl E, Reaven PD, Zvaifler NJ, Terkeltaub R, Pierangeli SS, Curtiss LK, Branch DW, Palinski W, and Witztum JL. Antiphospholipid antibodies are directed against epitopes of oxidized phospholipids: Recognition of cardiolipin by monoclonal antibodies to epitopes of oxidized low-density lipoprotein. J Clin Invest 1996; 98:815–825.
93. Hörkkö S, Miller E, Itabe H, Subbanagounder HG, Leitinger N, Berliner JA, et al. Monoclonal autoantibodies specific for oxidized phospholipids or oxidized phospholipid-protein adducts inhibit macrophage uptake of oxidized low-density lipoproteins. J Clin Invest 1999; 103:117–128.
94. Witztum JL and Palinski W. Autoimmunity to oxidized lipoproteins. In: G.K. Hansson and P. Libby (eds.). Immune functions of the vessel wall. Harwood Academic Publishers, Amsterdam 1996; 159–172.
95. Freigang S, Hörkkö S, Miller E,Witztum JL, and Palinski W. Immunization of LDL receptor-deficient mice with homologous malondialdehyde-modified and native LDL reduces progression of atherosclerosis by mechanisms other than induction of antibodies to oxidative neoepitopes. Arterioscler Thromb Vasc Biol 1999; 1998; 18:1972–1982.
96. Palinski W, Miller E, and Witztum JL. Immunization of LDL receptor-deficient rabbits with homologous malondialdehyde-modified LDL reduces atherogenesis. Proc Natl Acad Sci USA 1995; 92:821–825.
97. George J, Afek A, Gilburd B, Levkovitz H, Shaish A, Goldberg I, Kopolovic Y, Wick G, Shoenfeld Y, and Harats D. Hyperimmunization of apo-E-deficient mice with homologous malondialdehyde low-density lipoprotein suppresses early atherogenesis. Atherosclerosis 1998; 138:147–152.
98. Zhou X, Paulsson G, Stemme SD, and Hansson GK. Hypercholesterolemia is associated with a T helper (Th) 1/Th2 switch of the autoimmune response in atherosclerotic apoE-knockout mice. J Clin Invest 1998; 101:1717–1725.
99. Roselaar SE, Kakkanathu PX, and Daugherty A. Lymphocyte populations in atherosclerotic lesions of apoE-/- and LDL receptor-/- mice. Decreasing density with disease progression. Arterioscler Thromb Vasc Biol 1996; 16:1013–1018.
100. Tellides G, Tereb DA, Kirkiles-Smith NC, Kim RW, Wilson JH, Schechner JS, Lorber MI, and Pober JS. Interferon-gamma elicits arteriosclerosis in the absence of leukocytes. Nature 2000; 403:207–211.
101. George J, Shoenfeld Y, Afek A, Gilburd B, Keren P, Shaish A, Kopolovic J, Wick G, and Harats D. Enhanced fatty streak formation in C57BL/6J mice by immunization with heat shock protein-65. Arterioscler Thromb Vasc Biol 1999; 19:505–510.
102. George J, Afek A, Gilburd B, Blank M, Levy Y, Aron-Maor A, et al. Induction of early atherosclerosis in LDL-receptor-deficient mice immunized with beta2–glycoprotein I. Circulation 1998; 98:1108–1115.
103. Nicoletti A, Kaveri S, Caligiuri G, Bariâety J, and Hansson GK. Immunoglobulin treatment reduces atherosclerosis in apo E knockout mice. J Clin Invest 1998; 102:910–918.
104. Boring L, Gosling J, Chensue SW, Kunkel SL, Farese RV Jr, Broxmeyer HE, and Charo IF. Impaired monocyte migration and reduced type 1 (Th1) cytokine responses in C-C chemokine receptor 2 knockout mice. J Clin Invest 1997; 100:2552–2561.
105. Boring L, Gosling J, Cleary M, and Charo IF. Decreased lesion formation in CCR2-/- mice reveals a role for chemokines in the initiation of atherosclerosis. Nature 1998; 394:894–897.
106. Nakashima Y, Raines EW, Plump AS, Breslow JL, and Ross R. Upregulation of VCAM-1 and ICAM-1 at atherosclerosis-prone sites on the endothelium in the ApoE-deficient mouse. Arterioscler Thromb Vasc Biol 1998; 18:842–851.

107. Iiyama K, Hajra L, Iiyama M, Li H, DiChiara M, Medoff BD, and Cybulsky MI. Patterns of vascular cell adhesion molecule-1 and intercellular adhesion molecule-1 expression in rabbit and mouse atherosclerotic lesions and at sites predisposed to lesion formation. Circ Res 1999; 85:199–207.

108. Ramos CL, Huo Y, Jung U, Ghosh S, Manka DR, Sarembock IJ, and Ley K. Direct demonstration of P-selectin- and VCAM-1-dependent mononuclear cell rolling in early atherosclerotic lesions of apolipoprotein E-deficient mice. Circ Res 1999; 84:1237–1244.

109. Collins RG, Velji R, Guevara NV, Hicks MJ, Chan L, and Beaudet AL. P-Selectin or intercellular adhesion molecule (ICAM)-1 deficiency substantially protects against atherosclerosis in apolipoprotein E-deficient mice. J Exp Med 2000; 191:189–194.

110. Dong ZM, Chapman SM, Brown AA, Frenette PS, Hynes RO, and Wagner DD. The combined role of P- and E-selectins in atherosclerosis. J Clin Invest 1998; 102:145–152.

111. Patel SS, Thiagarajan R, Willerson JT, and Yeh ET. Inhibition of alpha4 integrin and ICAM-1 markedly attenuate macrophage homing to atherosclerotic plaques in ApoE-deficient mice. Circulation 1998; 97:75–81.

112. Suzuki H, Kurihara Y, Takeya M, Kamada N, Kataoka M, Jishage K, et al. A role for macrophage scavenger receptors in atherosclerosis and susceptibility to infection. Nature 1997; 386:292–296.

113. Sakaguchi H, Takeya M, Suzuki H, Hakamata H, Kodama T, Horiuchi S, et al. Role of macrophage scavenger receptors in diet-induced atherosclerosis in mice. Lab Invest 1998; 78:423–434.

114. Horvai A, Palinski W, Wu H, Moulton KS, Kalla K, and Glass CK. Scavenger receptor A gene regulatory elements target gene-expression to macrophages and to foam cells of atherosclerotic lesions. Proc Natl Acad Sci USA 1995; 92:5391–5395.

115. Smith JD, Trogan E, Ginsberg M, Grigaux C, Tian J, Miyata M. Decreased atherosclerosis in mice deficient in both macrophage colony-stimulating factor (op) and apolipoprotein E. Proc Natl Acad Sci USA 1995; 92:8264–8268.

116. Nishina PM, Naggert JK, Verstuyft J, and Paigen B. Atherosclerosis in genetically obese mice: the mutants obese, diabetes, fat, tubby, and lethal yellow. Metabolism 1994; 43:554–558.

117. Reaven P, Merat S, Casanada F, Sutphin M, and Palinski W. Effect of streptozotocin induced hyperglycemia on lipid profiles, formation of advanced glycation endproducts in lesions and extent of atherosclerosis in LDL receptor deficient mice. Arterioscler Thromb Vasc Biol 1997; 17:2250–2256.

118. Kunjathoor VV, Wilson DL, and LeBoeuf RC. Increased atherosclerosis in streptozotocin-induced diabetic mice. J Clin Invest 1996; 97:1767–1773.

119. Schmidt AM, Hori O, Chen JX, Li JF, Crandall J, Zhang J, Cao R, Yan SD, Brett J, and Stern D. Advanced glycation endproducts interacting with their endothelial receptor induce expression of vascular cell adhesion molecule-1 (VCAM-1) in cultured human endothelial cells and in mice. A potential mechanism for the accelerated vasculopathy of diabetes. J Clin Invest 1995; 96:1395–1403.

120. Merat S, Casanada F, Palinski W, and Reaven PD. Western-type diets induce insulin resistance in LDL receptor-deficient mice but do not increase aortic atherosclerosis, compared to normoinsulinemic mice in which similar plasma cholesterol levels are achieved by a fructose-rich diet. Arterioscler Thromb Vasc 1999; Biol 19:1223–1230.

121. Surwit RS, Wang S, Petro AE, Sanchis D, Raimbault S, Ricquier D, and Collins S. Diet-induced changes in uncoupling proteins in obesity-prone and obesity-resistant strains of mice. Proc Natl Acad Sci USA 1998; 95:4061–4065.

122. Schreyer SA. Chua SC, and LeBoeuf RC. Obesity and diabetes in TNF-alpha receptor-deficient mice. J Clin Invest 1998; 102:402–411.

123. Li AC, Brown KK, Silvestre MJ, Willson TM, Palinski W, Glass CK. PPARγ ligands inhibit the development of atherosclerosis in low density lipoprotein receptor-deficient mice. J Clin Invest 2000: 106; in press.

124. Marotti KR, Castle CK, Boyle TP, Lin AH, Murray RW, and Melchior GW. Severe atherosclerosis in transgenic mice expressing simian cholesteryl ester transfer protein. Nature 1993; 364:73–75.

125. Hayek T, Masucci-Magoulas L, Jiang X, Walsh A, Rubin E, Breslow JL, and Tall AR. Decreased early atherosclerotic lesions in hypertriglyceridemic mice expressing cholesteryl ester transfer protein transgene. J Clin Invest 1995; 96:2071–2074.

126. Seo HS, Lombardi DM, Polinsky P, Powell-Braxton L, Bunting S, Schwartz SM, and Rosenfeld ME. Peripheral vascular stenosis in apolipoprotein E-deficient mice. Potential roles of lipid deposition, medial atrophy, and adventitial inflammation. Arterioscler Thromb Vasc Biol 1997; 17:3593–3601.

127. Napoli C, D'Armiento FP, Mancini FP, Witztum JL, Palumbo G, and Palinski W. Fatty streak formation occurs in human fetal aortas and is greatly enhanced by maternal hypercholesterolemia. Intimal accumulation of LDL and its oxidation precede monocyte recruitment into early atherosclerotic lesions. J Clin Invest 1997; 100:2680–2690.

13 Rabbit Models of Atherosclerosis

Masanori Aikawa, MD, PhD,
Yoshihiro Fukumoto, MD, PhD,
Elena Rabkin, MD, PhD, and Peter Libby, MD

CONTENTS

INTRODUCTION

Epidemiologic and clinical studies thus far suggest that elevated plasma cholesterol levels increase the risk of coronary heart disease *(1)*. Recent clinical studies have demonstrated that lowered cholesterol plays a role in reducing

From: *Contemporary Cardiology: Vascular Disease and Injury: Preclinical Research*
Edited by: D. I. Simon and C. Rogers © Humana Press Inc., Totowa, NJ

acute coronary events *(2)*. In the early 20th century, Anitschkow found that a cholesterol-enriched diet could induce atherosclerosis in rabbit arteries, and established a relationship between cholesterol consumption and severity of atheroma *(3)*. Since then, hypercholesterolemic rabbits have been widely used for atherosclerosis research. Cholesterol-fed rabbits are the most commonly used model among three popular rabbit models of atherosclerosis. Watanabe heritable hyperlipidemic (WHHL) rabbits with endogenous hypercholester-olemia—which causes spontaneous atherosclerosis—are also widely used. A casein-rich diet can induce endogenous hypercholesterolemia and atheroscle-rosis in rabbits. This chapter provides profiles of each rabbit model of athero-sclerosis and discusses the similarities, differences, and advantages among these models. Effects of lipid lowering on rabbit atherosclerosis are also discussed.

LIPID PROFILE OF CHOLESTEROL-FED RABBITS

The New Zealand White is the most commonly used rabbit for studies in-volving consumption of a high-cholesterol diet. The total plasma cholesterol levels of rabbits fed a high-cholesterol diet show a positive correlation with dietary cholesterol intake *(4,5)*. Total cholesterol levels also become elevated with time *(5)*. Over a 10-wk period, rabbits fed a 0.9% cholesterol diet show extremely high cholesterol levels (>2,000 mg/dL), while animals fed a 0.3% cholesterol diet have moderately elevated cholesterol levels (approx 700 mg/dL) *(5)*. Moderate cholesterol supplementation is preferable, because extreme exogenous hypercholesterolemia causes liver dysfunction. For example, a diet of 0.9% cholesterol increases levels of hepatocellular enzymes within 6–9 wk *(5)*. If high cholesterol levels (>1,500–2,000 mg/dL) are maintained over sev-eral months, rabbits sometimes develop jaundice, ascites, or weight loss. It should also be noted that cholesterol levels vary depending on the individual animal, and that rabbits may be high or low responders to a cholesterol-en-riched diet. In high responders, even with moderate cholesterol content in the diet (i.e., 0.3%), total plasma cholesterol levels can increase to over 2,000 mg/dL. Under microscopic examination, the livers of these animals reveal features such as lipid deposition, disruption of the parenchymal architecture, fibrotic change, central-vein sclerosis, and cholestasis (Fig. 1). The use of animals with severe liver dysfunction to study atherogenesis of hypercholesterolemia is in-advisable because they have altered lipid metabolism, and because such liver damage can increase blood concentration of drugs (i.e., general anesthetic or lipid-lowering drugs). Liver damage can be limited by monitoring plasma cho-lesterol levels at least every month by adjusting cholesterol content in the diet individually, or by supplying the minimally required amount of diet daily. These procedures help limit the elevation of cholesterol levels and also reduce the variation of target cholesterol levels and lesion morphology and size *(6)*.

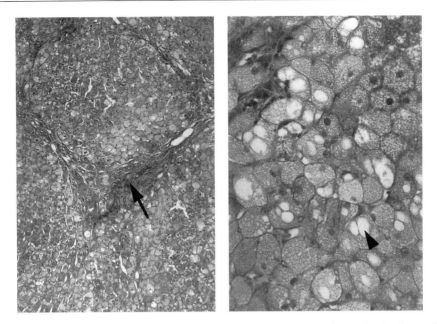

Fig. 1. The liver of cholesterol-fed rabbits with extensive hypercholesterolemia shows the disruption of parenchymal architecture and the fatty change (Masson trichrome staining). Increased fibrous tissue (arrow) forms broad septa that subdivide liver into small pseudolobules (*left*). Original magnification: ×100. Accumulation of lipid in the form of large cytoplasmic vacuoles indicated by arrowhead (*right*). Original magnification: ×400. (See color plate 3 appearing in the insert following p. 236).

In contrast to the most common type of human hypercholesterolemia in which LDL-cholesterol is the largest fraction, a large proportion of the total plasma cholesterol of cholesterol-fed rabbits is present as VLDL-cholesterol *(4,7)*. VLDL becomes the major carrier, especially when total cholesterol levels are above 800 mg/dL. Several studies have addressed whether this difference in lipid profile affects the nature of atherosclerotic lesions in comparison to WHHL and casein-fed rabbits, where the major fraction of plasma cholesterol is LDL-cholesterol. Rosenfeld and Tsukada et al. demonstrated similar qualitative morphogenesis of aortic lesions in 0.2% cholesterol-fed and 20% casein-fed rabbits to spontaneous atherosclerosis of WHHL rabbits *(8–10)*. More recently, Daley et al. reported quantitative analysis showing a difference in lesion area and volume between cholesterol-fed rabbits and casein-fed rabbits. The lesions in 0.125–0.5% cholesterol-fed rabbits had 1.9 times the surface area and 3.4 times the volume of the aortic lesion compared with the 27% casein-fed rabbits—although topographical distribution in the aorta was similar *(7)*. After 6 mo of feeding, cholesterol-fed rabbits had more advanced lesions (resembling human atherosclerosis) than those of casein-fed rabbits *(11)*.

NATURE OF ATHEROSCLEROSIS
OF CHOLESTEROL-FED RABBITS

The atherosclerosis of cholesterol-fed rabbits develops in proportion to cholesterol content in the diet and plasma cholesterol levels (4). Bocan et al. demonstrated that lesion coverage, cholesterol ester content, and extent of macrophage accumulation within the thoracic aorta of rabbits fed a cholesterol-rich diet for 9 mo were linearly related to total plasma cholesterol exposure (area under cholesterol time curve). The threshold level of total plasma cholesterol required for consistent lesion development in 9 mo was over 700 mg/dL.

Several studies have addressed topographic distribution of aortic atherosclerosis in cholesterol-fed rabbits (7,12). The proximal portion of the aorta tends to have greater involvement than its distal portion. Daley et al. reported that lipid staining with oil-red-O after 6 mo of cholesterol-enriched diet determined that 68% or 39%, respectively, of the surface areas in the thoracic or abdominal aorta covered with lesion (7). These data also suggest that spontaneous aortic atherosclerosis of hypercholesterolemic rabbits is inconsistent, and that intact areas remain where no intima is seen. This results in large variations, depending on the individual animal. This inhomogeneity can be minimized by the addition of mechanical injury.

The aortic lesion of cholesterol-fed rabbits contains various types of atherosclerotic changes including fatty streak, diffuse intimal thickening, fibrous plaque, and advanced atheromatous plaque. The abdominal aorta tends to have more fibrous plaques than the thoracic aorta, while the thoracic aorta is rich in foam cells compared with the abdominal aorta (11). These changes also depend on plasma cholesterol levels and length of feeding periods. Consumption by rabbits of a diet containing over 0.5% cholesterol causes lipid- and foam cell-rich lesions in a relatively short period of time, but the lesion resembles an early fatty streak of the human artery, not typical atherosclerosis (4). With moderate levels of cholesterol content in the diet (i.e., 0.2–0.3%) for relatively long periods of time (i.e., 6 mo–1 yr), the rabbit aorta can develop lesions containing all major components of human advanced atherosclerosis—such as macrophage accumulation and atheromatous debris covered by a fibrous cap consisting of smooth muscle cells (SMCs) and extracellular matrix (4). Thus, increasing the periods of cholesterol feeding with moderate content leads to creation of a lesion similar to that which occurs in advanced human atherosclerosis. Mechanical arterial injury accelerates lesion formation as discussed later.

In addition to cholesterol content in the diet, various sources of dietary fats can have different atherogenic effects (13). In general, saturated fats such as coconut oil are highly atherogenic in comparison to unsaturated fats such as corn oil. One exception is peanut oil, which is atherogenic yet relatively low in saturated fatty acids. The atherogenicity of dietary fats also depends on the fatty-acid spectrum. The atherogenicity of peanut oil may result from the content of long-chain fatty acids such as behenic (C22) and arachidic (C20) acids, which may possess particularly atherogenic properties. Cocoa butter is more saturated but less atherogenic than palm oil (rich in palmitic acid, C16), probably because of its high content of stearic (C18) acid.

MECHANICAL INJURY ACCELERATES FORMATION OF ATHEROSCLEROTIC LESIONS OF CHOLESTEROL-FED RABBITS

Mechanical injury to the rabbit artery can help produce lesions similar to advanced human atheroma in shorter periods of moderate cholesterol supplementation *(4,14)*. Medial injury accelerates intima formation in cholesterol-fed rabbits *(15)*. Aikawa et al. demonstrated that mechanical injury caused by Fogarty balloon catheter withdrawal through the aorta of New Zealand White rabbits (Millbrook Farm Inc., MA) and followed by an atherogenic diet (95% purified chow, 0.3% cholesterol, and 4.7% coconut oil, Research Diets Inc., NJ) for 4 mo created well-developed, thickened intima containing abundant macrophages underlying a layer of SMCs, which resembled advanced atherosclerosis of the human coronary artery *(14)* (Fig. 2). The balloon injury enhances formation of a fibrous cap, whereas cholesterol-feeding alone for a short period usually develops a foam cell-rich lesion resembling the human fatty streak. The balloon injury can also help to create more uniform lesions. Spontaneous atherosclerosis of hypercholesterolemic rabbits has considerably high variations in lesion distribution, size, and characteristics within an animal and between animals, which can affect quantitative analysis. Uniform lesions should help to obtain reproducible data and statistical significance for quantitative analyses. However, it should be noted that excessive injury such as overstretch by an oversized balloon often causes medial necrosis and aneurysmal change.

ATHEROSCLEROTIC LESIONS OF CHOLESTEROL-FED RABBITS EXPRESS ATHEROTHROMBOGENIC MOLECULES RELATED TO PATHOGENESIS OF HUMAN ATHEROSCLEROSIS

In addition to the morphological similarity between the arterial lesion in cholesterol-fed rabbits and human atherosclerosis, many other features of atherosclerosis—such as the presence of atherothrombogenic molecules—can be seen in hypercholesterolemic rabbits. For example, macrophages in rabbit aortic atherosclerosis express potent proteolytic enzymes, including matrix metalloproteinase-1 (MMP-1 or collagenase-1), which is overexpressed by macrophages in human atheroma *(14,16)* (Fig. 2). Proteolytic activity by other MMPs, including MMP-2, MMP-3, and MMP-9, was also detected by substrate zymography *(14)*. These matrix-degrading enzymes probably play an

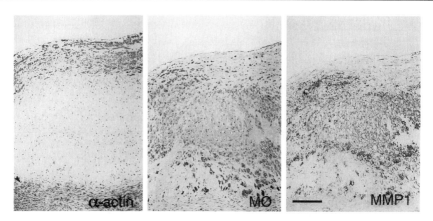

Fig. 2. Rabbit aortic lesions after 4 mo of a high-cholesterol diet contain numerous macrophages expressing MMP-1 (collagenase-1). Mouse MAb against rabbit macrophages (RAM11, Dako Corp., CA) detected abundant macrophages in the intima. A smooth-muscle layer (identified by anti-α-actin MAb, 1A4, Dako Corp., CA) overlies macrophage accumulation. This structure resembles macrophage-rich atheroma in the human coronary artery. Lesional macrophages express MMP-1 (collagenase-1) detected by antirabbit MMP-1 antibody (a gift from Dr. Michael W. Lark, Merck Research Laboratories). The arrowhead indicates the internal elastic lamina. Scale bar: 200 μm. Original magnification: ×100. Reproduced with permission from ref. *(14)*.

important role in plaque disruption, resulting in acute thrombotic complications of coronary atherosclerosis in patients *(17)*. Atheroma of cholesterol-fed rabbits contains tissue-factor activity, another key contributor to acute coronary events *(18,19)*.

Activation of vascular cells, a feature commonly found in human atherosclerosis, is also seen in rabbit atheroma. Within 1 wk after initiation of the atherogenic diet, the aortic endothelial cells of cholesterol-fed rabbits show activation gauged by overexpression of vascular cell-adhesion molecule 1 (VCAM-1), which may play a key role in monocyte recruitment into the arterial wall *(20,21)*. Rosenfeld et al. showed proliferation of macrophages in advanced lesions of hypercholesterolemic rabbits, suggesting another potential mechanism of macrophage accumulation in atheroma *(22)*. Vascular cells in rabbit atheroma express macrophage-colony-stimulating factor (M-CSF), an important molecule for macrophage survival and proliferation *(23,24)*. Activation of nuclear factor-κB (NF-κB) and increased expression of NF-κB-dependent proinflammatory factors such as monocyte chemoattractant protein 1 (MCP-1) were seen in the atheroma of cholesterol-fed rabbits *(25,26)*.

Macrophages   Collagenase-1 / MMP-1

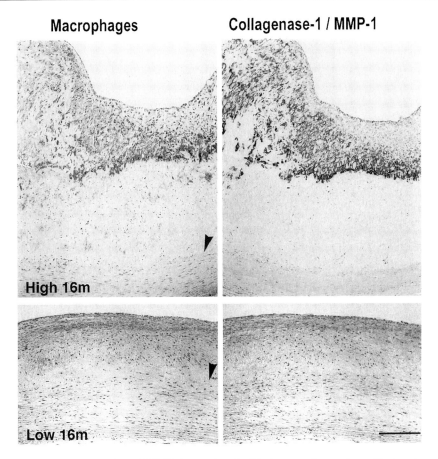

Fig. 3. Reduced expression of MMP-1 associated with decrease in number of lesional macrophages. (*top*) Macrophages within the lesion of the High group animal after an additional 16 mo of the atherogenic diet continue to express MMP-1 strongly; (*bottom*) 16 mo after cessation of the high-cholesterol diet, MMP-1 and macrophages are almot undetectable. Arrowheads indicate the internal elastic lamina. Scale bar: 200 μm. Original magnification: ×100. Adapted with permission from ref. *(14)*.

SMCs in human atherosclerotic lesions differ from those in the apparently normal media with respect to gene expression, function, and morphology *(27)*. In atheroma of humans and cholesterol-fed rabbits, activated SMCs overexpress MMPs, including MMP-3 and MMP-9, and tissue factor *(16,18,28,29)*. As a whole, these results support the relevance of using cholesterol-fed rabbits for further understanding of the regulatory mechanisms that effect expression of such atherogenic factors, and to investigate the molecular events that occur during therapeutic interventions.

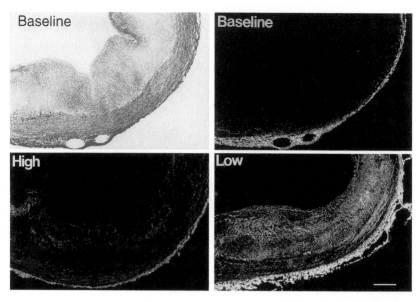

Fig. 4. Interstitial collagen content in the aortic intima detected by the picrosirius red polarization method. (*top left*) Picrosirius red staining without polarized light on the rabbit aorta after 4 mo of the atherogenic diet (baseline) shows the thickened intima of the aorta. (*top right*) The serial aortic section from the baseline lesion shows positive picrosirius red staining under polarized light in the media and adventitia only. (*bottom left*) The aortic lesion of the High group animal that continued the atherogenic diet for 16 mo shows some increase in interstitial collagen content with time. (*bottom right*) The aorta of the Low group animal after 16 mo of dietary lipid-lowering contains abundant interstitial collagen within the intima. Scale bar: 400 μm. Original magnification: ×40. Reprinted with permission from ref. *(14)*. (See color plate 4 appearing in the insert following p. 236).

AORTA OF A MECHANICALLY-INJURED, CHOLESTEROL-FED RABBIT: ANOTHER MODEL OF LIPID LOWERING ON UNSTABLE ATHEROSCLEROTIC PLAQUES

Recent clinical trials have established that lipid lowering with HMG-CoA reductase inhibitors reduces the incidence of acute coronary events. Because such treatment produces little improvement in fixed luminal stenosis, the clinical benefits may involve qualitative and functional changes in unstable atherosclerotic plaques ("stabilization") rather than quantitative changes ("regression") *(30,31)*. To improve mechanistic understanding, Aikawa et al. have recently studied the effects of dietary lipid lowering on atherosclerotic lesions of cholesterol-fed rabbits *(14,18,29)*. In rabbit atheroma created by both balloon injury and 0.3%-cholesterol feeding for 4 mo, lesional macrophages

α-Smooth Muscle Actin   Smooth Muscle Myosin

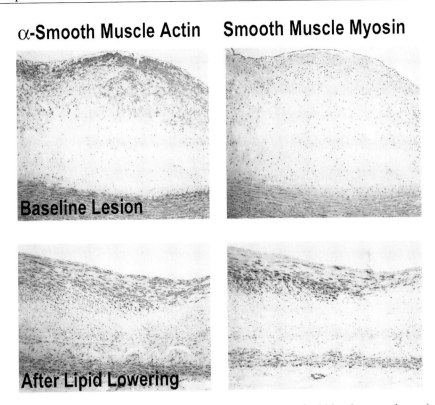

Fig. 5. Phenotype of intimal SMCs in plaque's fibrous cap of rabbit atheroma determined by expression of α-smooth-muscle actin and a myosin heavy-chain isoform (SM2) specific to mature SMCs. SM2–positive SMCs were less numerous than α-actin-positive cells, whereas medial SMCs stained positive for both α-actin and SM2. After 16 mo of lipid-lowering, many intimal SMCs stained positively for both α-actin and SM2, indicating that intimal SMCs exhibit a mature phenotype similar to medial SMCs. Scale bar: 200 μm. Original magnification: ×100. Adapted with permission from ref. *(29)*.

overexpressed collagenase-1 (MMP-1) (Fig. 2) However, after 16 mo of dietary lipid-lowering, macrophage number and collagenase expression decreased substantially, while the atheroma of rabbits maintained on the atherogenic diet for another 16 mo contained macrophages expressing collagenase *(14)* (Fig. 3). After 4 mo of cholesterol feeding, picrosirius red polarization in the atheroma detected only a small amount of interstitial collagen, a key determinant of plaque stability. There was slight increase in collagen content in the intima after 16 mo of continued hypercholesterolemia. However, 16 mo of lipid-lowering dramatically increased collagen accumulation in the intima, suggesting that a reduction in macrophages producing proteolytic activity permits accumulation of collagen *(14)* (Fig. 4). Increased accumulation of collagen in atheroma of cholesterol-fed rabbits during dietary lipid-lowering were also reported by Kockx et al *(32)*.

Dietary lipid-lowering also decreased tissue-factor expression and activity in rabbit atheroma associated with diminished macrophages *(18)*. SMCs in atheroma of humans and cholesterol-fed rabbits possess immature phenotype, as gauged by altered expression of smooth muscle myosin heavy chain isoforms *(29,33,34)*. Such immature SMCs express MMPs *(29)*. However, long-term dietary lipid lowering promoted accumulation of mature SMCs expressing smooth muscle myosin *(29)* (Fig. 5). These more mature smooth muscle cells expressed less MMPs. The reduction in proteolytic and thrombogenic macrophages and the accumulation of more normal SMCs in mechanically-injured, cholesterol-fed rabbit atheroma sheds new light on mechanisms by which lipid-lowering reduces acute thrombotic complications in patients at risk.

WHHL RABBITS: A MODEL OF ENDOGENOUS HYPERCHOLESTEROLEMIA

A line of WHHL rabbits with unprovoked hypercholesterolemia, increased blood levels of LDL, pronounced atherosclerosis, and skin xanthoma were developed by Watanabe et al *(35-37)*. In the absence of cholesterol feeding, these animals show serum cholesterol levels more than 10 times higher than normal rabbits, a characteristic caused by an inherited mutation in the gene encoding LDL-receptor. The features of the WHHL rabbits resemble those of familial hypercholesterolemia in humans *(38)*.

In WHHL rabbits, atherosclerosis in the aorta, coronary artery and other arteries, and xanthomas in digital joints begin to develop prematurely, and progress with age *(35,36,39)*. Mild lesions were found in 14% of 1–4-mo-old rabbits, and moderate to severe atherosclerotic changes were seen in all cases of 5- to 35-mo-old rabbits *(35)*. Kolodgie et al. demonstrated that the percentage of surface area covered by atherosclerotic changes in the aortic arch of WHHL rabbits increased with age (11%, 3–5 mo; 28%, 6–9 mo; 54%, 12–14 mo), and that only occasional lesions were found in the descending thoracic aorta *(40)*. The aortic arch of mature WHHL rabbits (22 mo) contains a prominent macrophage accumulation underlying a thin SMC layer (Fig. 6). Fibrous caps are less well-developed than those in the balloon-injured aorta of New Zealand White rabbits fed a 0.3% cholesterol diet for 4 mo (Fig. 2). Lesional macrophages in WHHL rabbits also express MMPs, including MMP-1, MMP-3, and MMP-9, and tissue factor, like those in cholesterol-fed rabbits *(41,42)*. Watanabe et al. demonstrated that at age of 5–36 mo, 30–35% of rabbits had atherosclerotic lesions of coronary arteries *(36)*.

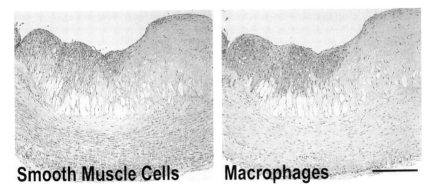

Smooth Muscle Cells   Macrophages   ⎯⎯⎯

Fig. 6. Atherosclerotic lesion of WHHL rabbits. In the intima of the aortic arch of 22-mo-old WHHL rabbit, RAM11–positive macrophages underlie a thin layer of SMCs detected by anti-smooth muscle actin antibody (1A4). Scale bar: 200 μm. Original magnification: ×100. (See color plate 5 appearing in the insert following p. 236).

The level of total plasma cholesterol in WHHL rabbits is 650–950 mg/dL on standard chow diet *(43)*, although their cholesterol levels decrease slightly with age *(9)* and vary depending on individual animals and colonies. Although atherosclerotic lesions of WHHL rabbits contain abundant foam cells, the liver does not show manifest lipid deposition, unlike cholesterol-fed rabbits *(37)*. The major fraction of plasma cholesterol in WHHL rabbits is LDL-cholesterol similar to familial hypercholesterolemia in humans, whereas cholesterol-fed rabbits have VLDL-hypercholesterolemia *(9,35)*. Tsukada and Rosenfeld demonstrated that the structure and cell composition of atherosclerotic lesions of WHHL and 0.2% cholesterol- and 20% casein-fed rabbits were qualitatively similar *(8–10)*. Their results may suggest that lack of LDL-receptor activity and different lipoprotein distribution between cholesterol-fed and WHHL rabbits do not influence the morphogenesis of atherosclerosis.

Several studies have used WHHL rabbits to determine the effects of lipid-lowering on atherosclerosis *(41,42,44–46)*. Watanabe and Shiomi et al. have extensively studied suppression of atherosclerosis by lipid-lowering with HMG-CoA reductase inhibitors on both the aorta and the coronary artery of WHHL rabbits *(44–46)*. Lipid-lowering with HMG-CoA reductase inhibitors reduces MMP expression in atherosclerotic lesions in both young and mature WHHL rabbits *(41,42)*. Rosenfeld et al. previously showed that macrophages in advanced lesions of both cholesterol-fed and WHHL rabbits proliferate, as mentioned earlier, comprising approx 30% of cells labeled with ^{3}H-methyl-thymidine *(22)*. Aikawa et al. have recently found that lipid-lowering with an HMG-CoA reductase inhibitor suppresses proliferation of macrophages in the aorta of WHHL rabbits *(41)*.

CASEIN-FED RABBITS: ANOTHER MODEL OF ENDOGENOUS HYPERCHOLESTEROLEMIA

A casein-enriched diet induces moderate levels of endogenous hypercholes-terolemia in rabbits, because of increased cholesterol absorption, increased VLDL secretion, delayed VLDL turnover, and decreased activities of LDL receptor and hepatic HMG-CoA reductase *(47,48)*. This results in atherosclerotic lesion formation *(49,50)*. Daley et al. reported that when rabbits were matched for moderate levels of total plasma cholesterol (approx 500 mg/dL), the main fraction of plasma cholesterol of 27% casein-fed rabbits was present as LDL-cholesterol, while 0.125–0.5% of cholesterol-fed rabbits had equal levels of VLDL-, IDL-, and LDL-cholesterol *(7)*. Despite matched total cholesterol, lesion area and volume in their study were greater in cholesterol-fed rabbits than casein-fed rabbits after 6 mo of the feeding period *(7)*. Furthermore, all stages of atherosclerosis from fatty streaks to advanced atheromatous plaques were equally observed in the aortas of casein-fed rabbits, while cholesterol-fed rabbits contained more advanced lesions *(11)*. These data suggest that different patterns of cholesterol fractions may influence the rate of progression of atherosclerosis. Casein-fed rabbits have been extensively used for studies of drugs related to lipid metabolism, because their lipid profiles are similar to that of humans and because they exhibit minimal liver damage *(51–53)*.

TRANSGENIC RABBITS AS NEW TOOLS FOR ATHEROSCLEROSIS RESEARCH

Genetically altered animals that overexpress or lack specific genes related to lipid disorders or atherogenesis are useful models for understanding the pathogenesis of atherosclerosis. A number of transgenic or gene-targeted mice have been produced for the study of human atherosclerosis *(54)*. Several transgenic rabbits overexpressing human apolipoproteins and lipid enzymes have also been developed *(55,56)*.

Both mice and rabbits have advantages and limitations. Mice differ from humans in some aspects of lipid metabolism. For example, unlike humans and rabbits, mice lack cholesteryl ester transfer protein (CETP), which plays an important role in atherogenesis. Also, HDL is predominant in mice plasma. Thus, mice are much less susceptible to diet-induced atherosclerosis than rabbits. Physiological procedures such as mechanical injury on the artery are more easily performed in rabbits than in mice. It is also easier to collect sufficient tissue specimens or blood samples for biochemical assays in rabbits than in mice. Rabbits are more suitable than mice for the study of the role of certain genes, such as human apolipoprotein (a) (apo [a]). Human apo (a) can bind to rabbit apo B to form lipoprotein (a) (Lp[a]), but it does not bind to mouse apoB

(57). Thus, the rabbit can be a useful alternative to the mouse. However, the technology of producing transgenic rabbits is not as well established as that of mice. Also, gene-targeting in rabbits (e.g., availability of embryonic stem cells) is not well developed, and knockout rabbits have not been established, while many mouse models with deficiency of genes related to atherogenesis have provided considerable knowledge in atherosclerosis research.

To date, overexpression of several human genes encoding apolipoproteins or lipid enzymes in rabbits have been reported. A human apoA-I transgene in cholesterol-fed New Zealand White and WHHL rabbits increased plasma levels of HDL-cholesterol and decreased surface areas of the thoracic aorta covered by lesions compared with those in nontransgenic controls *(58)*. New Zealand White rabbits that overexpress human apoE2, an ApoE variant associated with type III hyperlipoproteinemia, had higher VLDL-cholesterol levels and more aortic atherosclerosis than those of wild-type animals *(59)*. Overexpression of human lecithin:cholesterol acyltransferase (LCAT), a potential antiatherogenic enzyme, suppressed aortic lesion development in cholesterol-fed New Zealand White rabbits *(59)*. Human hepatic lipase transgenic rabbits consuming an atherogenic diet had decreased total cholesterol levels and attenuation of diet-induced atherosclerosis *(60,61)*.

CONCLUSION

Profiles of hypercholesterolemic rabbit models of atherosclerosis are controversial because they entail extreme hypercholesterolemia results in atheroma consisting predominantly of macrophage-foam cells, unlike advanced human atherosclerosis *(62,63)*. Swine or nonhuman primates may indeed develop lesions that morphologically resemble human atherosclerosis *(62,63)*. However, rabbits are less expensive and easier to handle than swine or nonhuman primates, although WHHL rabbits are expensive. These advantages have enabled the study of greater numbers of animals to increase statistical power. Furthermore, researchers have recently chosen lower cholesterol levels and longer feeding periods to create more fibrous, human-like lesions. Based on a number of previous studies, one can choose proper procedures (e.g., types of rabbit models, cholesterol content in the diet, feeding periods, additional mechanical injury, etc.) depending on the target plasma cholesterol levels and what types of lesions are needed. Recent studies indicate that macrophage-rich atheromatous plaques cause most acute coronary events in humans *(30)*. Thus, rabbit models may be useful and relevant for the study of molecular mechanisms of macrophage activation in such unstable plaques. Finally, increasing evidence has shown that rabbit atheroma express a number of molecules related to pathogenesis of human atherosclerosis, while limited information regarding molecular and cellular biology is available for other animals such as swine or nonhuman primates. In conclusion, we believe that hypercholesterolemic rabbits will continue to serve as useful models of atherosclerosis in the future.

ACKNOWLEDGMENT

The studies from the Cardiovascular Division cited here were supported by grants to Peter Libby from the National Heart, Lung, and Blood Institute (HL-34636, PO1 HL48743), a research award from the Japan Heart Foundation to Masanori Aikawa, and a Merck/Banyu Fellowship to Yoshihiro Fukumoto. We thank Ms. Karen E. Williams for her editorial expertise.

REFERENCES

1. LaRosa JC, Hunninghake D, Bush D, Criqui MH, Getz GS, Gotto AM Jr., et al. The cholesterol facts. A summary of the evidence relating dietary fats, serum cholesterol, and coronary heart disease. A joint statement by the American Heart Association and the National Heart, Lung, and Blood Institute. The Task Force on Cholesterol Issues, American Heart Association. Circulation 1990; 81:1721–1733.

2. Libby P, Aikawa M. New insights into plaque stabilisation by lipid-lowering. Drugs 1998; 56:9–13.

3. Anitschkow N, Chalatow S. Ueber experimentelle cholesterinsteatose und ihre bedeutehung einiger pathologischer prozesse. Centrbl Allg Pathol Pathol Anat 1913; 24:1–9.

4. Bocan TM, Mueller SB, Mazur MJ, Uhlendorf PD, Brown EQ, and Kieft KA. The relationship between the degree of dietary-induced hypercholesterolemia in the rabbit and atherosclerotic lesion formation. Atherosclerosis 1993; 102:9–22.

5. Libby P, Fleet JC, Salomon RN, Li H, Loppnow H, Clinton SK. Possible roles of cytokines in atherogenesis. In: Stein SEO, Stein Y, eds. Atherosclerosis IV: Proceedings of the Ninth International Symposium on Atherosclerosis. Creative Communications Ltd., Tel Aviv, Israel 1992; pp. 339–350.

6. Bocan TM, Mazur MJ, Mueller SB, Brown EQ, Sliskovic DR, O'Brien PM, et al. Antiatherosclerotic activity of inhibitors of 3–hydroxy-3—methylglutaryl coenzyme A reductase in cholesterol-fed rabbits: a biochemical and morphological evaluation. Atherosclerosis 1994; 111:127–142.

7. Daley SJ, Herderick EE, Cornhill JF, Rogers KA. Cholesterol-fed and casein-fed rabbit models of atherosclerosis. Part 1: Differing lesion area and vol despite equal plasma cholesterol levels. Arterioscler Thromb 1994; 14:95–104.

8. Tsukada T, Rosenfeld M, Ross R, Gown A.M. Immunocytochemical analysis of cellular components in atherosclerotic lesions. Use of monoclonal antibodies with the Watanabe and fat-fed rabbit. Arteriosclerosis 1986; 6:601–613.

9. Rosenfeld ME, Tsukada T, Gown AM, Ross R. Fatty streak initiation in Watanabe Heritable Hyperlipemic and comparably hypercholesterolemic fat-fed rabbits. Arteriosclerosis 1987; 7:9–23.

10. Rosenfeld ME, Tsukada T, Chait A, Bierman EL, Gown AM, Ross R. Fatty streak expansion and maturation in Watanabe heritable hyperlipemic and comparably hypercholesterolemic fat-fed rabbits. Arteriosclerosis 1987; 7:24–34.

11. Daley SJ, Klemp KF, Guyton JR, Rogers KA. Cholesterol-fed and casein-fed rabbit models of atherosclerosis. Part 2: Differing morphological severity of atherogenesis despite matched plasma cholesterol levels. Arterioscler Thromb 1994; 14:105–141.

12. Garbarsch C, Matthiessen ME, Helin P, Lorenzen I. Spontaneous aortic arteriosclerosis in rabbits of the Danish Country strain. Atherosclerosis 1970; 12:291–300.

13. Kritchevsky D. Dietary fat and experimental atherosclerosis. Int J Tissue React 1991; 13:59–65.

14. Aikawa M, Rabkin E, Okada Y, Voglic SJ, Clinton SK, Brinckerhoff CE, et al. Lipid lowering by diet reduces matrix metalloproteinase activity and increases collagen content of rabbit atheroma: a potential mechanism of lesion stabilization. Circulation 1998; 97:2433–2344.

15. Constantinides P. The role of arterial wall injury in atherogenesis and arterial thrombogenesis. Zentbl Allg Pathol 1989; 135:517–530.

16. Galis ZS, Sukhova GK, Lark MW, Libby P. Increased expression of matrix metalloproteinases and matrix degrading activity in vulnerable regions of human atherosclerotic plaques. J Clin Invest 1994; 94:2493–2503.

17. Libby P, Geng YJ, Aikawa M, Schoenbeck U, Mach F, Clinton SK, et al. Macrophages and atherosclerotic plaque stability. Curr Opin Lipidol 1996; 7:330–335.

18. Aikawa M, Voglic SJ, Sugiyama S, Rabkin E, Taubman MB, Fallon JT, et al. Dietary lipid-lowering reduces tissue factor expression in rabbit atheroma. Circulation 1999; 100:1215–1222.

19. Taubman MB, Fallon JT, Schecter AD, Giesen P, Mendlowitz M, Fyfe BS, et al. Tissue factor in the pathogenesis of atherosclerosis. Thromb Haemostasis 1997; 78:200–204.

20. Cybulsky MI, Gimbrone, MA, Jr. Endothelial expression of a mononuclear leukocyte adhesion molecule during atherogenesis. Science 1991; 251:788–791.

21. Li H, Cybulsky MI, Gimbrone, MA, Jr, Libby P. An atherogenic diet rapidly induces VCAM-1, a cytokine-regulatable mononuclear leukocyte adhesion molecule, in rabbit aortic endothelium. Arterioscler Thromb 1993; 13:197–204.

22. Rosenfeld M E, Ross R. Macrophage and smooth muscle cell proliferation in atherosclerotic lesions of WHHL and comparably hypercholesterolemic fat-fed rabbits. Arteriosclerosis 1990; 10:680–687.

23. Rosenfeld ME, Yla-Herttuala S, Lipton BA, Ord VA, Witztum JL, Steinberg D. Macrophage colony-stimulating factor mRNA and protein in atherosclerotic lesions of rabbits and humans. Am J Pathol 1992; 140:291–300.

24. Clinton SK, Underwood R, Hayes L, Sherman ML, Kufe DW, Libby P. Macrophage colony-stimulating factor gene expression in vascular cells and in experimental and human atherosclerosis. Am J Pathol 1992; 140:301–316.

25. Hernandez-Presa MA, Bustos C, Ortego M, Tunon J, Ortega L, Egido J. ACE inhibitor quinapril reduces the arterial expression of NF-kappaB-dependent proinflammatory factors but not of collagen I in a rabbit model of atherosclerosis. Am J Pathol 1998; 153:1825–1837.

26. Hernandez-Presa MA, Gomez-Guerrero C, Egido J. In situ non-radioactive detection of nuclear factors in paraffin sections by Southwestern histochemistry. Kidney Int 1999; 55:209–214.

27. Schwartz SM, deBlois D, O'Brien ER. The intima. Soil for atherosclerosis and restenosis. Circ Res 1995; 77:445–465.

28. Wilcox JN, Smith KM, Schwartz SM, Gordon D. Localization of tissue factor in the normal vessel wall and in the atherosclerotic plaque. Proc Natl Acad Sci USA 1989; 86:2839–2843.

29. Aikawa M, Rabkin E, Voglic SJ, Shing H, Nagai R, Schoen FJ, et al. Lipid lowering promotes accumulation of mature smooth muscle cells expressing smooth muscle myosin heavy chain isoforms in rabbit atheroma. Circ Res 1998; 83:1015–1026.

30. Libby P. Molecular bases of the acute coronary syndromes. Circulation 1995; 91:2844–2850.

31. Brown BG, Zhao XQ, Sacco DE, Albers JJ. Lipid lowering and plaque regression. New insights into prevention of plaque disruption and clinical events in coronary disease. Circulation 1993; 87:1781–1791.

32. Kockx MM, De Meyer GR, Buyssens N, Knaapen MW, Bult H, Herman AG. Cell composi-
    tion, replication, and apoptosis in atherosclerotic plaques after 6 mo of cholesterol withdrawal.
    Circ Res 1998; 83:378–387.

33. Kuro-o M, Nagai R, Nakahara K, Katoh H, Tsai RC, Tsuchimochi H, et al. cDNA cloning of
    a myosin heavy chain isoform in embryonic smooth muscle and its expression during vascular
    development and in arteriosclerosis. J Biol Chem 1991; 266:3768–3773.

34. Aikawa M, Sivam PN, Kuro-o M, Kimura K, Nakahara K, Takewaki S, et al. Human smooth
    muscle myosin heavy chain isoforms as molecular markers for vascular development and
    atherosclerosis. Circ Res 1993; 73:1000–1012.

35. Watanabe Y. Serial inbreeding of rabbits with hereditary hyperlipidemia (WHHL-rabbit).
    Atherosclerosis 1980; 36:261–268.

36. Watanabe Y, Ito T, Shiomi M. The effect of selective breeding on the development of coronary
    atherosclerosis in WHHL rabbits. An animal model for familial hypercholesterolemia. Ath-
    erosclerosis 1985; 56:71–79.

37. Aliev G, Burnstock G. Watanabe rabbits with heritable hypercholesterolaemia: a model of
    atherosclerosis. Histol Histopathol 1998; 13:797–817.

38. Goldstein JL, Kita T, Brown MS. Defective lipoprotein receptors and atherosclerosis. Lessons
    from an animal counterpart of familial hypercholesterolemia. N Engl J Med 1983; 309:288–296.

39. Buja LM, Kita T, Goldstein JL, Watanabe Y, Brown MS. Cellular pathology of progressive
    atherosclerosis in the WHHL rabbit. An animal model of familial hypercholesterolemia.
    Arteriosclerosis 1983; 3:87–101.

40. Kolodgie FD, Virmani R, Rice HE, Mergner WJ. Vascular reactivity during the progression
    of atherosclerotic plaque. A study in Watanabe heritable hyperlipidemic rabbits. Circ Res
    1990; 66:1112–1126.

41. Aikawa M, Rabkin E, Sugiyama S, Voglic SJ, Fukumoto Y, Furukawa Y, et al. Cerivastatin,
    an HMG-CoA reductase inhibitor suppresses growth of macrophages expressing matrix
    metalloproteinases and tissue factor in vivo and in vitro. Circulation (in press).

42. Fukumoto Y, Aikawa M, Rabkin E, Shiomi M, Enomoto M, Hirouchi Y, et al. Prolonged
    pravastatin treatment increases collagen synthesis and smooth muscle and collagen accumu-
    lation in atheroma of WHHL rabbits [abstract] Circulation 1999; 100:I–753.

43. Tanzawa K, Shimada Y, Kuroda M, Tsujita Y, Arai M, Watanabe H. WHHL-rabbit: a low
    density lipoprotein receptor-deficient animal model for familial hypercholesterolemia. FEBS
    Lett 1980; 118:81–84.

44. Watanabe Y, Ito T, Shiomi M, Tsujita Y, Kuroda M, Arai M, et al. Preventive effect of
    pravastatin sodium, a potent inhibitor of 3- hydroxy-3-methylglutaryl coenzyme A reductase,
    on coronary atherosclerosis and xanthoma in WHHL rabbits. Biochim Biophys Acta 1988;
    960:294–302.

45. Shiomi M, Ito T, Tsukada T, Yata T, Watanabe Y, Tsujita M, et al. Reduction of serum
    cholesterol levels alters lesional composition of atherosclerotic plaques. Effect of pravastatin
    sodium on atherosclerosis in mature WHHL rabbits. Arterioscler Thromb Vasc Biol 1995;
    15:1938–1944.

46. Shiomi M, Ito T. Effect of cerivastatin sodium, a new inhibitor of HMG-CoA reductase, on
    plasma lipid levels, progression of atherosclerosis, and the lesional composition in the plaques
    of WHHL rabbits. Br J Pharmacol 1999; 126:961–968.

47. Beynen AC, Van der Meer R, West CE. Mechanism of casein-induced hypercholesterolemia:
    primary and secondary features. Atherosclerosis 1986; 60:291–293.

48. Pfeuffer M. Differences in the underlying mechanisms of cholesterol- and casein-induced
    hypercholesterolemia in rabbit and rat. Atherosclerosis 1989; 76:89–91.

49. Richardson M, Kurowska EM, Carroll KK. Early lesion development in the aortas of rabbits fed low-fat, cholesterol-free, semipurified casein diet. Atherosclerosis 1994; 107:165–178.
50. Kratky RG, Ivey J, Rogers KA, Daley S, Roach MR. The distribution of fibro-fatty atherosclerotic lesions in the aortae of casein- and cholesterol-fed rabbits. Atherosclerosis 1993; 99:121–131.
51. Chao Y, Yamin TT, Alberts AW. Effects of cholestyramine on low density lipoprotein binding sites on liver membranes from rabbits with endogenous hypercholesterolemia induced by a wheat starch-casein diet. J Biol Chem 1982; 257:3623–3627.
52. Krause BR, Pape ME, Kieft K, Auerbach B, Bisgaier CL, Homan R, et al. ACAT inhibition decreases LDL cholesterol in rabbits fed a cholesterol-free diet. Marked changes in LDL cholesterol without changes in LDL receptor mRNA abundance. Arterioscler Thromb 1994; 14:598–604.
53. Auerbach BJ, Krause BR, Bisgaier CL, Newton RS. Comparative effects of HMG-CoA reductase inhibitors on apo B production in the casein-fed rabbit: atorvastatin versus lovastatin. Atherosclerosis 1995; 115:173–180.
54. Faraci FM, Sigmund CD. Vascular biology in genetically altered mice: smaller vessels, bigger insight. Circ Res 1999; 85:1214–1225.
55. Brousseau ME, Hoeg JM. Transgenic rabbits as models for atherosclerosis research. J Lipid Res 1999; 40:365–375.
56. Fan J, Challah M, Watanabe T. Transgenic rabbit models for biomedical research: current status, basic methods and future perspectives. Pathol Int 1999; 49:583–594.
57. Rouy D, Duverger N, Lin SD, Emmanuel F, Houdebine LM, Denefle P, et al. Apolipoprotein(a) yeast artificial chromoome transgenic rabbits. Lipoprotein(a) assembly with human and rabbit apolipoprotein B. J Biol Chem 1998; 273:1247–1251.
58. Duverger N, Kruth H, Emmanuel F, Caillaud JM, Viglietta C, Castro G, et al. Inhibition of atherosclerosis development in cholesterol-fed human apolipoprotein A-I-transgenic rabbits. Circulation 1996; 94:713–717.
59. Huang Y, Schwendner SW, Rall SC Jr, Sanan DA, Mahley RW. Apolipoprotein E2 transgenic rabbits. Modulation of the type III hyperlipoproteinemic phenotype by estrogen and occurrence of spontaneous atherosclerosis. J Biol Chem 1997; 272:22,685–22,694.
60. Fan J, Wang J, Bensadoun A, Lauer SJ, Dang Q, Mahley RW, et al. Overexpression of hepatic lipase in transgenic rabbits leads to a marked reduction of plasma high density lipoproteins and intermediate density lipoproteins. Proc Natl Acad Sci USA 1994; 91:8724–8728.
61. Taylor JM. Transgenic rabbit models for the study of atherosclerosis. Ann NY Acad Sci 1997; 811:146–152.
62. Vesselinovitch D. Animal models and the study of atherosclerosis. Arch Pathol Lab Med 1988; 112:1011–1017.
63. Armstrong ML, Heistad DD. Animal models of atherosclerosis. Atherosclerosis 1990; 85:15–23.

14 Atherosclerosis in Nonhuman Primates

David Kritchevsky, PHD and Robert J. Nicolosi, PHD

CONTENTS

INTRODUCTION

Nonhuman primates represent an ideal animal model for human atherosclerosis. They develop arterial lesions which resemble those seen in humans, and often respond to lipidemic stimulus with the production of lipoproteins resembling those seen in man. The disadvantages are that nonhuman primates are expensive to purchase and maintain, and they are often difficult to handle. Nevertheless, there has been considerable activity in this area of research. The extent of the research effort is a function of consistent availability, and there are now some locally-based breeding colonies which assure a reliable, steady supply and which allow for testing of genetic characteristics through selective breeding. Since not all strains react similarly, they will be treated individually in the following discussion.

NEW WORLD MONKEYS

Lofland, Clarkson, and their colleagues *(1–3)* pioneered studies in these primates until they discovered that their chronic renal disease modulated both lipoprotein metabolism and atherosclerosis *(1,2)*. Clarkson et al. described this

From: *Contemporary Cardiology: Vascular Disease and Injury: Preclinical Research*
Edited by: D. I. Simon and C. Rogers © Humana Press Inc., Totowa, NJ

Table 1
Serum Lipids and Spontaneous Atherosclerosis in New World Monkeys[a]

Species	No.	Cholesterol (mg/dL)		Atherosclerosis index (%)	
		Total	β-Lipoprotein	Thoracic	Abdominal
Squirrel (Saimiri sciureus)	270	105	74	4.95	2.64
Capuchin (Cebus appella)	21	98	76	0.0	0.0
Ringtail (Cebus albifrons)	57	90	67	1.88	0.96
Spider (ateles)	29	130	118	1.88	0.60
Woolly (Lagothrix lagothrix)	20	133	118	0.38	0.63
Marmoet (Sanguinis nigricollis)	44	69	50	0.65	0.0

[a] Adapted from ref. (4).

model (3). Nevertheless, they demonstrated that the level of cholesterolemia did not always reflect the severity of atherosclerotic lesions (4) (Table 1).

Cebus Monkey (Cebus albifrons)

Mann et al. (5) were able to induce atherosclerosis in cebus monkeys by feeding them diets high in cholesterol and low in sulfur-containing amino acids for 18–30 wk. Hypercholesterolemia can be prevented by feeding 1g/d of dl-methionine or L-cystine. Cholesterol levels can be restored to normal by feeding 1g of dl-methionine daily. Wissler et al. (6) fed cebus monkeys diets containing 0.5% cholesterol and 25% butterfat, coconut oil, or corn oil. Aortas from all the coconut oil-fed monkeys contained lesions, compared to 75% and 0% incidence for the butterfat and corn oil-fed monkeys, respectively.

OLD WORLD MONKEYS
Rhesus Monkeys (Macaca mulatta)

Almost a half-century ago, Mann and Andrus (7) found that when adult rhesus monkeys were fed a diet high in fat and cholesterol for almost 4 yr, they exhibited extensive atherosclerosis of the aorta and all its major branches. The diet was based on dried egg yolk (45%) plus 5% added cholesterol (providing 6.5 g cholesterol per 100 g diet) and 10% corn oil as fat. After 10 mo of this diet, serum cholesterol had risen to 1200 mg/dL (31 mM/L) and remained elevated for the duration of the study. The serum β-lipoproteins (S_f 12–20) were also grossly elevated. The vascular lesions were similar to those seen in human atherosclerosis.

Taylor and colleagues published a series of studies of atherosclerosis in rhesus monkeys (8–14). Eighteen monkeys (10F, 8 M)) were fed a daily stock diet containing 3 g of cholesterol and 15 g of corn oil for 28–105 wk. Five monkeys were characterized as hyporesponders (average blood cholesterol rising by 99% over 50 ± 14 wk of feeding); seven were characterized as average responders (blood cholesterol rising by 159% over 47 ± 9 wk of feeding) and six as hyperresponders (blood cholesterol rising by 333% after 52 ± 12 wk on the diet). This observation prestaged the continuing interest in genetics of cholesterol response *(15)*. They also saw seasonal fluctuation of blood cholesterol levels—results which have also been observed in cynomolgus *(16)* and vervet *(17)* monkeys. The variable cholesterolemic responses were associated with average severity of aortic atherosclerosis of 2.43 ± 0.27. (Graded on a 0–4 basis). Another study with rhesus monkeys revealed that a combination of cholesterol, vitamin D, and nicotine resulted in more severe atherosclerosis than treatment with any of the three factors individually *(18)*.

Wissler et al. *(19)* fed adult male rhesus monkeys table-prepared rations (using real foods) designed to reflect the average American diet (27% fat; 175 mg cholesterol; 560 calories/d) and compared them with monkeys fed a prudent diet (*PD*) (14% fat; 81 mg cholesterol; 360 calories/d) for 2 yr. Average cholesterol levels were 383 ± 35 mg/dL (9.92 ± 0.91 mM/L) in monkeys fed the "American" diet compared to 199 ± 13 mg/dL (5.15 ± 0.35 mM/L) in those fed the PD. Average atherosclerosis (0–4 scale) was 0.2 ± 0.1 in monkeys fed the PD compared to 1.1 ± 0.9 in those fed the "American" diet.

Pigtail Macaque (Macaca nemestrina)

This strain of monkey was fed a diet that promoted a low-level hypercholesterolemia. The monkeys were autopsied at 2,3, or 3.5 years. The findings by Masuda and Ross *(20,21)* together with earlier observations by this group *(22, 23)* formed the basis of Ross' elegant hypothesis regarding the formation of atheromatous plaques.

Cynomolgus Monkeys (Macaca fascicularis) Macaca irus

The cynomolgus monkey exhibits naturally-occurring atherosclerotic lesions *(24)*. These lesions are present in the aortic arch, as well as in the thoracic and abdominal aorta. Diet-induced atherosclerosis in this species has been observed by Armstrong *(25)*, Kramsch and Hollander *(26)*, and Malinow et al. *(27)*, among others. Wagner et al. *(28)* have found that compared to rhesus monkeys, aortic lesions in cynomolgus monkeys show greater intimal thickening, more extracellular lipid, a greater fibrogenic response, and higher mineral content. Bond et al. *(29)* also observed myocardial infarctions in cynomolgus monkeys fed a diet containing 25% lard and 0.5% cholesterol.

Alderson et al. *(30)* reported that peanut oil—an unsaturated fat—reduced the severity of diet-induced atherosclerosis in cynomolgus monkeys. In this study, the monkeys were fed 0.1% cholesterol and a mixture (20%) of butter, olive oil, and corn oil, or a butter, olive oil, corn-oil mix of 15% or 10% with 5% or 10% added peanut oil. The iodine values (calculated) of the three fats were 72, 81, and 90, respectively.

Soy protein has been shown to prevent diet-induced coronary-artery atherosclerosis in male cynomolgus monkeys *(31)*. The effect was attributed to the phytoestrogen content of soy protein.

The cynomolgus monkey has also been used to assess the effects of social stress on atherosclerosis. Kaplan et al. *(32)* reported that socially stressed adult male cynomolgus monkeys developed more extensive coronary-artery atherosclerosis than unstressed controls. The monkeys were all fed a low-fat, low-cholesterol diet. The monkeys were stressed by being introduced into a new social environment. It was later shown that social stress elicited a similar response in female cynomolgus monkeys *(33)*. Part of the stress syndrome is related to an increased heart rate *(34,35)*. These findings implicate aggressiveness and sympathetic arousal in the pathogenesis of atherosclerosis, *(36)* and may yield important clues relating to behavioral issues in human atherosclerosis.

African Green (Vervet) Monkey (Circopithecus aethriops)

The aortic lesions and lipoprotein changes elicited by diet in this model resemble those seen in man *(37–39)*. There is a growing body of literature regarding diet and atherosclerosis in the vervet. Much of the data regarding effects of dietary fat on cholesterolemia and atherosclerosis have been accumulated by Rudel and his colleagues *(40–43)*. They fed vervet monkeys an atherogenic diet (0.8 mg/kcal cholesterol and 40 cal% as saturated fat) for 11 wk, and then divided them into groups of roughly equal plasma cholesterol and saturated, monounsaturated, or polyunsaturated fat (35 cal%). There were two phases in the study—one in which monkeys were fed fat mixtures and the other in which they were fed individual fats. Total plasma cholesterol levels were maintained on the saturated fat, and fell when the monkeys were fed either mono- or polyunsaturated fat. The relative percentages of LDL and HDL cholesterol were generally the same on either the mono- or polyunsaturated fat diets, with LDL/HDL cholesterol ratios between 2.40 and 3.96. In monkeys fed the mixture providing polyunsaturated fat, the LDL/HDL ratio rose to 3.23 (suggesting a drop in HDL cholesterol levels), whereas in monkeys fed the oleic acid-rich safflower oil, it fell to 1.32—suggesting a reduction in the percentage of LDL and a substantial rise in the percentage of HDL *(40)*. Another experiment *(41)* showed that fish oil, fed for 2.5 – 3.0 yr led to lower plasma cholesterol levels (231 ± 37 mg/dL; 5.97 ± 0.96 mM/L), compared to lard 360 ± 44 mg/dL (9.31 ± 1.14 mM/L). Aortic atherosclerosis was significantly less severe in the mon-

Table 2
Effect of Transunsaturated Fat on Experimental Atherosclerosis
in Vervet Monkeys[b]

Group[a]	Atherosclerosis		Arteriosclerosis	
	Incidence	% of Surface	Incidence	% of Surface
3T	6/8	2.47	3.8	1.30
3R	6/8	5.09	3.8	1.35
6T	5/8	5.29	3/8	0.41
6R	6/7	2.95	5.7	1.43
Control	12/15	6.55	5/15	0.50

[a] 3T—fed 3.2% trans fat for 12 mo; 3R—fed 3.2% trans fat for 6 mo, then control diet; 6T—fed 6.0% trans fat for 12 mo; 6R—fed 6.0% trans fat for 6 mo, then control diet.
[b] Adapted from ref. (48).

keys given fish oil. Subsequent studies showed that feeding polyunsaturated fat from an early age reduced the risk of coronary-artery atherosclerosis (42, 43).

The lipidemic and atherogenic effects of trans-unsaturated fats (trans fats) have been a concern of nutritionists since the 1960s. In the early 1960s, McMillan's group showed that trans fats were hyperlipidemic, but not more atherogenic than corresponding cis fats in cholesterol-fed rabbits (44–46). The same was true for rabbits fed cholesterol-free, atherogenic diets (47). Vervet monkeys were fed semipurified, cholesterol-free diets containing 3.2% or 6.0% trans fat for either 6 or 12 mo. Some animals fed trans fat for 6 mo were returned to a control diet for 6 mo. There were no significant differences in either lipidemia or atherosclerosis between the control and trans fat-fed monkeys (Table 2) (48).

Vervet monkeys (6/gp) were fed a semipurified, cholesterol-free diet containing 25% casein, 14% coconut oil, and 15% fiber for 23 wk (49). Average sudanophilia (% area) was 3.8 ± 1.5 when the fiber was cellulose, 1.5 ± 0.4 when it was wheat straw, and 4.1 ± 2.9 when it was alfalfa. Although one of the monkeys fed alfalfa exhibited severe sudanophilia (18.1%), the average for the other five monkeys was 1.2 ± 0.6.

In another study (50), effects of dietary fiber were assessed in vervets (7/gp) fed a "Western" diet (WD) actually composed of everyday foodstuffs. The diet contained 46.2% calories as fat, 39.8% as carbohydrates, and 14.0% as protein. A third group (control) was fed commercial monkey ration augmented with fruit and bread. Average serum cholesterol levels over the 34-wk feeding period were cellulose, 300 ± 30 mg/dL (7.76 ± 0.78 mM/L), pectin 223 ± 16 mg/

dL (5.77 ±0.41 mM/L) and control 113 ± 9 mg/dL (2.92 ± 0.23 mM/L). LDL/ HDL cholesterol ratios in the three groups were cellulose, 4.78; pectin, 2.67; and control, 1.62. Average aortic sudanophilia in the three groups was 10.6 ± 4.6 cellulose, 8.1 ± 2.5 pectin, and 1.1 ± 0.4 control.

In another study, adult female vervet monkeys were fed a control (commercial) monkey diet, a high-calorie *WD*, or a prudent Western diet (PD). The Western diets were prepared by cooking and combining real food. The diets were maintained for 4 yr, and yielded highly significant data *(51–55)*. Two groups were fed the WD or PD diets for 47 mo; a third was fed the WD for 20 mo and the PD for the next 27 mo. The starting cholesterol level was 147 mg/ dL (3.8 mM/L) and increased to 174 mg/dL (4.50mM/L) on PD and 376 mg/dL (9.72 mM/L) on the WD. Reversal from WD to PD quickly led to lowered serum cholesterol. Increases in blood calcium, zinc, and Vitamin E, and decreases in Vitamin B$_6$ were associated with WD relative to PD. There were no effects on triglycerides, glucose, vitamin A, insulin, glucagon, copper, or magnesium *(51)*. The total aortic surface containing lesions was (% ± SD); WD –53.2 ± 27; PD –27.8 ± 27; and WD/PD –22.3 ± 20. Surface lipid area was (% ± SD); WD –43.8 ± 24; PD – 27.4 ± 26; and WD/PD 21.0 ± 21. In every other aortic parameter, the WD resulted in the most severe injury, PD the least, and WD/PD was intermediate *(52)*. The plasma LDL pool was expanded because of a threefold increase of LDL particles of relatively normal composition. The LDL esters contained more arachidonic and less linoleic acid. Multivariate analysis showed that the severity of atherosclerosis was highly dependent on lecithin and sphingomyelin in LDL *(53)*. After 40 mo, the kinetics of LDL apo B were measured in 10 animals on each dietary regimen. The fractional catabolic rate (pools per d) was 0.45 ± 0.11 on WD, 0.59 ± 0.11 on PD, and 0.61 ± 0.11 on the control high-carbohydrate diet (HCD) ($p<0.0125$). LDL turnover rate (mg/24 h) was WD = 57.0 ± 27.0, PD = 28.0 ± 11.2, and HCD = 29.7 ± 9.8 ($p<0.005$). Synthetic rate (mg/kg/d) was WD =13.8 ± 4.5, PD =7.4 ± 3.2, and HCD = 8.6 ± 2.4 ($p<0.0025$) *(54)*. Analysis of the total aortic lipids revealed that lipid levels were significantly elevated throughout the aortic intima, suggesting that atherosclerosis may be developing in the entire aorta rather than at focal points. Aortic lesions were correlated significantly with aortic total, free, and esterified cholesterol, sphingomyelin, lecithin, and lysolecithin concentrations and with the oleic and palmitic acid content of aortic esterified cholesterol *(55)*.

Baboons (Papio ursinus)

Whereas extensive studies have examined baboons, cholesterol, lipoprotein metabolism, and the factors affecting them, relatively few studies have addressed atherosclerosis in baboons. Gillman and Gilbert *(56)* published a study of 59 female and 26 male baboons (*Papio ursinus*) between three and fifteen yr,

Table 3
Serum Lipids and Aortic Sudanophilia in Baboons Fed Semipurified
Diets for 12 mo: Effect of Carbohydrates[a]

Carbohydrate source	Serum cholesterol (mg/dL)	Sudanophilia (%)
Fructose	162 ± 10	11.2 ± 5/7
Sucrose	152 ± 9	6.7 ± 4.7
Starch	156 ± 8	9.3 ± 4.3
Glucose	151 ± 11	6.2 ± 4.8
Control	113 ± 11	0.02 ± 0.02

[a] Adapted from ref. 65. Diets contain 40% carbohydrate, 25% casein, 14% coconut oil, 15% cellulose.

subsisting on a diet low in cholesterol. From their study they concluded: (1) a one-to-one relationship does not exist between level of dietary fat and serum lipids or between serum lipids and atherosclerosis; (2) accumulation of aortic fat is not necessarily dependent on blood lipids, but appears to be secondary to alterations in the aortic tissue which favor binding fat and calcium; and (3) the functional and structural integrity of the intima and media are determined not only by their intrinsic properties but also by factors arising beyond the vascular tree.

McGill et al. (57) examined the arteries of 163 free-ranging Kenya baboons and found that about 75% of the adults exhibited some degree of fatty streaking in the aorta. The amount of streaking increased with age. Strong and McGill (58) fed baboons high-cholesterol diets for 2 yr. Serum cholesterol increased moderately, and some fatty streaks were observed, but no advanced lesions. A 4-yr experiment involving a diet high in fat and cholesterol (59) led to moderate cholesterolemia, but on necropsy, the principal lesion was still only a fatty streak. Cholesterol-fed baboons exhibited a positive relationship between aortic fatty streaks and elevated serum levels of LDL and VLDL-cholesterol. There was also a negative relationship between HDL-cholesterol levels and aortic fatty streaks (60).

In another study, baboons were fed a semipurified diet containing 40% carbohydrate from different sources, 25% casein, 14% coconut oil, and 15% cellulose (61). The baboons were fed diets in which the carbohydrate was fructose, sucrose, starch, or glucose for 12 mo. A control group was fed the usual baboon regimen of commercial ration augmented with fruit, vegetables, and bread. There were 3 male and 3 female baboons in each group. There were no differences among the average serum cholesterol levels of the test groups. Aortic sudanophilia was most severe in the baboons fed fructose, and the least severe in those fed glucose (61) (Table 3). This type of diet is atherogenic for rabbits,

Table 4
Serum Lipids and Aortic Sudanophilia in Baboons Fed Semipurified Diets
for 17 Mo: Effects of Carbohydrates and 0.1% Cholesterol[a]

Carbohydrate	Serum cholesterol (mg/dL)	Sudanophilia (%)
Fructose	144 ± 5	11.3 ± 4.2
Sucrose	143 ± 3	10.4 ± 5.4
Starch	155 ± 5	21.3 ± 8.9
Glucose	155 ± 6	17.2 ± 10.3
Lactose	170 ± 5	65.8 ± 13.6
Control	117 ± 3	1.4 ± 0.4

[a] Adapted from ref. 61. Diets contain 40% carbohydrate, 25% casein, 14% coconut oil, 15% cellulose.

Table 5
Effect of Feeding a Semipurified Diet Containing 40% Lactose ± 0.1%
Cholesterol for 8.5 Mo: on Serum Lipids and Aortic Sudanophilia in Baboons[a]

	Group		
	Lactose	Lactose plus cholesterol	Control
Serum lipids (mg/dL)			
Cholesterol	149 ± 4[a]	171 ± 9[b]	98 ± 2[ab]
Triglycerides	144 ± 13[c]	130 ± 8[d]	68 ± 7[cd]
Aortas			
% Sudanophilia	2.2 ± 0.7[ef]	20.8 ± 7.4[eg]	0.3 ± 0.2[fg]
Plaques	0/6	1/6	0/6

[a] Adapted from ref. 65. Diets contain 40% carbohydrate, 25% casein, 14% coconut oil, 15% cellulose. Values in horizontal row bearing same letter are significantly different ($p<0.05$).

(62) and the severity of atherosclerosis is a function of the carbohydrate (63,64). In a second study in baboons, (65) a similar study was carried out, but another carbohydrate group (lactose) was added, the diets contained 0.1% cholesterol, and the feeding period was 17 mo. The group fed lactose and 0.1% cholesterol exhibited severe sudanophilia, and a few atherosclerotic lesions were observed (Table 4). When lactose was fed without added cholesterol, aortic sudanophilia was mild and in the same range of severity as that observed in the first study (65) (Table 5). A comparison of the lactose ± 0.1% cholesterol diets is shown in Table 5. This model for atherogenesis would appear to be a useful one, but it has not been reported.

These results suggest that primate models of atherosclerosis are variable and can be influenced by diet and stress. A major goal of human studies is to effect regression of preestablished lesions. Regression of atherosclerosis in primates has been reviewed by Stary *(66)* and Malinow *(67).* Reversion of primates from an atherogenic diet to one low in fat and cholesterol will lead to diminution of lesion severity in rhesus and cynomolgus monkeys. Wagner et al. *(68)* fed rhesus monkeys an atherogenic diet for 19 mo. Twelve animals were necropsied at 19 mo to provide baseline data. The remaining 36 monkeys were fed diets designed to maintain their plasma cholesterol levels at about 200 or 300 mg/dL for an additional 48 mo. More cholesterol was lost from arteries of monkeys maintained at 200 mg/dL than those kept at 300 mg/dL. Eggen et al. *(69)* have shown that preestablished lesions in rhesus monkeys can regress even when fed a diet free of cholesterol but high in saturated fat for 30 or 52 wk. Vesselinovitch et al. *(70)* have demonstrated that rhesus monkeys fed a *PD* exhibit about 70% fewer aortic lesions than those fed an atherogenic diet for 14 mo, and 77% fewer lesions than monkeys fed the same diet for 48 mo. Addition of a hypocholesterolemic drug (cholestyramine) to the *PD* results in 65% fewer lesions than *PD* alone. The primate model is useful for the study of both progression and regression of atherosclerosis, and is closer to man than the other available models.

ACKNOWLEDGMENT

The authors wish to thank Susan Ralls for manuscript preparation and the support of Dr. Kritchevsky's NIH Research Career Award HL-00734.

REFERENCES

1. Middleton CC, Clarkson TB, Lofland HB, et al. Atherosclerosis in the squirrel monkey. Naturally occurring lesions of the aorta and coronary arteries. Arch Path 1964; 78:16–23.
2. Stills HF, Bullock BC. Renal disease in squirrel monkeys (Saimiri sciureus). Vet Pathol 1981; 18(Suppl):38–44.
3. Clarkson TB, Lehner MD, Bullock BC, et al. Atherosclerosis in new world monkeys. Primates Med 1976; 9:90–144.
4. Lofland HB, St. Clair RW, Macnintch JE, et al. Atherosclerosis in new world primates. Biochemical Studies. Arch Path 1967; 83:211–214.
5. Mann GV, Andrus SB, McNally A, et al. Experimental atherosclerosis in cebus monkeys. J Exp Med 1953; 98:195–218.
6. Wissler RW, Frazier LE, Hughes RH, et al. Atherogenesis in the cebus monkey I. A comparison of three food fats under controlled dietary conditions. Arch Path 1962; 74:312–322.
7. Mann GV, Andrus SB. Xanthomatosis and atherosclerosis produced by diet in an adult rhesus monkey. J Lab Clin Med 1956; 48:533–550.
8. Cox GE, Taylor CB, Cox LG, et al. Atherosclerosis in rhesus monkeys I. Hypercholesterolemia induced by dietary fat and cholesterol. Arch Path 1958; 66:32–52.

9. Taylor CB, Cox GE, Manalo-Estrella P, et al. Atherosclerosis in rhesus monkeys II. Arterial lesions associated with hypercholesterolemia induced by dietary fat and cholesterol. Arch Path 1962; 74:16–34.

10. Taylor CB, Trueheart RE, Cox GE. Atherosclerosis in rhesus monkeys III. The role of increased thickness of arterial walls in atherogenesis. Arch Path 1963; 76:14–28.

11. Cox GE, Trueheart RE, Kaplan J, et al. Atherosclerosis in rhesus monkeys IV. Repair of arterial injury—An important secondary atherogenic factor. Arch Path 1963; 76:166–176.

12. Taylor CB, Manalo-Estella P, Cox GE. Atherosclerosis in rhesus monkeys V. Marked diet-induced hypercholesterolemia with xanthomatosis and severe atherosclerosis. Arch Path 1963; 76:239–249.

13. Taylor CB, Patton DE, Cox GE. Atherosclerosis in rhesus monkeys VI. Fatal myocardial infarction in a monkey fed fat and cholesterol. Arch Path 1963; 76:404–412.

14. Manalo-Estella P, Cox GE, Taylor CB. Atherosclerosis in rhesus monkeys VII. Mechanism of hypercholesterolemia: hepatic cholesterolgenesis and the hypercholesterolemic threshold of dietary cholesterol. Arch Path 1963; 76:413–423.

15. Myers LH, Bhattacharyya AK, Eggen DA, et al. Changes in plasma lipoprotein concentrations and compositions upon feeding cholesterol in high- and low-responding monkeys. Ann Nutr Metab 1990; 34:317–326.

16. Kritchevsky D, McCandless RFJ. Weekly variations in serum cholesterol levels of monkeys. Proc Soc Exp Biol Med 1957; 95:152–154.

17. Kritchevsky D, Davidson LM, Goodman GT. Seasonal variation in serum lipids in the vervet monkey. Atherosclerosis 1987; 68:151–157.

18. Liu LB, Taylor CB, Peng SK, et al. Experimental arteriosclerosis in rhesus monkeys induced by multiple risk factors: cholesterol, vitamin D and nicotine. Paroi Arterielle/Arterial Wall 1979; 5:25–38.

19. Wissler RW, Vesselinovitch D, Hughes R, et al. Arterial lesions and blood lipids in rhesus monkeys fed human diets. Exp Molec Path 1983; 38:117–136.

20. Masuda J, Ross, R. Atherogenesis during low level hypercholesterolemia in the nonhuman primate I. Fatty streak formation. Arteriosclerosis 1990; 10:164–177.

21. Masuda J, Ross, R. Atherogenesis during low level hypercholesterolemia in the nonhuman primate II. Fatty streak conversion to fibrous plaque. Arteriosclerosis 1990; 10:178–187.

22. Faggioto A, Ross R, Harker, L. Studies of hypercholesterolemia in the nonhuman primate I. Changes that lead to fatty streak formation. Arteriosclerosis 1984; 4:323–340.

23. Faggiotto A, Ross R. Studies of hypercholesterolemia in the nonhuman primate II. Fatty streak conversion to fibrous plaque. Arteriosclerosis 1984; 4:341–356.

24. Pathap K. Spontaneous aortic lesions in wild adult Malaysian long-tailed monkeys (*Macaca irus*) J Path 1973; 110:135–143.

25. Armstrong ML. Atherosclerosis in rhesus and cynomolgus monkeys. Primates Med 1976; 9:16–40.

26. Kramsch D, Hollander W. Occlusive atherosclerotic disease of the coronary arteries in monkeys (Macaca irus) induced by diet. Exp Molec Path 1968; 9:1–22.

27. Malinow MR, McLaughlin P, Papworth L, et al. A model for therapeutic interventions on established coronary atherosclerosis in a nonhuman primate. Adv Exp Med Biol 1976; 67:3–31.

28. Wagner WD, St. Clair RW, Clarkson TB. Angiochemical and tissue cholesterol changes in *Macaca fascicularis* fed an atherogenic diet for three years. Exp Mol Path 1978; 28:140–153.

29. Bond MG, Bullock BC, Bellinger DA, et al. Myocardial infarction in a large colony of nonhuman primates with coronary artery atherosclerosis. Am J Path 1980;101:675–692.

30. Alderson LM, Hayes KC, Nicolosi RJ. Peanut oil reduces diet-induced atherosclerosis in cynomolgus monkeys. Arteriosclerosis 1986; 6:465–474.

31. Anthony MS, Clarkson TB, Bullock BC, et al. Soy protein versus soy phytoestrogens in the prevention of diet-induced coronary artery atherosclerosis in male cynomolgus monkeys. Arterioscler Thromb Vasc Biol 1997; 17:2524–2531.

32. Kaplan JR, Manuck SB Clarkson TB, et al. Social stress and atherosclerosis in normo-cholesterolemic monkeys. Science 1983; 220:733–735.

33. Manuck SB, Kaplan JR, Adams MR, et al. Behaviorally elicited heart rate reactivity and atherosclerosis in female cynomolgus monkeys (*Macaca fascicularis*) Psychosom Med 1989; 51:306–318.

34. Kaplan JR, Manuck SB, Gatsonis C. Heart rate and social status among male cynomolgus monkeys (*Macaca fascicularis*) housed in disrupted social groups. Am J Primatol 1990; 21:175–187.

35. Kaplan JR, Manuck SB, Clarkson TB. The influence of heart rate on coronary artery athero-sclerosis, J Cardiovasc Pharmacol 1987; 10 (Suppl):s100–s102.

36. Kaplan JR, Manuck SB. Monkeys, aggression and the pathobiology of atherosclerosis. Aggress Behav 1998; 24:323–334.

37. Clarkson TB. Arteriosclerosis of African green and stump-tailed macaque monkeys. Schettler G, Weizel A, eds. J Atheroscler III: 1974; 291–294.

38. Bullock BC, Lehner NDM, Clarkson TB, et al. Comparative primate atherosclerosis I. Tissue cholesterol concentrations and pathologic anatomy. Exp Molec Path 1975; 22:151–175.

39. Wagner WD, Clarkson TB. Comparative primate atherosclerosis II. A biochemical study of lipids, calcium and collagen in atherosclerotic arteries. Exp Molec Path 1975; 23:96–121.

40. Rudel LL, Haines JL, Sawyer JK. Effects on plasma lipoproteins of monounsaturated, satu-rated, and polyunsaturated fatty acids in the diet of African green monkeys. J Lipid Res 1990; 31:1873–1882.

41. Parker JS, Kaduck-Sawyer J, Bullock BC, et al. Effects of dietary fish oil on coronary artery and aortic atherosclerosis in African green monkeys. Arteriosclerosis 1990;10:1102–1112.

42. Wolfe MS, Parks JS, Morgan TM, et al. Childhood consumption of dietary polyunsaturated fat lowers risk for coronary artery atherosclerosis in African green monkeys. Arterioscler Thromb 1993; 13:863–875.

43. Rudel LL, Parks JS, Sawyer, JK. Compared with dietary monounsaturated and saturated fat, polyunsaturated fat protects African green monkeys from coronary artery atherosclerosis. Arteroscler Thromb Vasc Biol 1995; 15:2101–2110.

44. Weigensberg BI, McMillan GC, Ritchie AC. Elaidic acid-effect on experimental atheroscle-rosis. Arch Path 1961; 72:358–366.

45. McMillan GC, Silver MD, Weigensberg BI. Elaidinized olive oil and cholesterol atheroscle-rosis. Arch Path 1963; 76:105–112.

46. Weigensberg BI, McMillan GC. Lipids in rabbits fed elaidinized olive oil. Exp Molec Path 1964; 3:210–214.

47. Ruttenberg H, Davidson LM, Little NA, et al. Influence of trans unsaturated fats on experi-mental atherosclerosis in the rabbit. J Nutr 1983; 113:835–844.

48. Kritchevsky D, Davidson LM, Weight M, et al. Effect of trans unsaturated fats on experimen-tal atherosclerosis in vervet monkeys. Atherosclerosis 1984; 51:123–133.

49. Kritchevsky D, Davidson LM, Krendel DA, et al. Influence of dietary fiber on aortic sudano-philia in vervet monkeys. Ann Nutr Metab 1981; 25:125–136.

50. Kritchevsky D, Davidson LM, Scott DA, et al. Effects of dietary fiber in vervet monkeys fed "western" diets. Lipids 1988; 23:164–168.

51. Fincham JE, Faber M, Weight MJ, et al. Diets realistic for westernized people significantly effect lipoproteins, calcium, zinc, vitamins C, E, B_6 and hematology in vervet monkeys. Atherosclerosis 1987; 66:191–203.

52. Fincham JE, Woodroof CW, vanWyk MJ, et al. Promotion and regression of atherosclerosis in vervet monkeys by diets realistic for westernized people. Atherosclerosis 1987; 66:205–213.

53. Benadé AJS, Fincham JE, Smuts CM, et al. Plasma low density lipoprotein composition in relation to atherosclerosis in nutritionally defined vervet monkeys. Atherosclerosis 1988; 74:157–168.

54. Weight MJ, Benadé AJS, Lombard CJ, et al. Low density lipoprotein kinetics in African green monkeys showing variable cholesterolemic responses to diets realistic for westernized people. Atherosclerosis 1988; 73:1–11.

55. Fincham JE, Benadé AJS, Kruger M, et al. Atherosclerosis: aortic lipid changes induced by diets suggest diffuse disease with focal severity in primates that model human atheromas. Nutr 1998; 14:17–22.

56. Gillman J, Gilbert C. Atherosis in the baboon (Papio ursinus). Its pathogenesis and etiology. Exp Med Surg 1957; 15:181–221.

57. McGill HC, Jr., Strong JP, Holman RL, et al. Arterial lesions in the Kenya baboon. Circ Res 1960; 8:670–679.

58. Strong JP, McGill HC, Jr. Diet and experimental atherosclerosis in baboons. Am J Path 1967; 50:669–690.

59. Strong JP, Eggen DA, Jirge SK. Atherosclerotic lesions produced in baboons by feeding an atherogenic diet for four years. Exp. Molec Path 1976; 24:320–332.

60. McGill HC, Jr, McMahan CA, Kruski AW, et al. Relationship of lipoprotein cholesterol concentrations to experimental atherosclerosis in baboons. Arteriosclerosis 1981; 1:3–12.

61. Kritchevsky D, Davidson LM, Kim HK, et al. Influence of type of carbohydrate on atherosclerosis in baboons fed semipurified diets plus 0.1% cholesterol. Am J Clin Nutr 1980; 33:1869–1887.

62. Kritchevsky D, Tepper SA. Factors affecting atherosclerosis in rabbits fed cholesterol-free diets. Life Sci 1965; 4:1467–1471.

63. Kritchevsky D, Sallata P, Tepper SA. Experimental atherosclerosis in rabbits fed cholesterol-free diets. Influence of various carbohydrates. J Atheroscler Res 1968; 8:697–703.

64. Kritchevsky D, Tepper SA, Kitagawa M. Experimental atherosclerosis in rabbits fed cholesterol-free diets. Comparison of fructose and lactose with other carbohydrates. Nutr Rep Int 1973; 7:193–202.

65. Kritchevsky D, Davidson LM, Shapiro IL, et al. Lipid metabolism and experimental atherosclerosis in baboons: influence of cholesterol-free, semi synthetic diets. Am J Clin Nutr 1974; 27:29–50.

66. Stary HC. Regression of atherosclerosis in primates. Virchows Arch A Path Anat Histol 1979; 383:117–134.

67. Malinow MR. Atherosclerosis. Regression in nonhuman primates. Circ Res 1980; 46:311–320.

68. Wagner WD, St. Clair RW, Clarkson TB, et al. A study of atherosclerosis regression in Macaca mulatta. Am J Path 1980; 100:633–650.

69. Eggen DA, Strong JP, Newman WP, et al. Regression of experimental atherosclerotic lesions in rhesus monkeys consuming a high saturated fat diet. Arteriosclerosis 1987; 7:125–134.

70. Vesselinovitch D, Wissler RW, Schaffner TJ. Quantitation of lesions during progression and regression of atherosclerosis in rhesus monkeys. In: Naito HK, ed. Nutrition and heart disease SP Medical and Scientific Books, New York, 1982, pp. 121–149.

IV Vascular Disease in Transplanted Vessels

15 Murine Carotid Loop Model of Transplant Vascular Disease

Victor Chengwei Shi, MD and Jennifer L. Hoover, BA

INTRODUCTION

Although immunosuppression largely prevents acute rejection of transplanted organs, transplant-associated arteriosclerosis—defined by a diffuse neointimal formation in vessels of transplanted organs—remains a major obstacle to long-term graft survival (1–3). This disease does not respond to current immunosuppressive therapy and its underlying pathogenesis is not fully understood. Indeed, animal models represent an invaluable determinant in biological and pathologic studies which correlate to clinical observations. In particular, the mouse provides an excellent model system for defining the role of genetic variables in transplant-associated arteriosclerosis by use of murine transgenic and gene manipulation technologies. As described here, the role of genes or molecules thought to be involved in transplant arteriosclerosis can be directly examined in mutant mice. As such, a mouse model of transplant-asso-

From: Contemporary Cardiology: Vascular Disease and Injury: Preclinical Research
Edited by: D. I. Simon and C. Rogers © Humana Press Inc., Totowa, NJ

ciated arteriosclerosis was developed based on the transplantation of a carotid-artery loop between pairs of mice crossing histocompatibility barriers *(4)*. This model offers the following advantages:

(1) An operative mortality rate of less than 5% because the thorax or peritoneum are not entered.
(2) An overall initial patency rate of more than 95%.
(3) The investigator can perform up to six transplants during each working day.
(4) Syngeneic grafts show almost no neointimal formation and resemble normal arteries at d 30 after transplantation.
(5) In allografts, a nearly occlusive neointima developed in a highly reproducible manner by d 30 after transplantation.
(6) Histomorphological studies can focus on a particular segment of the transplanted loop—such as the region of the anastomosis, which is characterized by turbulent blood flow—or the center loop, a site of less turbulent blood flow.
(7) Each donor animal can contribute two genetically identical grafts.
(8) Finally, the development of transplant-associated arteriosclerosis can be evaluated within a single vessel in a highly reproducible and quantitative manner. However, the nature of the surgery is technically demanding, and is thus a limitation to the model.

SURGERY (TRANSPLANTATION)

The operation was performed on anesthetized (ketamine and zylaxine cocktail) mice under a surgical or dissecting microscope. The donor/recipient was fixed in a supine position with its neck extended. A midline incision was made on the ventral side of the neck from the suprasternal notch to the chin. In preparation of the donor graft, the left and right carotid arteries were gently dissected from the aortic arch to the internal/external bifurcation. Arterial segments were perfused with normal saline to remove all residual blood components. Both ends of the graft were trimmed to achieve a 50–60 degree angle when connected to the recipient carotid artery. Harvested arteries were preserved in 4°C isotonic saline solution prior to transplantation. In preparation of the recipient, the left (or right) carotid artery was dissected from the bifurcation in the distal end toward the proximal end, as far as technically possible. The artery was then occluded with two microvascular clamps, one at each end, and two longitudinal arteriotomies (0.5 mm–0.6 mm) were performed with a fine needle (30-gauge) and scissors. The carotid artery graft is paratopically sutured into the recipient carotid artery in an end-to-side anastomosis as a loop (Fig. 1) with an 11/0 continuous nylon suture under 16× or 25× magnification. Prior to the second (distal) anastomosis, the microvascular clamp at the proximal end was released temporarily (1–2 s) to flush away any residual blood inside the graft lumen and to assess the patency of the proximal anastamosis. At this time, the distal anas-

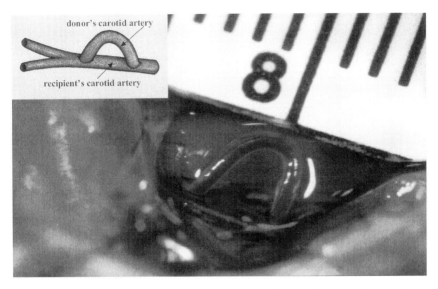

Fig. 1. Photograph of the surgical field showing the left carotid artery of the recipient to which the donor artery loop has been sutured via end-to-side anastomosis. Inset: A schematic drawing of the murine carotid loop model as described in the surgery section. Briefly, a donor carotid artery loop is grafted into the recipient carotid artery as illustrated; blood flow is directed mainly through the donor artery.

tomosis was performed (as described above) to complete the graft procedure. Both clamps were released to evaluate vessel patency. During such a procedure, prominent pulsation should be visible in both the transplanted loop and the native vessel. If there was no pulsation or if it was diminished within a few minutes of restoration of blood flow, clot formation at the anastomosis was assumed, and the procedure was terminated and considered a surgical failure. If successful, the skin incision was closed with a 5/0 or 6/0 interrupted suture. The transplanted carotid artery can be harvested at different time points (day 3, 7, 15, 30, and 45, up to 90 days) after surgery based on the purpose of each experiment.

TECHNICAL CONSIDERATIONS

Surgically, this model can be constructed from the following two alternative methods:

Donor Carotid Artery Grafting as a Loop with Native Carotid Artery Ligation (Fig. 2)

In order to increase the blood flow through the transplanted donor carotid artery, which may influence the process of lesion development, the recipient carotid artery can be ligated permanently between the two anastomoses after

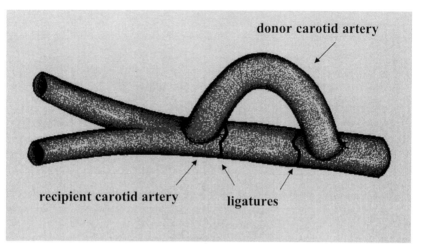

Fig. 2. A representative drawing of the donor carotid artery graft as a loop with native carotid artery ligation as indicated in the technical considerations section. Herein, the recipient carotid artery is permanently ligated at the anastomoses (ligatures) of the donor graft such that blood flow is directed through the grafted loop (donor artery) only.

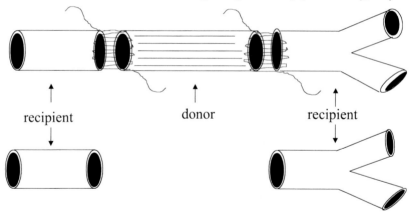

Fig. 3. A schematic drawing depicting the interposition graft described in the technical considerations section. This particular graft procedure incorporates a small portion of the donor carotid artery into a portion of the recipient carotid artery to form an interposition graft.

the donor carotid artery has been sutured into the recipient carotid artery in a loop formation as described in the above section. The recipient artery is ligated with two nylon ligatures (8/0 or 9/0) placed close to the anastomosis to direct blood flow exclusively through the grafted loop. Although practical, this alternative may increase the risk of focal thrombosis around the ligatures, which may complicate neointimal formation.

Interposition Graft (Fig. 3)

In order to minimize turbulence and shear stress within the carotid artery graft, the donor carotid artery can be sutured into the native carotid artery as an interposition graft by an interrupted or continuous suture. Briefly, a small portion (2–3 mm) of the native vessel is removed and replaced with a segment of the donor carotid artery, as depicted in Fig. 3, to form an interposition graft. Although similar to the carotid-loop model, this procedure is more technically demanding, and the amount of tissue available for histopathological analysis is limited.

HISTOLOGY

Morphologically, the neointima formed in this model is characterized by 2–4 accumulated cell layers in the lumen of the donor vessel by d 7 after transplantation. At this time CD45 positive leukocytes predominant within the developing neointima. Immunohistochemical localization confirmed the presence of CD4+, CD8+ T cells and F4/80+ monocyte/macrophages. Alpha-actin positive smooth muscle cells (SMCs) begin to migrate into the lumen by d 15 after transplantation, although a number of inflammatory cells still persist in the developing neointima. By d 30, a florid, nearly occlusive lesion—comprised predominantly of SMCs and extracellular matrix—is formed (Fig. 4).

RELEVANCE TO CLINICAL INVESTIGATION

Immunologic components in recipient mice needed for the development of transplant arteriosclerosis have been identified by applying this model to several mutant mouse strains with immunologic defects (5). The significance of donor major histocompatibility complex (MHC) and adhesion molecules have also been evaluated in this model (6). Several risk factors which may contribute to the disease have been determined (7, 8). Many features of human disease are well mimicked, so that this model not only provides a valuable tool to investigate molecular mechanisms of transplant-associated arteriosclerosis, but also has potential application in the development of novel immunosuppressive agents.

MATERIALS

Animals

The following combinations have been tested; selection of different strain combinations should be based on the goals of study:

1. B10.A(2R)>>>C57BL/6;
2. B10.A(2R)>>>B10.BR;

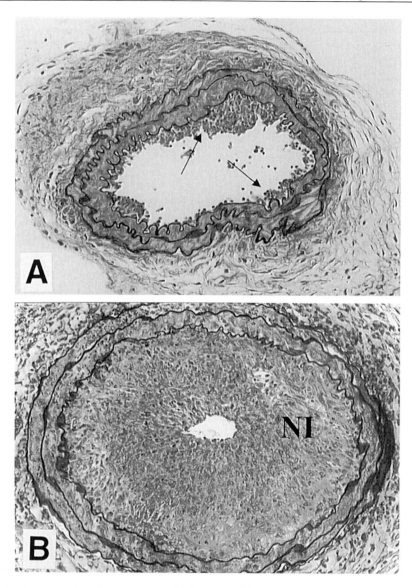

Fig. 4. Representative photomicrographs from carotid-artery loop allografts at d 7 **(A)** and day 30 **(B)** following transplantation. Note formation of an early neointima (2–4 cellular layers) along the lm of the donor vessel (arrows) at day 7. By d 30, a florid, nearly occlusive neointima has formed (NI), comprised predominantly of vascular SMCs and extracellular matrix as indicated by immunohistochemistry. Elastic lamina is stained in black (paraffin embedded, 50×).

3. B10.A(2R)>>>B6/129;
4. C57BL/6>>>> CBA/ca;
5. B6/129>>>>>>CBA/ca; and
6. 129SV>>>>>>CBA/ca.

All mice listed above should be available through Jackson Laboratory. An age range from 8–12 wk is preferred.

MICROSCOPE

Surgical microscopes (Carl Zeiss or Leica) are highly recommended. Dissecting microscope is optional. Light source: cold light source.

MICROSURGICAL INSTRUMENTS

Surgical instruments were purchased from Roboz Surgical Instrument Company Inc., Rockville, MD, as described here:

1. One pair #5 Dumont Tweezers (Roboz-RS-5065);
2. One pair #7 Dunont tweezers (Roboz-RS-4982);
3. One microdissecting spring scissors (Roboz-RS-5618);
4. One microdissecting spring scissors (Roboz-RS-5658);
5. One microdissecting scissors (Roboz-RS-5882);
6. One microsuturing needle holder (Roboz-RS-6416;
7. One needle holder (Roboz-RS-7800);
8. One microdissecting forceps (Roboz-RS-5236);
9. One microclip setting forceps (Roboz-RS-6496); and
10. Two microvascular clips (Roboz-RS-6470).

SURGICAL SUPPLIES

1. B-D 30 G1/2 needle for arteriotomy (Becton Dickson and Company, Franklin Lakes, NJ);
2. B-D 26G1/2 syringe (Becton Dickson and Company, Franklin Lakes, NJ) 11/0 Dermalon on a TE 50 (Davis & Geck, Division of AMERICAN CYANAMID, Wayne, NJ);
3. 6/0 or 5/0 Dermalon (Davis & Geck, Division of AMERICAN CYANAMID, Wayne, NJ);
4. 2 × 2–4ply Nu Gauze (Baxter Healthcare Corporation, Deerfield, IL).
5. High-temperature surgical cautery; fine tip (General Medical Corporation, Tewsbury, MA);
6. Oster Professional cord/cordless trimmer; and
7. Two dissecting boards.

ANESTHETICS AND OTHER REAGENTS

1. Ketamine and zylaxine cocktail;
2. 100 U/mL (of saline) heparin sulfate solution for in vivo treatment, organ perfusion and storage;
3. Sodium chloride irrigation, USP;
4. Alcohol for skin preparation; and
5. Betadine for skin preparation.

REFERENCES

1. Sharples LD, Caine N, Mullins JP Scott, et al. Risk factor analysis for the major hazards following heart transplantation-rejection, infection and coronary occlusive disease. Transplantation 1991; 52:244–252.
2. Billingham ME. Graft coronary disease: the lesions and the patients. Transplant Proc 1989; 21:3665–3666.
3. Sarris GE, Moore KA, Schroeder JS et al. Cardiac transplantation: the Stanford experience in the cyclosporine era. J Thorac Cardiovasc Surg 1994; 108:240–252.
4. Shi C, Russell ME, Bianchi C, Newell JB, et al. Murine model of accelerated transplant arteriosclerosis. Circ Res 1994; 75:199–207.
5. Shi C, Lee WS, He Q, et al. Immunologic basis of transplant-associated arteriosclerosis. Proc Natl Acad Sci USA 1996; 93:4051–4056.
6. Shi C, Feinberg MW, Zhang D, et al. Donor MHC and adhesion molecules in transplant aterosclerosis. J Clin Invest 1998; 103:469–474.
7. Shi C, Lee WS, Russell ME, et al. Hypercholesterolemia exacerbates transplant arteriosclerosis via increased neointimal smooth muscle cell accumulation: studies in apolipoprotein E knockout mice. Circulation 1997; 96:2722–2728.
8. Moons L, Shi C, Ploplis V, Plow E, Haber E, Colleen D, Carmeliek P. Reduced transplant arteriosclerosis in plasminogen-deficient mice. J Clin Invest 1998; 102:1788–1797.

16 Murine Heterotopic Model of Transplant Arteriopathy

Richard N. Mitchell, MD, PhD

CONTENTS

INTRODUCTION

In human heart transplantation, graft arteriosclerosis (GA, also called transplant-associated arteriopathy and transplant vascular sclerosis) is the single most important long-term limitation to graft and patient survival *(1)*. Angiography results indicate that GA is present in 14% of patients by 1 yr posttransplant a percentage that rises to 40% by 5 yr. *(2)*. Using more sensitive intravascular ultrasound (IVUS) imaging modalities, significant disease in large epicardial arteries can be detected as early as 4 wk. IVUS has detected GA in up to 60–70% of patients by 1 yr posttransplant, and this condition is significant in 25% of them *(3)*. Patients with GA typically present with congestive failure caused by silent ischemic injury, and/or sudden cardiac death *(4)*. Because of the diffuse nature of the disease, allograft recipients are not usually amenable to surgical coronary bypass intervention, and retransplant remains the only viable treatment option.

From: *Contemporary Cardiology: Vascular Disease and Injury: Preclinical Research*
Edited by: D. I. Simon and C. Rogers © Humana Press Inc., Totowa, NJ

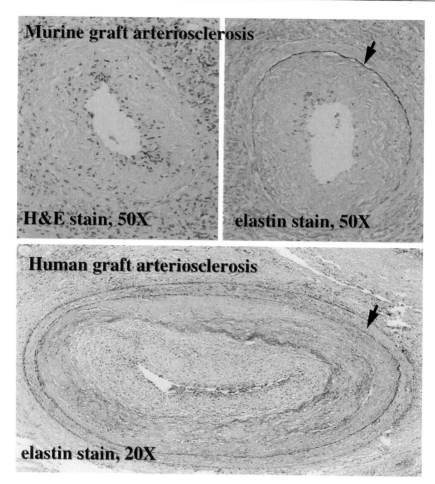

Fig. 1. Histologic appearance of graft arteriosclerosis (GA) in humans and mice. Shown are hematoxylin and eosin (H & E) or elastin-stained sections of GA lesions from an ortho-topic human heart allograft 3.5 yr posttransplantation (20× magnification), or a heterotopic mouse-heart allograft 12 wk posttransplantation (50× magnification). The arrows on the elastin-stained section indicate the internal elastic lamina (IEL) on these arteries. In nor-mal arteries, the intima (between the IEL and the vessel lumen) is only 1–2 cell layers thick. In these arteries, the intimal hyperplasia has encroached on the vessel lumen and resulted in variable degrees of graft ischemia. GA lesions may have variable amounts of extracellular matrix and cells; the cellularity is composed of SMCs, fibroblasts, macroph-ages, and T-lymphocytes. (See color plate 6 appearing in the insert following p. 236).

Unfortunately, GA does not correlate with incidence or severity of acute parenchymal rejection, and clearly arises in the setting of immunosuppression adequate to prevent graft failure caused by acute parenchymal rejection (PR) *(5)*. Potential contributory (and confounding) factors in the evolution of GA include perioperative ischemic injury, infection, and host factors such as body-mass index or hypercholesterolemia *(6)*. Clear-cut parameters for risk assessment are unknown, and even diagnosing the extent of GA is problematic. Thus, current imaging modalities almost certainly underestimate the severity of GA. Since the majority of involved vasculature is intramyocardial, it is not amenable to IVUS analysis, and coronary angiography may miss diffuse, concentric narrowing of vessels *(3,7)*. Although dobutamine stress echocardiography has been suggested as a diagnostic tool, it has yet to be widely adopted *(8)*.

Although some progress has been made in the pharmacologic amelioration of GA using alternate immunosuppressive regimens *(9)* or HMG-CoA reductase inhibitors, *(10)* results are far from ideal. Clearly, a better understanding of the pathogenic mechanisms underlying the disease is necessary—including the role of antibodies vs cells in the etiopathogenesis, the contribution of alloantigen nonspecific mediators such as macrophages or cytokine networks, and the effects of ischemia and thrombosis.

MURINE HETEROTOPIC CARDIAC TRANSPLANTATION

Murine heterotopic cardiac transplantation is an excellent model to dissect the interconnected pathologic mechanisms underlying GA. Importantly, the histology and composition of the parenchymal rejection and GA lesions in mice accurately recapitulate those seen in humans (Fig. 1) *(11,12)*. Moreover, GA lesions evolve over 8–12 wk in the murine model (vs months to years in humans), making it practical and affordable to use in the laboratory setting. Among the other benefits of the model—relative to human studies—is the availability of a large number of inbred mouse strains with defined differences in major histocompatibility (MHC) and non-MHC molecules, including congenic lines with isoforms of surface molecules (e.g., Thy-1) that can be used to clearly identify selected cell populations. A wealth of well-characterized and commercially available murine reagents are available, including cytokines and monoclonal antibodies (mAbs) both for blocking experiments and analysis. Although pharmacologic agents may have different efficacy in mice vs humans the animal model nevertheless permits well-controlled comparative studies of the actions of selected agents. Finally, and perhaps most importantly, recent advances in molecular biology have permitted the generation of an impressive menagerie of congenitally-deficient ("knockout") or transgenic animals with altered repertoires of selected cytokines, chemokines, receptors, or entire cell populations. Thus, animals deficient in mature B cells (Ig-/-;) *(13)* or interferon-γ, *(12,14)*

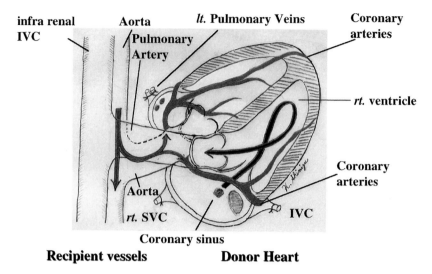

Fig. 2. Schematic of heterotopic grafts. Donor hearts are perfused with chilled, heparinized 0.9% saline, or heparinized Stanford solution via the inferior vena cava, and are harvested after ligation of the vena cavae and pulmonary veins. The aorta and pulmonary artery of the donor heart are anastomosed to the infrarenal abdominal aorta and the inferior vena cava of the recipient mouse, respectively using microsurgical technique. The aortic valve is initially competent following surgery; it therefore does not allow retrograde flow. The blood flows into the allograft at aortic pressures via the coronary arteries, perfusing the myocardium, and returning to the right atrium at the coronary sinus. With time, the aortic valve becomes regurgitant, allowing formation of a thrombus in the relatively static left ventricle lumen. Drawing courtesy of Koichi Shimizu, MD, Department of Cardiothoracic Surgery, Tokyo Medical and Dental University. (See color plate 7 appearing in the insert following p. 236).

for example, may be used to specifically assess the role of antibodies or the major cytokine driving macrophage activation. Allografts have also been successfully transplanted into immunodeficient recipients lacking all mature T and B lymphocytes (e.g., SCID or recombinase-deficient mice), thus permitting the adoptive transfer of defined antibody or cell preparations

TECHNICAL ASPECTS

The procedure was originally described by Corry, et al., *(15)* and is schematically drawn in Fig. 2. Donor and recipient mice are usually 8–12-wk-old male mice (25–30 g); younger mice are too small for surgery; older animals tend to accrue too much adipose tissue, making dissection difficult. Male mice are routinely used as both recipients and donors to avoid potential confounding H–Y antigen mismatches, and because the uterus and ovarian vessels in female recipients tend to limit the surgical field. We find that certain mouse strains (e.g., C57BL/6) tolerate the procedure extremely well, while others (e.g., BALB/c) are much less hearty as graft recipients. Yet with practice, we have been able to use a wide variety of strains. We have focused on a rather restricted number of mouse strains (Table 1), in part due to the well-defined MHC I, MHC II, total MHC, and non-MHC mismatches in this collection of animals. In addition, the majority of knockout and transgenic mice are initially derived in the 129/J strain, with subsequent back-breeding onto the C57BL/6 background; our extensive experience with 129/J and C57BL/6 donors and recipients, enables us to take immediate advantage of newly generated mouse knockouts.

Mice may be anesthetized by methoxyfluorane, or isofluorane inhalation. Methoxyfluorane (Metofan; Pittman-Moore, Mundelein, IL) is preferable because of its slower and more easily regulated anesthesia; we have also found lesser strain variation in dosing. Donor hearts are perfused with chilled, heparinized 0.9% saline or heparinized Stanford solution (16) via the inferior vena cava, and are harvested after ligation of the vena cavae and pulmonary veins. The aorta and pulmonary artery of the donor heart are anastomosed to the infrarenal abdominal aorta and the inferior vena cava of the recipient mouse, respectively, using microsurgical technique and 10–0 Ethilon (Ethicon, Somerville, NJ). Typically, the aortic anastomosis is performed first using two separate running sutures, each of 6–7 throws. The pulmonic anastomosis is performed next with one continuous suture and 10–12 throws. Surgical loops do not provide adequate magnification, and we find that a dissecting microscope with 2.5–4x magnification is required.

Ischemic time during the procedure is routinely 30 min, with greater than 90% initial graft and recipient survival; grafts resume spontaneous beating prior to closure. Fig. 3 shows the gross appearance of the heterotopic transplant in the abdomen at the time of closure. Grafts that do not resume spontaneous beating are considered to be surgical failures, and are not used in any analyses. While the procedure *is* technically difficult, we have found that untrained but motivated personnel can typically achieve viable grafts by the 5th–10th animal, and develop routine success by the 25th–30th transplant. Surgically adept individuals can master the technique much sooner. We typically have new trainees practice with isografts in relatively robust outbred Swiss mice, and assess their expertise by histologic measurement of the extent of ischemic injury 1 wk posttransplant. When only mild ischemic injury (less than 10% surface area) is seen on routine transverse sections, the trainee may proceed to more challenging strains and allograft combinations.

As shown in Fig. 2, because the aortic valve is initially competent following surgery, it does not allow retrograde flow. The blood flows into the allograft at aortic pressures via the coronary arteries, perfusing the myocardium and returning to the right atrium at the coronary sinus. Flow patterns (if not volumes) are thus normal through the tricuspid and pulmonic valves, exiting into the in-

Table 1
Mouse Strain Combinations and Immunosuppression Regimens[a]

Mismatch	Graft survival without immunosuppression	Immunosuppression required for long-term graft survival
Isograft (no mismatch) e.g., C57BL/6 (H2^b) C57BL/6 (H2^b)	>12 wk	None
Non-MHC mismatch e.g., 129/J (H2^b) C57BL/6 (H2^b)	>12 wk	None
MHC I mismatch e.g., bm1 (H2^{bm1}) C57BL/6 (H2^b)	>12 wk	None
MHC II mismatch e.g., bm12 (H2^{bm12}) C57BL/6 (H2^b)	4–8 wk	Anti-CD4/anti-CD8 pretransplant, 15 mg/kg QD cyclosporine A, or 1 mg/kg QOD rapamycin
Total mismatch (non-MHC, MHC I, MHC II) e.g., BALB/c (H2^d) C57BL/6 (H2^b)	7–10 d	anti-CD4/anti-CD8 pre-and/or posttransplant, or 1 mg/kg QOD rapamycin

[a]Other strain combinations have been used, particularly across complete MHC mismatches or non-MHC mismatches (30,35,36). Long-term immunosuppression in total allo-mismatches is achieved by various regimens of CD4 and CD8 MAbs, antiadhesion molecule antibodies, or by anti-CD40 ligand antibodies (11,30,35). We have focused on the particular combinations outlined above in part because of the defined MHC I, MHC II, or non-MHC mismatches. In addition, the majority of knockout mice are initially generated in 129/J mice, with most being rapidly backbred onto the C57BL/6 MHC background. Thus, transplant combinations making use of C57BL/6 mice are most amenable to rapid translation into engineered strains.

ferior vena cava anastomosis. To date, no successful orthotopic (i.e., donor heart replacing the recipient heart) murine cardiac transplantation has been reported. The fact that the grafts in this model are heterotopic and are therefore not necessary for host survival also permits the development of severe graft rejection that could not be sustained if the recipient depended on graft function.

Allograft function is followed by routine daily palpation of the heterotopic graft; loss of beating activity is defined as the date of rejection. Typically, grafts beat less vigorously and at a slower rate as rejection proceeds, until all activity ceases. Assessment by this method also requires some practice, and the skill of the observer will influence whether weak heartbeats are appreciated. It is particularly difficult to distinguish heartbeats from respirations. Usually, transient

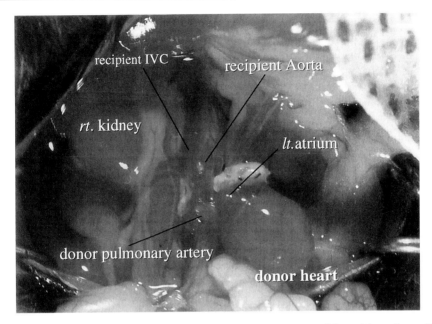

Fig. 3. Photograph of the heterotopic graft after surgery. Loops of bowel have been displaced for this photograph, but are returned before closure. The metallic retractors at the edge of the photograph are paper clips. Photograph courtesy of Koichi Shimizu, MD, Department of Cardiothoracic Surgery, Tokyo Medical and Dental University.

gentle squeezing of the animal will suppress breathing for the period of time necessary to palpate heartbeat. Although cardiac ultrasonography has been used as a diagnostic tool in a variety of mouse experimental models, animals must be anesthetized to obtain accurate readings, and the technique requires equipment not available to most laboratories. Since the results by echocardiography roughly correlate with the manual assessment technique (M. Russell, personal communication), we use palpable graft beat as our sole criteria for graft function. Nevertheless, it is extremely important to always corroborate the manual assessment with the histology of failed allografts. Survival data based exclusively on palpable beat is subject to observer variation, and is not by itself a reliable indicator of allograft injury. Moreover, the pathology of failed grafts may also provide insight into the mechanism of failure (e.g., predominantly parenchymal rejection and injury vs vasculitis with thrombosis and coagulation necrosis).

EVALUATION OF THE ALLOGRAFTS

Parenchymal rejection is apparent by 3–4 d posttransplant, while mature GA lesions only develop after 8–12 wk *(11,12)*. At earlier time points (e.g., 4 wk), vessels may show an intense perivascular and/or intralumenal collection of mononuclear inflammatory cells. However, these are not the characteristic intimal hyperplastic lesions of GA containing smooth-muscle-cells (SMCs) and increased extracellular matrix. Although these almost certainly represent precursor lesions to GA, they should not properly be identified as graft arteriosclerosis (12).

Grafts may be explanted at the time of beat cessation, or—to evaluate the pathology prior to end-stage failure—at any intermediate interval. However, it is important to note that even a single day's delay in removing failed nonbeating allografts will result in necrosis artifact that will render the specimen useless for analysis. We routinely evaluate grafts through a variety of modalities. Thus, freshly explanted allografts are sectioned transversely into thirds. The most **basal third**, with larger-diameter coronary vessels, is fixed in phosphate-buffered 10% formalin, and embedded in paraffin, and serial 5–6 μ sections are stained by routine histologic techniques. Hematoxylin and eosin are used for grading rejection, and Weigert's elastic fiber stain is used to identify the internal elastic lamina of arteries for assessing the extent of GA. Parenchymal rejection is graded using a scale modified from the International Society for Heart and Lung Transplantation: (0) no rejection; (1) focal mononuclear cell infiltrates without necrosis; (2) focal mononuclear cell infiltrates with necrosis; (3) multifocal infiltrates with necrosis; (4) widespread infiltrate with hemorrhage and/or vasculitis (12,17). The GA score is calculated from the number and severity of involved vessels: 0, vascular occlusion <10%; (1) 10–25% occlusion; (2) 25–50% occlusion; (3) 50–75% occlusion; (4) >75% occlusion. Typically, 10 or more vessels are scored for each heart, and the degree of vascular occlusion for each is averaged. Scores for each specimen uniformly fall within a range of one grade for 2–3 blinded observers, and are averaged (12). In long-term grafts, mesenteric adipose tissue, loops of bowel, and/or pancreas will frequently be attached to the epicardial surface by postsurgical adhesions; we have found no evidence that these influence parenchymal rejection or GA.

The **intermediate third** of each heart is frozen in OCT compound (Ames Co., Division of Miles Laboratories, Elkhart, IN) and stored at –80°C for immunohistochemistry. Staining can be performed for a variety of markers, including adhesion molecules (e.g., vascular cell-adhesion molecule-1, intercellular adhesion molecule-1), costimulatory molecules (e.g., CD40, B7), inflammatory cell subsets (e.g., CD4 or CD8 T cells, B cells, and macrophages), cytokines, and MHC molecules (11,12,18–20).

The most **apical third** is either collagenase digested to recover infiltrating inflammatory cells for flow cytometric analysis, (21,22) or solubilized in TRIzol (Gibco BRL/Life Technologies, Grand Island, NY), following the manufacturer's recommendations for extracting RNA for polymerase chain reaction or RNase protection assay analysis of cytokine message production (22).

IMMUNOSUPPRESSION

Without immunosuppression, total allogeneic mismatched grafts (e.g., BALB/c hearts into C57BL/6 hosts, with MHC I, MHC II, and non-MHC antigen differences) will cease functioning by 7–10 d posttransplantation, *(19)* (Table 1). Isografts (e.g., between animals of the same inbred strain) and non-MHC-mismatched grafts (e.g., 129/J grafts into C57BL/6 recipients) will typically function for long periods of time without immunosuppression. Likewise, MHC I-disparate grafts (e.g., bm1 into C57BL/6 hosts) will function indefinitely without treatment. On the other hand, MHC II-mismatched grafts (e.g., bm12 into C57BL/6 hosts) may occasionally function for extended periods (when there is minimal perioperative ischemia), but will typically fail by 5–6 wk posttransplant. Thus, to consistently yield the long-term functioning grafts necessary to develop GA lesions (8–12 wk), some form of immunosuppression is usually required.

We have adopted and extended the MAb-induced T-cell depletion model originally developed by Russell, et al. *(11)*. This involves ip administration of anti-CD4 (hybridoma line GK1.5, a rat IgG2b antibody) and anti-CD8 (hybridoma line 2.43, also a rat IgG2b antibody) MAbs prepared as ascites in nude mice (0.2 mL combined vol) at days 6, 3, and 1 before transplant. No further immunosuppression is administered. As ascites preparations are fairly labor-intensive (requiring frequent harvest from inoculated host animals), and vary somewhat in antibody concentrations, we have adopted high-density cell culture techniques to generate the same MAbs. Two culture systems that we have experience with are CELLMAX from Cellco, Incorporated, Germantown, MD, and the CL-1000 incubators from Integra BioSciences, Bedford, NH. Both yield comparable amounts of antibody, although the CL-1000 system is more convenient to use. The MAbs obtained from the culture systems are purified by ammonium sulfate precipitation and size exclusion chromatography, and 0.1 mL each of 1.5 mg/mL soln are administered. After a single injection of these MAbs, peripheral CD4+ and CD8+ T cell depletion is 98% at 1 wk and approx 88% at 2 wk. After three injections (analogous to days 6, 3, and 1 pretransplant), peripheral blood T-cell depletion is >98% at 2 wk, and approx 87% at 4 wk *(19)*. The MAb approach also has the potential to permit selective depletion of CD4+ helper or CD8+ cytolytic T cells to assess their relative contributions to rejection.

With this MAb immunosuppression protocol, we achieve consistent long-term survival (routinely ≥12 wk) of all but total allo-mismatched grafts; characteristic GA lesions are evident by 8–12 wk posttransplantation. Occasionally, total allo-mismatched grafts will also survive long-term with this protocol, but we typically find that they fail by 4–5 wk, concurrent with the recovery of peripheral CD4+ and CD8+ T cells. Additional weekly administration of MAbs

Table 2
Efficacy of Cyclosporine (CsA) and/or Rapamycin (RPM) Immunosuppression
in Total Allo-Mismatched Grafts: Scores for Parenchymal Rejection (PR) and GA

	BALB/c into C57BL/6 Allografts			
	no treatment	CsA alone	RPM alone	RPM+CsA
Number of animals	10	6	7	6
Duration	8.4 +/–1.5 d	4–8 wk	12 wk	12 wk
PR grade (0–4)	2.8 +/–0.4	3.2 +/–0.3	2.1 +/–0.2	1.7 +/–0.3
GA grade (0–4)	0.3 +/–0.1	1.9 +/–0.5[a]	1.6 +/–0.4	0.7 +/–0.3[b]

Values represent mean +/–SEM
[a]For CsA alone, vascular lesions at 4–8 wk are predominantly composed of mononuclear inflammatory cells and do not represent true GA lesions; the GA grade shown represents the degree of vascular occlusion.
[b]$p < 0.05$ vs RPM alone

posttransplant in the total allo-mismatch combinations (in addition to the three doses pretransplant) does result in long-term allograft survival, but with no parenchymal rejection or GA *(19)*. Thus, to achieve a satisfactory model for GA in total allo-mismatched combinations, we developed a protocol where grafts are transplanted without prior immunosuppression and are allowed to reject for four d. At that point, weekly anti-CD4 and anti-CD8 MAb administration is initiated, completely eliminating any further T-cell-mediated responses. In addition to reliably inducing GA in total allo-mismatched strain combinations, this protocol also makes the important point that a single episode of rejection is sufficient to recruit and activate secondary effectors that can eventually result in GA *(19)*.

We have also developed alternate, more "human-like" immunosuppression protocols (Hasegawa, et al., unpublished) as models for evaluating the mechanisms of GA (Table 2). Thus, 15 mg/kg/d of cyclosporine A (CsA) or 1 mg/kg every other d of rapamycin administered by sc injection yield long-term (12 wk) survival of MHC II-mismatched allografts, with concomitant development of GA. However, CsA alone—even at 30 mg/kg/d—does not permit long-term survival of total allo-mismatched hearts (grafts cease beating at 3–4 wk) *(23,24)*. It is not clear whether this is caused by accelerated murine catabolism of CsA or some other intrinsic in vivo resistance to CsA immunosuppression. Nevertheless, we find that rapamycin alone at 1 mg/kg every other d does result in long-term survival of total allo-mismatched grafts, which then also develop GA lesions. Interestingly, CsA and rapamycin in combination prevented both PR and GA in total allo-mismatched strain combinations (Hasegawa, et al., unpublished).

ADVANTAGES OF HETEROTOPIC CARDIAC TRANSPLANTATION RELATIVE TO OTHER MURINE TRANSPLANT ARTERIOPATHY MODELS

The vascularized heterotopic model has distinct advantages over non-vascularized grafts implanted on the neck or ear pinna *(25)*. In the non-vascularized model, the grafts invariably suffer extensive infarction before new vessel ingrowth restores flow (days to a week), and early alloresponses may be overwhelmed by antigen nonspecific ischemic injury. The heterotopic cardiac transplant model also has certain advantages over carotid or aortic interposition vascular grafts in mice, *(26,27)* in that the contribution of parenchymal rejection to the development of GA may be assessed. Indeed, we have seen that PR precedes GA, with the initial site of inflammatory cells in the myocardium, presumably as effector cells egress into the allograft via postcapillary venules, and then attack arterial-wall cells from the ablumenal aspect *(12)*. With inter-position grafts, inflammatory cells must attach and initiate injury directly beginning at the lumenal aspect of the vessel wall. In addition, with nonperfused vasa vasora in vessel allografts, a variable and frequently confounding degree of vascular-wall necrosis and scarring occurs, unrelated to the alloresponse.

DISADVANTAGES OF THE HETEROTOPIC TRANSPLANT MODEL

A hypothetical drawback to the model is the absence of left ventricular hemodynamic loading. While the effects of myocardial pressure and vol loading on allograft rejection have not been formally investigated, the reduction of left ventricular work could conceivably affect the metabolic demands placed on the myocardium, and result in less ischemic injury with worsening GA. Although we have noted that extremely long-term isografts (20–44 wk) show myocyte atrophy, our typical 4–12-wk isografts do not. A further frequent artifact of this model is the formation of a thrombus in the left ventricle when the aortic root dilates with subsequent aortic insufficiency. In the pathological evaluation of the specimen, it is important not to mistake the inflammation associated with the organizing thrombus for rejection.

TRANSLATION TO CLINICAL INVESTIGATION

The murine transplant model permits experimental approaches to questions not readily amenable to investigation in human transplant recipients. Given the caveat that metabolism in experimental animals may not necessarily reflect that seen in humans, the effects of particular drugs and interventions on both parenchymal rejection and GA can be tested.

Hearts may be transplanted across well-defined MHC incompatibilities, with selective depletion of particular inflammatory cell subsets (using either MAbs or knockouts). Because of these strain differences and the availability of highly specific antibodies, we have demonstrated that donor endothelium and vascular SMCs persist in long-term allografts *(20)*. The allograft vessel-wall cells are not replaced to any significant extent by host cells, and thus can continue to engender ongoing immune responses.

The number and severity of rejection episodes can also be modulated experimentally, and the effects of prolonged ischemia can be examined critically. For example, we have demonstrated that a single early episode of rejection is sufficient to induce the chain of events that culminate in GA *(19)*. This result is in agreement with experiments performed in the rabbit heterotopic transplant model, where a transient absence of CsA immunosuppression led to more severe GA lesions *(28)*. These results also suggest that more aggressive immunosuppression (limited by the complications of infection and malignancy) could conceivably reduce the incidence and/or severity of GA. Indeed, the efficacy of combined treatment with CsA and rapamycin in reducing GA may be attributable to enhanced immunosuppression with a more favorable therapeutic index (Hasegawa, unpublished; *9,29*)). We have also examined the relative effects of 4–h cold ischemia (comparable to the upper limit of cold ischemia allowable for human cardiac transplants) on the development of GA. We find that although 4–h cold ischemia can induce very mild GA in isografts, the contribution of the alloresponse to GA far overwhelms any cold ischemia effect (Furukawa, et al., submitted). Thus, any transient responses induced by ischemia alone are unlikely—by themselves—to significantly affect GA development.

Hearts may be explanted at intermediate time points to assess the pathologies that ultimately give rise to vascular lesions. In this manner we demonstrated that parenchymal rejection predominates at early time points (days to 4 wk), progressing to a coalescence of inflammation around arteries, with a lesser component of intralumenal inflammation *(12)*. As time progresses (8–12 wk), parenchymal rejection lessens, while the vascular lesions show reduced inflammation and an increased component of extracellular matrix *(12)*. Thus, by only examining the endpoint of GA pathology, intermediate states potentially amenable to intervention may be overlooked. This point is also important because the inflammatory cells and mediators present at later time points may not be at all indicative of the cells and effectors that initiated or drove the development of GA.

If hearts are transplanted into congenitally immunodeficient recipients (e.g., SCID or recombinase-deficient {Rag-/-} hosts), the grafts will survive indefinitely without immunosuppression; purified allospecific T cells or antiserum *(18)* can then be added back ("adoptive transfer") to identify relevant contributors to the rejection and/or GA pathways. Others have shown that allospecific antiserum raised in appropriately sensitized hosts can induce GA in allografts in the absence of host animal responses, suggesting that humoral immunity may play a role in the disease process *(18,30)*. Using adoptive transfer of allospecific CD4+ T cells only, we have also shown that GA lesions can be induced in grafts in Rag-/- hosts, in the complete absence of B cells or cytotoxic T cells (Becker, et al., submitted).

Finally, the availability of multiple knockout and transgenic strains can unambiguously establish the contribution of a wide range of cytokines, costimulatory molecules, and cell populations. Thus, we find that allografts in hosts congenitally lacking interferon-γ (IFNγ) do not develop GA *(12,19,31)*. The same effect is observed when blocking antibodies to IFNγ are administered at weekly intervals, demonstrating that the effect is not attributable to some developmental anomaly in animals congenitally lacking the cytokine *(12,32)*. In these IFNγ-deficient hosts, the lack of GA may be caused primarily by diminished macrophage recruitment and activation *(12,19)*; however, we also see reduced MHC II and CD40 costimulator expression, and diminished adhesion molecule expression. Similarly, roles for other inflammatory cytokines (e.g., interleukin-10 and interleukin-12) have been inferred using knockout animals or exogenously administered cytokines and MAbs, demonstrating the strength of this approach *(33,34)*.

REFERENCES

1. Hosenpud J, Novick R, Bennett L, Keck B, Fiol, B, Daily, O. 1996. The Registry of the International Society for Heart and Lung Transplantation: thirteenth official report—1996. J Heart Lung Transplant 1996; 15:655–674.
2. Gao S-Z., Alderman E, Schroeder J, Silverman J, Hunt S. Accelerated coronary vascular disease in the heart transplant patient: coronary angiographic findings. J Am Coll Cardiol 1988; 12:334–340.
3. Yeung A, Davis S, Hauptman P, Kobashigawa J, Miller L, Valantine H, et al. Incidence and progression of transplant coronary artery disease over 1 year: results of a multicenter trial with use of intravascular ultrasound. J Heart Lung Transplant 1995; 14:S215–S220.
4. Schoen F, Libby P. Cardiac transplant graft arteriosclerosis. Trends Cardiovasc Med 1991; 1:216–223.
5. Hauptman P, Nakagawa T, Tanaka H, Libby P. Acute rejection: Culprit or coincidence in the pathogenesis of cardiac graft vascular disease? J Heart Lung Transplant 1995; 14:S173–S180.
6. Hauptman P, Davis S, Miller L, Yeung A. The role of nonimmune risk factors in the development and progression of graft arteriosclerosis: preliminary insights from a multicenter intravascular ultrasound study. J Heart Lung Transplant 1995; 14:S238–S242.
7. Tuzcu E, deFranco A, Hobbs R, Rincon G, Bott-Silverman C, McCarthy P, et al. Prevalence and distribution of transplant coronary artery disease: insights from intravascular ultrasound imaging. J Heart Lung Transplant 1995; 14:S202–S206.
8. Akosah K, McDaniel S, Hanrahan J, Mohanty P. Dobutamine stress echocardiography early after heart transplantation predicts development of allograft coronary artery disease and outcome. J Am Coll Cardiol 1998; 31:1607–1614.

 9. Geerling R, DeBruin R, Scheringa M, Bonthuis F, Jeekei J, Izjermanns J, et al. Suppression of acute rejection prevents graft arteriosclerosis after allogeneic aorta transplantation in the rat. Transplantation 1994; 58:1258–1263.

10. Kobashigawa J, Katznelson S, Laks H, Johnson J, Yeatman L, Wang X, et al. Effect of pravastatin on outcomes after cardiac transplantation. N Engl J Med 1995; 333:621–627.

11. Russell P, Chase C, Win H, Colvin R. Coronary atherosclerosis in transplanted mouse hearts. I. Time course and immunogenetic and immunopathological considerations. Am J Pathol 1994; 144:260–274.

12. Nagano H, Mitchell R, Taylor M, Hasegawa S, Tilney N, Libby P. Interferon-γ deficiency prevents coronary arteriosclerosis but not myocardial rejection in transplanted mouse hearts. J Clin Investig 1997; 100:550–557.

13. Kitamura D, Roes J, Kuhn R, Rajewsky K. B cell-deficient mouse by targeted disruption of the membrane exon of the immunoglobulin μ chain gene. Nature 1991; 350:423–426.

14. Dalton D, Pitts-Meek S, Keshav S, Figari I, Bradley A, Stewart T. Multiple defects of immune cell function in mice with disrupted interferon-gamma genes. Science 1993; 259:1739–1742.

15. Corry, R, Winn H, Russell P. Primary vascularized allografts of hearts in mice. Transplantation 1973; 16:343–350.

16. Drinkwater D, Rudis E, Laks H, Ziv E, Marino J, Stein D, et al. University of Wisconsin solution versus Stanford cardioplegic solution and the development of cardiac allograft vasculopathy. J Heart Lung Transplant 1995; 14:891–896.

17. Billingham M, Cary N, Hammond M, Kemnitz J, Marboe C, McCallister H, et al. A working formulation for the standardization of nomenclature in the diagnosis of heart and lung rejection: heart Rejection Study Group. The international Society for Heart Transplantation. J Heart Transplant 1990; 9:587–593.

18. Russell P, Chase C, Winn H, Colvin R. Coronary atherosclerosis in transplanted mouse hearts. II. Importance of humoral immunity. J Immunol 1994; 152:5135–5141.

19. Nagano H, Libby P, Taylor M, Hasegawa S, Stinn J, Becker G, et al. Coronary arteriosclerosis after T-cell-mediated injury in transplanted mouse hearts. Role of Interferon-γ. Am J Pathol 1998; 152:1187–1197.

20. Hasegawa S, Becker G, Nagano H, Libby P, Mitchell R. Pattern of graft- and host-specific MHC class II expression in long-term murine cardiac allografts. Origin of inflammatory and vascular wall cells. Am J Pathol 1998; 153:1–11.

21. O'Garra A, Murphy K. Role of cytokines in determining T cell function (mouse). In: Weir D, ed. Handbook of Experimental Immunology, Vol. 4. Blackwell Science, Cambridge, 1996; pp. 210–221.

22. Stinn J, Taylor M, Becker G, Nagano H, Hasegawa S, Furukawa Y, et al. Interferon-γ-secreting T-cell populations in rejecting murine cardiac allografts: assessment by flow cytometry. Am J Pathol 1998; 153:1383–1392.

23. Morris R, Wu J, Shorthouse R. A study of the contrasting effects of cyclosporine, FK-506, and rapamycin on the suppression of allograft rejection. Transplantation Proc 1990; 22:1638–1641.

24. Mollison, K, Fey T, Krause R, Thomas V, Mehta A, Luly R. Comparison of FK-506, rapamycin, ascomycin, and cyclosporine in mouse models of host-versus-graft disease and heterotopic heart transplantation. Ann NY Acad Sci 1993; 685:55–57.

25. Judd, K, Trentin J. Cardiac transplantation in mice. I. Factors influencing the take and survival of heterotopic grafts. Transplantation 1971; 11:298–302.

26. Shi C, Russell M, Bianchi C, Newell J, Haber E. A murine model of accelerated transplant arteriosclerosis. Circ Res 1994; 75:199–207.

27. Chow L, Huh S, Jiang J, Zhong R, Pickering J. Intimal thickening develops without humoral immunity in a mouse aortic allograft model of chronic vascular rejection. Circulation 1996; 94:3079–3082.

28. Nakagawa T, Sukhova G, Rabkin E, Winters G, Schoen F, Libby P. Acute rejection accelerates graft coronary disease in transplanted rabbit hearts. Circulation 1995; 92:987–993.

29. Wasowska B, Hancock W, Onodera K, Korom S, Stadlbauer T, Zheng X, et al. Rapamycin and cyclosporine A treatment: a novel regimen to prevent chronic allograft rejection in sensitized hosts. Transplantation Proc 1997; 29:333.

30. Hancock W, Buelow R, Sayegh M, Turka L. Antibody-induced transplant arteriosclerosis is prevented by graft expression of anti-oxidant and anti-apoptotic genes. Nat Med 1998; 4:1392–1396.

31. Raisanen-Sokolowski A, Glysing-Jensen T, Koglin J, Russell M. Reduced transplant arteriosclerosis in murine cardiac allografts placed in interferon-gamma knockout recipients. Am J Pathol 1998; 152:359–365.

32. Russell P, Chase C, Winn H, Colvin B. Coronary atherosclerosis in transplanted mouse hearts. III. Effects of recipient treatment with a monoclonal antibody to interferon-gamma. Transplantation 1994; 57:1367–1371.

33. Piccotti J, Chan S, Goodman R, Magram J, Eichwald E, Bishop D. IL-12 antagonism induces T helper 2 responses yet exacerbates cardiac allograft rejection. Evidence against a dominant protective role for T helper 2 cytokines in alloimmunity. J Immunol 1996; 157:1951–1957.

34. Raisanen-Sokolowski A, Glysing-Jensen T, Russell M. Leukocyte-suppressing influences of interleukin(IL)-10 in cardiac allografts: insights from IL-10 knockout mice. Am J Pathol 1998; 153:1491–1500.

35. Isobe M, Yagita H, Okumura K, Ihara A. Specific acceptance of cardiac allograft after treatment with antibodies to ICAM-1 and LFA-1. Science 1992; 255:1125–1127.

36. Hirozane T, Matsumori A, Furukawa Y, Sasayama S. Experimental graft coronary artery disease in a murine heterotopic cardiac transplant model. Circulation 1995; 91:386–392.

17 Hyperacute Vascular Rejection
Lessons from Pig-to-Primate Xenotransplantation

Raymond H. Chen, MD, DPHIL and David H. Adams, MD

CONTENTS

INTRODUCTION
MATERIALS AND METHODS
MECHANISM OF HYPERACUTE REJECTION
EXPERIMENTAL STRATEGIES
CONCLUSION
ACKNOWLEDGMENT
REFERENCES

INTRODUCTION

Solid-organ transplantation has become a feasible treatment option for many patients with organ failure. The availability of organs, however, has not kept up with the increasing number of patients on the waiting list. In order to expand the supply of organs, many investigators have suggested the use of animal donors. Primates are man's closest evolutionary relatives and share many immunological traits. Yet primates rarely achieve human size, and thus simian heart xenografts cannot generate adequate cardiac output. The ethical issues surrounding their use and the fear of cross-species viral transmission have also prevented their acceptance as organ donors. Instead, pigs have emerged as the most promising candidate for organ donation. They grow to human size in a short period of time, and are easy to raise in large numbers. Their long history of domestication and their integral presence in the human diet decrease the likelihood of transmitting endogenous viruses previously unknown to man. Moreover, clinical medicine has long utilized swine as the source of insulin and

From: *Contemporary Cardiology: Vascular Disease and Injury: Preclinical Research*
Edited by: D. I. Simon and C. Rogers © Humana Press Inc., Totowa, NJ

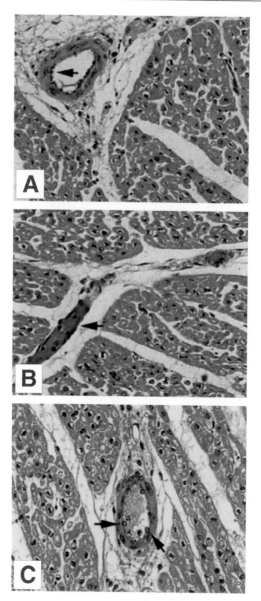

Fig. 1. Hyperacute rejection: wild-type pig heart transplanted into baboon, 60 min after implantation, (H and E, 320×). The heart is characterized by diffuse interstitial edema. Arrowheads show **(A)** activated enodthelium; **(B)** multiple thrombi within vessels; **(C)** polymorphonuclear leucocytes bound to the endothelium. (See color plate 8 appearing in the insert following p. 236).

heart valves. Consequently, pigs are the most medically feasible candidates from the list of potential animal donors, and are more ethically acceptable *(1)*. Porcine organs, however, are rapidly rejected within minutes of transplantation into primates. Upon the establishment of circulation, the graft—whether a kidney, heart or liver—becomes congested and cyanotic, and quickly fails within minutes *(2)*. The gross appearance and timing of graft rejection are similar to that observed in ABO incompatibility transplantation. Microscopic examination of a hyperacutely-rejected porcine heart in an olive baboon reveals signs of interstitial hemorrhage, intravascular thrombosis, perivascular edema, polymononuclear cellular adherence, endothelial-cell activation, and myocyte vacuolization (Fig. 1) *(3)*. Similarly, a porcine kidney transplanted into a baboon shows tubular vacuolization, peritubular edema, and glomeruli collapse. In this chapter we review the mechanism responsible for porcine hyperacute rejection, and discuss the current experimental strategies directed toward controlling this phenomenon.

MATERIALS AND METHODS

Experimental Animals

Olive baboons (*Papio Anubis*) served as transplant recipients. Transgenic pigs constitutively expressing the combination of human CD59/DAF were developed at Nextran (Princeton, NJ). Briefly, large genomic clones encompassing the genes encoding human CD59 and DAF were microinjected into fertilized porcine oocytes to develop transgenic pigs using standard technique *(4)*. Both clones are approx 90 Kb and contain 10–20 Kb of the 5' and 3' flanking sequences of their respective genes. G1 offspring from one founder that was transgenic for both human CD59 and DAF were used as heart donors. Wild-type pigs served as control donors. All animals received humane care in accordance with the guidelines of the Harvard University Animal Care Committee, and the "Guide for the Care and Use of Laboratory Animals" prepared by the Institute of Laboratory Animal Resources and published by the National Institutes of Health (NIH publications No. 86–23, revised 1985).

For invasive procedures and anesthesia induction, sedation was achieved using ketamine hydrochloride (10 mg/kg im) in baboons and telazol (5mg/kg im) in pigs. Respiratory secretions were controlled with atropine sulfate (0.03 mg/kg). Anesthesia was maintained with inhalational isoflurane (1.3–2.0%). Intraoperatively, both pigs and baboons were monitored with electrocardiography, noninvasive blood-pressure monitoring, and pulse-oximetry. All baboons received antibiotic coverage with cefazolin (20mg/kg im bid) and pain control with butrenorphine (0.005 mg/kg bid) postoperatively for 5 d. In the event of diminished fluid or caloric intake, recipients received their calculated daily needs as iv crystalloid soln or ensure tube feeds.

Heterotopic Heart Transplantation

Heart transplantation was performed in the neck as previously described *(5)*. Pigs were anesthetized and received systemic anticoagulation with heparin (100 IU/kg iv). The heart was then harvested in a standard fashion after protection by 500 cc of antegrade cold crystalloid cardioplegic soln (dextrose 2.5%, NaCl 0.45%, potassium 30 meq/L, bicarbonate 5 meq/L). Transplant organ ischemic time varied between 45–55 min.

Immunosuppression

The transgenic (n = 4) and control heart (n = 3) recipients received daily immunosuppression starting 7 d (d –7) prior to transplantation (d 0). The immunosuppressive regimen consisted of cyclosporine (7 mg/kg im) titrated to maintain a trough level 400–600 ng/mL, methylprednisolone (10 mg/kg im), and leflunomide (n = 2) (20 mg/kg p.o. or 10 mg/kg im) or mofetil mycophenolate (n = 5) (70 mg/kg p.o.).

Evaluation of Transplant Organ Function

Hearts were inspected 4 × per day. Daily echocardiography was performed, and open biopsies obtained on every third day and at the time of organ failure.

Termination of Experiment

Xenograft explant was performed at the time of graft failure. Cardiac failure was defined as the cessation of beating, as confirmed with palpation or ultrasound.

Histopathologic Studies of the Xenograft Heart

Biopsies were fixed in formalin and paraffin, or mounted in OCT media, and quick-frozen in liquid nitrogen for storage at –80°C. Paraffin sections were stained with hematoxylin and eosin. Cryostat sections were immunostained using standard indirect immunoperoxidase avidin-biotin techniques previously described, *(6)* with MAbs specific for CD59, DAF, IgM, IgG (all from Biodesign International, Kennebunk, ME), and membrane attack complex (Dako, Carpinteria, CA).

MECHANISM OF HYPERACUTE REJECTION

The hyperacute rejection mechanism that attacks xenotransplants—but not crossmatched-negative, ABO-compatible allografts—is mediated by antibodies *(7)*. The xenoreactive antibodies (XNA) are mainly of the IgM isotype and are predominantly directed against the galactose α *(1,3)* galactose disaccharide (Gal) *(8–11)*. This Gal terminal sugar moiety is added on to the cellular surface proteins by the enzyme α-1,3–galactosyltransferase. Since humans, apes, and

Old World monkeys are the only mammals that do not possess the enzyme, they are also the ones with circulating XNA against Gal *(12)*.

The importance of these XNA in hyperacute rejection has been demonstrated over the years in different models. Newborn humans and baboons without xeno-reactive antibodies do not hyperacutely reject xenotransplants *(13,14)*. Hyper-acute rejection is attenuated in adult baboons if IgM is first depleted by plasmapheresis *(15)*. Enzymatic removal of the Gal sugar from porcine cells prevents hyperacute attacks from human or cynomolgus monkey serum *(16)*. In the model where the heart from an α-1,3–galactosyltransferase knockout mouse was perfused with human serum, the significantly decreased deposition of XNA is consistent with its avoidance of hyperacute rejection *(17)*.

XNA are called preformed natural antibodies because they were once con-sidered to be synthesized with no previous history of sensitization to the xenoantigen *(18)*. Recently, however, it has been suggested that XNA may be synthesized as the result of previous priming sensitization to either food anti-gen or the ubiquitous microbial flora. The new thinking is supported by the observation that newborn piglets, if reared in a pathogen-free environment, do not produce XNA *(19)*. Similarly, dogs raised in isolated environments also do not synthesize antisheep XNA *(19)*.

As opposed to the guinea pig to rat xenotransplant model, in which hyper-acute rejection is mediated via the alternative complement pathway, the pres-ence of XNA is required for hyperacute rejection in baboons *(20)*. Baboon XNA binds to Gal moiety on the xenograft and activates the complement cascade. It has been shown that the binding XNA, on pig endothelium, does not induce downregulation of the Gal antigen. Consequently, even if XNA is first depleted by plasmapharesis, the persistence of Gal provides a target for antibody-medi-ated rejection once the level of XNA returns *(21)*. Although Chopek et al. had reported the phenomenon of "accommodation," in which ABO-incompatible transplantations survive after initial antibody depletion despite the return and deposition of ABO antibody, there is yet convincing evidence for "accommo-dation" in the hyperacute transplant setting *(22)*.

In humans and baboons, XNA include both the IgM and the IgG isotypes. Over the years it has been shown that it is IgM, not IgG, that is responsible for hyperacute rejection. Although anti-Gal IgG antibodies are often detected in the peripheral circulation of Old World monkeys, their deposition is not always present on hyperacutely-rejected xenografts *(3,7)*. In addition, the deposition of IgM—but not IgG—correlates with the severity of hyperacute rejection *(23,24)*. Because of their inefficiency in complement activation, *(25)* IgG do not con-tribute significantly to the immediate hyperacute rejection of xenotransplants.

On the other hand, IgM can initiate the hyperacute rejection via the comple-ment cascade *(26,27)*. Complements are circulating proteins which can be acti-vated by either exposed tissue factor (alternative pathway) or through bound

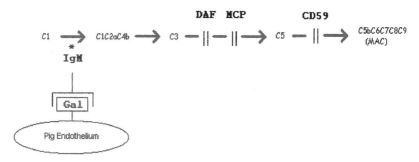

Fig. 2. Hyperacute rejection and complement regulatory proteins. During a pig-to-baboon xenotransplantation, baboon natural antibodies bind to the Gal on porcine cells. The bound XNA IgM can activate the complement cascade via the classical pathway. The human complement regulatory proteins transfected into the porcine cells can arrest the complement cascade at different stages. Whereas MCP (CD46) and DAF (CD55) can interrupt the pathway at the C3 activation level, CD59 disrupts the assembly of the final step—the membrane attack complex (MAC).

IgM (classical pathway). The Fc region of IgM cleaves and activates C1, which then cleaves and binds to C4. The activated complex of IgM-C1s-C4b binds and activates C2 and then C3 (28). The now-activated complex of C4–2a-3b then cleaves C5, with the split C5b fragment binding to C6 and C7. The C5b-C6–C7 complex is stabilized via the membrane bilayer (29). The complex then binds to C8 and C9 and assembles the membrane attack complex (MAC).

The function of MAC in xenotransplant has been the subject of various studies. Because MAC forms osmotically active pores across the cellular membrane and induces cytolysis via ionic efflux and water influx, it was hypothesized that endothelial cytolysis may be the mechanism of graft demise (7). However, it is now evident that MAC may also induce endothelium to undergo cellular changes that are responsible for hyperacute rejection. MAC can open the intercellular gap via endothelium retraction. As such, the endothelial barrier on the vasculature is broken down and allows vascular content to infiltrate the graft (30). MAC also induces the release of heparin sulfate from the endothelium and promotes platelet aggregation and thrombosis formation (31).

Even during hyperacute rejection, complements are closely regulated by complement regulatory proteins (CRP), such as the decay-accelerating factor (DAF, CD55), (32–34) the membrane cofactor protein (MCP, CD46), (35) and the complement inhibitor (CD59) (36,37). DAF acts on the early step of complement activation by preventing the activation of C3. Similarly, MCP is a cofactor for serine protease factor I, which cleave activated C3 and C4. CD59 acts on the final stage of complement cascade by inhibiting the assembly of MAC (Fig. 2).

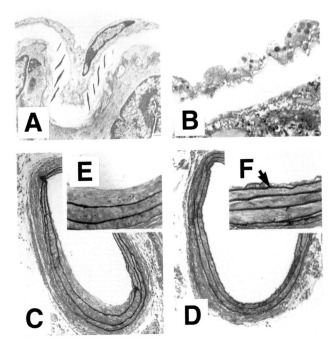

Plate 1, Fig. 2. (*See* discussion in Chapter 7 and full caption on p. 91). Photomicrographs of mouse carotid arteries after arterial dilation and endothelial denudations.

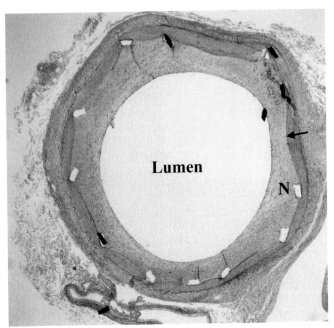

Plate 2, Fig. 2. (*See* discussion in Chapter 4 and full caption on p. 59). Photomicrograph of monkey iliac artery 28 d after stent implantation (Verhoeff tissue elastin stain).

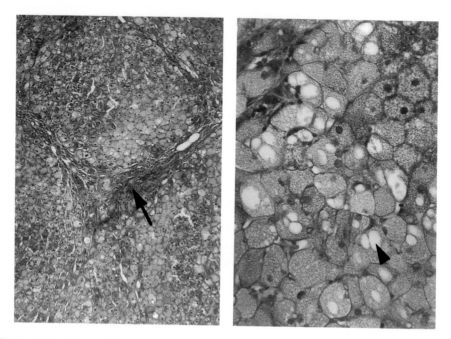

Plate 3, Fig. 1. (*See* discussion in Chapter 13 and full caption on p. 177). The liver of cholesterol-fed rabbits with extensive hypercholesterolemia shows the disruption of parenchymal architecture and the fatty change (Masson trichrome staining).

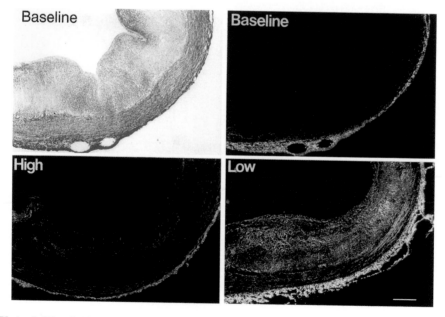

Plate 4, Fig. 4. (*See* discussion in Chapter 13 and full caption on p. 182). Interstitial collagen content in the aortic intima detected by the picrosirius red polarization method.

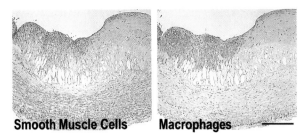

Plate 5, Fig. 6. (*See* discussion in Chapter 13 and full caption on p. 185). Atherosclerotic lesion of WHHL rabbits.

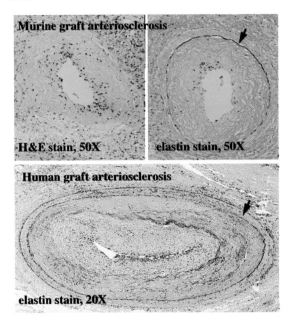

Plate 6, Fig. 1. (*See* discussion in Chapter 16 and full caption on p. 216). Histologic appearance of graft arteriosclerosis **(GA)** in humans and mice.

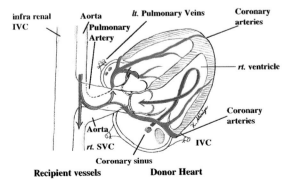

Plate 7, Fig. 2. (*See* discussion in Chapter 16 and full caption on p. 218). Schematic of heterotopic grafts.

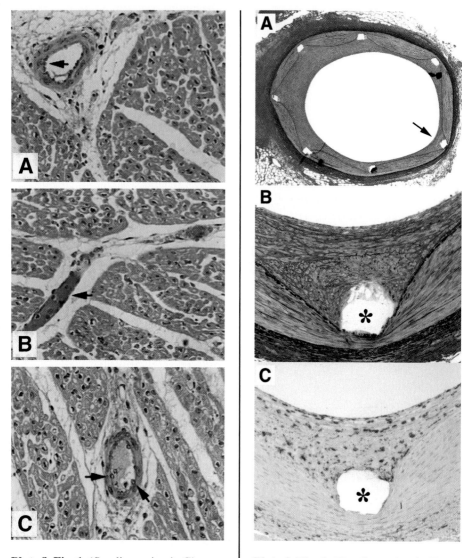

Plate 8, Fig. 1. (*See* discussion in Chapter 17 and full caption on p. 232). Hyperacute rejection: wild-type pig heart transplanted into baboon, 60 min after implantation.

Plate 9, Fig. 1. (*See* discussion in Chapter 22 and full caption on p. 332). Endovascular stainless-steel stent-implanted pig coronary artery, 28 d post implantation.

Complement regulatory proteins, however, are species-restricted such that porcine CRP fail to downregulate primate complements *(38–40)*. The absence of regulatory mechanisms contributes to the explosive destruction of xenograft during hyperacute rejection. *(41)*.

EXPERIMENTAL STRATEGIES
Recipient Modification

A number of strategies have been devised to overcome hyperacute rejection. The standard immunosuppressive regimen for allograft transplantation—i.e., cyclosporine, steroid, imuran or mycophenylate moefitil—fails to curtail hyperacute rejection. The addition of cyclophosphamide has been partially successful in curtailing the secretion of XNA, but often at the expense of pancytopenia and gastrointestinal hemorrhage. The prolongation of graft survival with plasmapheresis alone has been disappointing *(42)*. Using a Gal-column, Taniguchi et al. were able to reduce the titer of peripherally circulating XNA in baboons *(43)*. However, the circulating antibody quickly restored to pretreatment level after the cessation of treatment.

Cobra venom factor is a protein substrate that consumes and depletes C3. As such, it has been included as part of the immunosuppressive regimen in xenotransplantation. However, the baboon recipient quickly develops anticobra venom factor antibody after repeated treatments. Not only does the efficacy decrease with the neutralizing antibody, the bound antigen-antibody complex may induce anaphylaxis. In addition, since cobra venom factor contains the Gal sugar, its repeated use actually induces anti-galactose antibody in baboons *(44–47)*. Cobra venom factor thus fails as a long-term treatment for clinical xenotransplantation.

An alternative method of inhibiting the complement cascade is the human recombinant soluble complement receptor type 1 (rsCR1) *(44,48)*. rSCR1 is a soluble recombinant protein of the human complement receptor, and it inactivates both C3 and C5 convertases. As such it has been shown to increase the survival of porcine graft perfused with human blood. Alternatively, a plasma inhibitor of human C1 (C1 inh) has been used in combination with sol complement receptor type I. C1 inh is a serine protease that inactivates C1. As such, it has been shown to reduce the level of C3a and C5a. Its administration shows partial protection of porcine aortic endothelium from human serum *(49)*. Both the rsCRi and the C1 inh were shown to be synergistic with CD59 in their protection against complement lysis in perfused endothelium. Similarly, the combination of cyclosporine, cyclophosphamide, and steroid with continuous infusion of rsCR1 prolonged pig-heart survival in cynomolgus monkeys from 38 min to 11 d *(50)*.

Since natural antibodies are directed against the sugar moiety on the cellular surface, IV carbohydrates as competitive inhibitors to membrane Gal sugar has been attempted *(8,51)*. Using soluble Gal α-(1–3)Gal and Gal α-(1–3)Gal β-(1–4)GlcNAc, Cairns et al. showed incomplete inhibition of hyperacute rejection in vitro *(52)*. In addition, neutral oligosaccharides derived from porcine stomach mucin (PSM) are effective inhibitors of human anti-α-Gal IgG in vitro *(53)*. Alternatively, Sandrin et al. transfected xenogenic cells with the human α-1,2–fucosyltransferase, which shifts the production of sugar moiety from Gal to the nonantigenic human blood group O antigen—the α-1,2–fucosyl lactosamine moiety. As such, it reduces the target for XNA and prolongs graft survival in the pig-to-baboon heart transplant model *(54)*.

The other method of preventing the XNA-mediated hyperacute rejection is by neutralizing circulating anti-Gal antibodies. Koren et al. immunized mice against human anti-Gal antibody. Mouse serum showed antiidiotypic activity against human XNA, and the serum was able to protect porcine cells in culture from hyperacute rejection *(55)*.

Another method of blocking complement activation is the selective inactivation of C5. Murine antiprimate C5 MAb blocks the cleavage of C5 and the aggregation of MAC. As such, it prevents hyperacute rejection in porcine hearts perfused with human blood *(56)*. Humanized anti-C5 MAb is now available with retained binding specificity and capacity. The antibody may offer a new addition to the current xenotransplant immunosuppressive regimen.

Genetic Modification of the Donor

All of the methods of immunosuppression described here involve short-term modification of the recipient. A more promising approach is the genetic modification of the pig donor. The most obvious solution would have been the selective deletion of the swine α-1,3–galactosyltransferase gene to prevent the expression of pig GAL antigen. The technology, however, is still in an embryonic stage of development. Consequently, the current genetic strategies have focused on transfecting pigs with genes for human complement regulatory proteins to control hyperacute rejection. Initially, human CD59 and DAF genes were inserted in α- and β-globin cassettes for expression on erythrocytes, which then translocate to endothelium via intercellular transfer *(32,57)*. Transgenic mouse heart experienced decreased hyperacute rejection when perfused with human serum. The technology was applied to swine so that hearts from these transgenic pigs were able to survive for up to 30 h in baboons *(58)*. The grafts were subsequently rejected, because the endothelium failed to replenish the shed CD59 and DAF proteins.

In order to obtain better endothelial CD59 and DAF protein concentration in pig hearts, Byrne et al. expressed the human CD59 cDNA in a human α-globin gene cassette. Similarly, the human DAF cDNA was inserted between mouse

H2Kb promoter and polyadenylation signal sequences *(59)*. The direct endothelial expression of CRP conferred better survival of up to 69 h, a result consistent with decreased MAC deposition on the xenograft. However, since the cDNA clones lack the native regulatory signals, the resultant CD59/DAF pigs expressed these proteins at a lower level than that observed in human. In order to obtain better physiologic expression, 70 Kb-pair genomic clones of the CD59 and DAF genes—the ones that include all 5' and 3' regulatory elements—were used for transgenic pig synthesis. Hearts from these CD59/DAF transgenic pigs showed levels of expression comparable to those found in hearts as determined by immunohistochemistry *(60)*. These porcine grafts were able to survive for up to 6 d in baboons.

With recent improvements in heterotopic heart transplantation survival as shown above, Schmoeckel et al. performed orthotopic heart transplants from DAF transgenic pigs into baboons *(61)*. One animal survived for 9 d, then succumbed to pancytopenia and was euthanized. Autopsy and light microscopy revealed no sign of hyperacute rejection. Similarly, Zaidi et al. orthotopically transplanted DAF transgenic pig kidneys into cynomolgus monkeys. The recipients had a median survival of 13 d, with the longest period extending to 35 d. *(62)*. However, cynomolgus monkeys may not be the most compatible model for xenotransplantation in human, since the wild-type pig hearts usually did not experience hyperacute rejection, and survived an average of 6.5 d.

CONCLUSION

With improved transgenic technology and better immunosuppressive regimens, it now appears that hyperacute rejection can be adequately controlled in the pig-to-primate model. However, these grafts invariably fail in days to weeks, even in the absence of hyperacute rejection. Because of the delayed timing of graft demise as compared to the traditional immediate hyperacute rejection, the mechanism of graft failure has been called acute vascular xenograft rejection *(7)* or delayed xenograft rejection *(63)*. Histological studies of the failed grafts show XNA deposition, endothelial activation, intravascular thrombosis, and platelet aggregation. The mechanism behind the delayed graft rejection is still unclear. It has been hypothesized that XNA may play a role via the Fc-mediated cellular infiltration of NK cells. Alternatively, XNA may activate endothelium and induce the upregulation of adhesion molecules for neutrophil transmigration. Endothelium may also upregulate tissue factors, and it triggers the clotting cascade, which is responsible for graft thrombosis and ischemia. Delayed xenotransplant rejection remains the barrier preventing the clinical application of xenotransplantation, and further studies are needed in the pig-to-baboon model to overcome this obstacle.

ACKNOWLEDGMENT

Raymond H. Chen is the recipient of NIH Grant 1F32HL0996601 and American College of Surgeons Research Award.

REFERENCES

1. Cooper D, Ye Y, Rolf J, Zuhdi N. The pig as a potential organ donor for man. In: Cooper D, Kemp E, Reemtsma K, White D, eds. Xenotransplantation: the transplantation of organs and tissues between species. Springer-Verlag, Berlin, Germany, 1991, p. 481.
2. Calne R. Organ transplantation between widely disparate species. Transplant Proc 1970; 2:550.
3. Platt JL, Fischel RJ, Matas AJ, Reif SA, Bolman RM, Bach FH. Immunopathology of hyperacute xenograft rejection in a swine-to-primate model. Transplantation 1991; 52:214–220.
4. Logan J, Martin M. Transgenic swine as a recombinant production for human hemoglobulin. Methods Enzymol 1994:435.
5. Michler RE, McManus RP, Smith CR, Sadeghi AN, Rose EA. Technique for primate heterotopic cardiac xenotransplantation. J Med Primatol 1985; 14:357–362.
6. Adams D, Wyner L, Karnovsky M. Experimental graft arteriosclerosis II. Immunocytochemical analysis of lesion development. Transplantation 1993; 56:794.
7. Lawson JH, Platt JL. Molecular barriers to xenotransplantation. Transplantation 1996; 62:303–310.
8. Cooper DK, Koren E, Oriol R. Oligosaccharides and discordant xenotransplantation. Immunol Rev 1994; 141:31–58.
9. Palmetshofer A, Galili U, Dalmasso AP, Robson SC, Bach FH. Alpha-galactosyl epitope-mediated activation of porcine aortic endothelial cells: type II activation. Transplantation 1998; 65:971–978.
10. Vaughan HA, McKenzie IF, Sandrin MS. Biochemical studies of pig xenoantigens detected by naturally occurring human antibodies and the galactose alpha(1–3)galactose reactive lectin. Transplantation 1995; 59:102–109.
11. Sandrin M, Vaughan H, Dabkowski P, Mcenzie I. Anti-pig IgM antibodies in human serum reacts predominantly with Gal (alpha 1,3) epitopes. Proc Nat Acad Sci USA 1993; 90:11,391.
12. Larsen RD, Rivera-Marrero CA, Ernst LK, Cummings RD, Lowe JB. Frameshift and nonsense mutations in a human genomic sequence homologous to a murine UDP-Gal: beta-D-Gal(1,4)-D-GlcNAc alpha(1,3)—galactosyltransferase cDNA. J Biol Chem 1990; 265:7055–7061.
13. Kaplon RJ, Michler RE, Xu H, Kwiatkowski PA, Edwards NM, Platt JL. Absence of hyperacute rejection in newborn pig-to-baboon cardiac xenografts. Transplantation 1995; 59:1–6.
14. Xu H, Edwards NM, Chen JM, Dong X, Michler RE. Natural antipig xenoantibody is absent in neonatal human serum. J Heart Lung Transplant 1995; 14:749–754.
15. Lin SS, Weidner BC, Byrne GW, et al. The role of antibodies in acute vascular rejection of pig-to-baboon cardiac transplants. J Clin Invest 1998; 101:1745–1756.
16. LaVecchio JA, Dunne AD, Edge AS. Enzymatic removal of alpha-galactosyl epitopes from porcine endothelial cells diminishes the cytotoxic effect of natural antibodies. Transplantation 1995; 60:841–847.
17. Tearle RG, Tange MJ, Zannettino ZL, et al. The alpha-1,3–galactosyltransferase knockout mouse. Implications for xenotransplantation. Transplantation 1996; 61:13–29.
18. Boyden S. Natural antibodies and the immune response. Adv Immunol 1966; 5:1–28.

19. Cramer D. Natural antibodies. In: Tilney N, Strom T, Paul L, eds. Transplantation Biology. Lippincott-Raven, Philadelphia, 1996; 473.

20. Miyagawa S, Hirose H, Shirakura R, et al. The mechanism of discordant xenograft rejection. Transplantation 1988; 46:825–839.

21. Parker W, Holzknecht ZE, Song A, et al. Fate of antigen in xenotransplantation: implications for acute vascular rejection and accommodation. Am J Pathol 1998; 152:829–839.

22. Chopek M, Simmons R, Platt J. ABO incompatible renal transplantation: initial immuno-pathologic evaluation. Transplant Proc 1987; 19:4553.

23. Platt J, Lindman B, Geller R, et al. The role of natural antibodies in the activation of xenogenic endothelial cells. Transplantation 1991; 52:1037.

24. Parker W, Bruno D, Holzknecht Z, Platt J. Xenoreactive naural antibodies: isolation and initial characterization. J Immunol 1994; 153:3791.

25. Magee JC, Collins BH, Harland RC, et al. Immunoglobulin prevents complement-mediated hyperacute rejection in swine-to-primate xenotransplantation. J Clin Invest 1995; 96:2404–2412.

26. Leventhal JR, Dalmasso AP, Cromwell JW, et al. Prolongation of cardiac xenograft survival by depletion of complement. Transplantation 1993; 55:857–865; discussion 865–866.

27. Leventhal JR, John R, Fryer JP, et al. Removal of baboon and human antiporcine IgG and IgM natural antibodies by immunoadsorption. Results of in vitro and in vivo studies. Transplantation 1995; 59:294–300.

28. Roserberg J, Hawkins E, Rector F. Mechanisms of imunological injury during antibody-mediated hyperacute rejection of renal heterografts. Transplantation 1971; 11:151.

29. Mathieson P, Fearon D, Moore F, Jr. Complement. In: Tilney N, Strom T, Paul L, eds. Transplantation Biology. Lippincott-Raven, Philadelphia, 1996; 163.

30. Saadi S, Platt JL. Transient perturbation of endothelial integrity induced by natural antibodies and complement. J Exp Med 1995; 181:21–31.

31. Platt JL, Dalmasso AP, Vercellotti GM, Lindman BJ, Turman MA, Bach FH. Endothelial cell proteoglycans in xenotransplantation. Transplant Proc 1990; 22:1066.

32. Byrne GW, McCurry KR, Kagan D, et al. Protection of xenogeneic cardiac endothelium from human complement by expression of CD59 or DAF in transgenic mice. Transplantation 1995; 60:1149–1156.

33. Davitz MA. Decay-accelerating factor (DAF): a review of its function and structure. Acta Med Scand Suppl 1987; 715:111–121.

34. Schmoeckel M, Nollert G, Shahmohammadi M, et al. Prevention of hyperacute rejection by human decay accelerating factor in xenogeneic perfused working hearts. Transplantation 1996; 62:729–734.

35. Liszewski MK, Post TW, Atkinson JP. Membrane cofactor protein (MCP or CD46): newest member of the regulators of complement activation gene cluster. Annu Rev Immunol 1991; 9:431–455.

36. Miyagawa S, Shirakura R, Matsumiya G, et al. Possibility of prevention of hyperacute rejection by DAF and CD59 in xenotransplantation. Transplant Proc 1994; 26:1235–1238.

37. Brooimans RA, van Wieringen PA, van Es LA, Daha MR. Relative roles of decay-accelerating factor, membrane cofactor protein, and CD59 in the protection of human endothelial cells against complement-mediated lysis. Eur J Immunol 1992; 22:3135–3140.

38. Hansch G, Hammer G, Vanguri P, Shin M. Homologous species restriction in lysis of erythrocytes by terminal complement proteins. Proc Natl Acad Sci USA 1981; 78:5118.

39. Rollins SA, Zhao J, Ninomiya H, Sims PJ. Inhibition of homologous complement by CD59 is mediated by a species-selective recognition conferred through binding to C8 within C5b-8 or C9 within C5b-9. J Immunol 1991; 146:2345–2351.

40. Shin M, Hansch G, Hu V, Nicholson-Weller A. Membrane factors responsible for homologous species restriction of complement mediated lysis: evidence for a factor other than DAF operating at the stage of C8 and C9. J Immunol 1986; 136:1777.
41. Lachmann PJ. The control of homologous lysis. Immunol Today 1991; 12:312–315.
42. Kroshus TJ, Dalmasso AP, Leventhal JR, John R, Matas AJ, Bolman RM, 3rd. Antibody removal by column immunoabsorption prevents tissue injury in an ex vivo model of pig-to-human xenograft hyperacute rejection. J Surg Res 1995; 59:43–50.
43. Taniguchi S, Neethling FA, Korchagina EY, et al. In vivo immunoadsorption of antipig antibodies in baboons using a specific Gal(alpha)1–3Gal column. Transplantation 1996; 62:1379–1384.
44. Candinas D, Lesnikoski BA, Robson SC, et al. Soluble complement receptor type 1 and cobra venom factor in discordant xenotransplantation. Transplant Proc 1996; 28:581.
45. Kobayashi T, Taniguchi S, Neethling FA, et al. Delayed xenograft rejection of pig-to-baboon cardiac transplants after cobra venom factor therapy. Transplantation 1997; 64:1255–1261.
46. Mohiuddin M, Kline G, Shen Z, Ruggiero V, Rostami S, DiSesa VJ. Experiments in cardiac xenotransplantation. Response to intrathymic xenogeneic cells and intravenous cobra venom factor. J Thorac Cardiovasc Surg 1993; 106:632–635.
47. Taniguchi S, Kobayashi T, Neethling FA, et al. Cobra venom factor stimulates anti-alpha-galactose antibody production in baboons. Implications for pig-to-human xenotransplantation. Transplantation 1996; 62:678–681.
48. Pruitt SK, Kirk AD, Bollinger RR, et al. The effect of soluble complement receptor type 1 on hyperacute rejection of porcine xenografts. Transplantation 1994; 57:363–370.
49. Heckl-Ostreicher B, Wosnik A, Kirschfink M. Protection of porcine endothelial cells from complement-mediated cytotoxicity by the human complement regulators CD59, C1 inhibitor, and soluble complement receptor type 1. Analysis in a pig-to-human in vitro model relevant to hyperacute xenograft rejection. Transplantation 1996; 62:1693–1696.
50. Davis EA, Pruitt SK, Greene PS, et al. Inhibition of complement, evoked antibody, and cellular response prevents rejection of pig-to-primate cardiac xenografts. Transplantation 1996; 62:1018–1023.
51. Cooper DK, Ye Y, Niekrasz M, et al. Specific intravenous carbohydrate therapy. A new concept in inhibiting antibody-mediated rejection—experience with ABO-incompatible cardiac allografting in the baboon. Transplantation 1993; 56:769–777.
52. Cairns T, Lee J, Goldberg L, et al. Inhibition of the pig to human xenograft reaction, using soluble Gal alpha 1–3Gal and Gal alpha 1–3Gal beta 1–4GlcNAc. Transplantation 1995; 60:1202–1207.
53. Li SF, Neethling FA, Taniguchi S, et al. Glycans derived from porcine stomach mucin are effective inhibitors of natural anti-alpha-galactosyl antibodies in vitro and after intravenous infusion in baboons. Transplantation 1996; 62:1324–1331.
54. Sandrin MS, Fodor WL, Mouhtouris E, et al. Enzymatic remodelling of the carbohydrate surface of a xenogenic cell substantially reduces human antibody binding and complement-mediated cytolysis (see comments). Nat Med 1995; 1:1261–1267.
55. Koren E, Milotic F, Neethling FA, et al. Monoclonal antiidiotypic antibodies neutralize cytotoxic effects of anti-alphaGal antibodies. Transplantation 1996; 62:837–843.
56. Kroshus TJ, Rollins SA, Dalmasso AP, et al. Complement inhibition with an anti-C5 monoclonal antibody prevents acute cardiac tissue injury in an ex vivo model of pig-to-human xenotransplantation. Transplantation 1995; 60:1194–1202.
57. McCurry K, Kooyman D, Diamond L, Byrne G, Logan J, Platt J. Transgenic expression of human complement regulatory proteins in mice results in diminished complement deposition during organ xenoperfusion. Transplantation 1995; 59:1177.

58. McCurry KR, Kooyman DL, Alvarado CG, et al. Human complement regulatory proteins protect swine-to-primate cardiac xenografts from humoral injury (see comments). Nat Med 1995; 1:423–427.

59. Byrne GW, McCurry KR, Martin MJ, McClellan SM, Platt JL, Logan JS. Transgenic pigs expressing human CD59 and decay-accelerating factor produce an intrinsic barrier to complement-mediated damage. Transplantation 1997; 63:149–155.

60. Chen RH, Naficy S, Logan JS, Diamond LE, and Adams DH. Hearts from transgenic pigs constructed with CD59/DAF genomic clones demonstrate improved survival in primates. Xenotransplantation 1999; 6:194–200.

61. Schmoeckel M, Bhatti FN, Zaidi A, et al. Orthotopic heart transplantation in a transgenic pig-to-primate model. Transplantation 1998; 65:1570–1577.

62. Zaidi A, Schmoeckel M, Bhatti F, et al. Life-supporting pig-to-primate renal xenotransplantation using genetically modified donors. Transplantation 1998; 65:1584–1590.

63. Dorling A, Riesbeck K, Warrens A, Lechler R. Clinical xenotransplantation of solid organs. Lancet 1997; 349:867–871.

V VASCULAR DISEASE IN MODELS OF ARTERIAL HYPERTENSION

18 Methods for Examining Cerebrovascular Disease in Experimental Models of Hypertension

Gary L. Baumbach, MD

INTRODUCTION

Chronic hypertension alters several characteristics of the cerebral circulation. Diameter of cerebral vessels is reduced, (1,2) autoregulation of cerebral blood flow is shifted to a higher range of blood pressure, (3–6) and responses of cerebral vessels to dilator stimuli are diminished (3,7). Associated with these alterations are important changes in structural and mechanical characteristics of the vessel wall. At the time we began our studies of cerebral blood vessels 15 yr ago, many of the concepts regarding effects of chronic hypertension on cerebral vascular structure and mechanics were based on findings in large arteries. Thus, a major focus of our laboratory from its inception has been to increase our understanding of these structural and mechanical alterations at the arteriolar level of cerebral circulation.

The purpose of this chapter is to consider some of the methods that we have used to examine the effects of chronic hypertension on cerebral blood vessels. The main body of this chapter is divided into three sections and each focuses on a method that has permitted us to define and further explore several new con-

From: *Contemporary Cardiology: Vascular Disease and Injury: Preclinical Research*
Edited by: D. I. Simon and C. Rogers © Humana Press Inc., Totowa, NJ

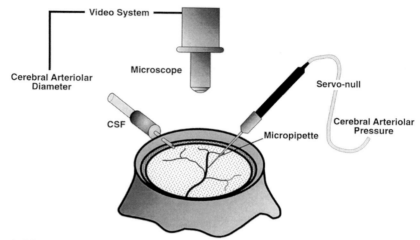

Fig. 1. Measurement of Cerebral Arteriolar Pressure and Diameter. The brain is exposed through a craniotomy. Physiological conditions are maintained by suffusing the brain surface with artificial CSF. Pressure is measured in cerebral arterioles on the brain surface through a micropipette attached to a servo-null pressure-measuring device. Diameter of cerebral arterioles is measured through a video microscope. We emphasize that the servo-null system allows for accurate measurements of pulse pressure as well as mean pressure.

cepts. The three sections are (1) the *servo-null system* for measuring pressure in cerebral arterioles, (2) the *unilateral carotid ligation* method for lowering arterial pressure to one side of the brain, and (3) the *arteriovenous (AV) fistula* method for selectively increasing pulse pressure to cerebral blood vessels. Each section begins by considering the rationale that led to our adaptation and development of a particular method. These introductory remarks are followed by a description of the method with an emphasis on previously unpublished details that are often crucial to successful implementation of the method. Finally, each section concludes with a brief discussion of the new concepts that have resulted from the method.

THE SERVO-NULL SYSTEM

We performed our initial studies of effects of chronic hypertension on mechanics and composition of cerebral arterioles in the mid-1980s. Many of the prevailing theories regarding effects of chronic hypertension on cerebral vascular mechanics at this time were based on findings in large arteries. We postulated, however, that effects of chronic hypertension on vascular mechanics probably vary with vessel size. This supposition was based on the observations that pressure during chronic hypertension is less in cerebral arterioles than in large arteries, *(2,8)* and that composition of the arterial wall varies with vessel size *(9)*.

Our ability to pursue studies of cerebral vascular mechanics at the level of arterioles in their in vivo state was greatly enhanced by the introduction of the servo-null pressure measuring system into our laboratory. The basic parameters of the method we use to measure pressure and diameter in cerebral arterioles on the surface of the brain are shown in Fig. 1. The concept for using a servo-null system for measuring pressure in the microvasculature was developed and put into practice over 30 yr ago by Curt Wiederhielm *(10)*. Modifications in the early 1970s by Marcos Intaglietta *(11)* and Benjamin Zweifach *(12)* made the servo-null pressure measuring system more reliable, and contributed to development of a commercially available system through Instruments for Medicine and Physiology (IMP), Inc. Unfortunately, IPM went out of business several years ago. Recently, however, Vista Electronics (23461 Vista Vicente Way, Ramona, CA 92065) purchased the inventory of IPM, and now makes an updated version of the system.

Before measuring pressure and diameter in cerebral arterioles on the surface of the brain, it is necessary to create a craniotomy. Although we have previously published many of the basics of craniotomies in rats, *(13,14)* there are still some important details that have not yet appeared in print. Two of the more important ones are minimization of brain swelling and opening the dura without significant injury to the brain surface.

We discovered early in our studies that the brain would often swell to the point of pronounced extrusion of cerebral tissue above the craniotomy opening shortly after completion of a craniotomy. We initially assumed that brain swelling was related to overheating of the skull during the drilling process used to create the craniotomy. However, the problem persisted—although not as pronounced—even after doubling the amount of high-pressure air used to cool the drilling site. With additional experimentation, we discovered that brain swelling is essentially eliminated by firmly securing the rat's head in the stereotactic head holder. The ear bars that are used to hold the head in place should be tightened until absolutely no back-and-forth movement of the head can be detected in the coronal plane. We postulate that any head movement during drilling translates to brain tissue in the form of vibrational energy, and results in a traumatic form of brain injury with subsequent edema.

The first difficulty encountered when opening the dura is to grasp the dura to make the opening without bruising the underlying brain. One might assume that this could be accomplished with a fine-tip forceps and a fine-spring scissors. A much easier and more reliable method is to use a fine-gauge needle with its tip bent to an angle of approx 45° (Fig. 2). The dura can be snagged, lifted, and opened with the tip of the bent needle in one motion with no force applied to the underlying brain.

Once the dura is opened, the next problem that usually arises is bleeding from the cut ends of dural-based blood vessels. The extent of bleeding can be

Before   **After**

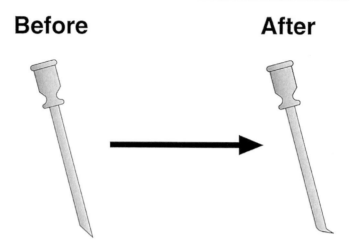

Fig. 2. Illustration of needle used to open dura. The tip of the needle is bent to an angle of about 30–45° using a forceps. The bent tip is used to snag the surface of the dura. After the dura is snagged, it can be lifted to allow penetration of the dura with the needle tip without disturbing the brain surface. The initial opening in the dura can then be easily extended with the needle.

limited by opening only the dura immediately over the vessels of interest. Nevertheless, one is often forced to cut through a dural vessel to achieve optimal exposure. When bleeding does become a problem, it is inadvisable to cauterize cut vessels either electrically or chemically, because irreversible damage to the underlying brain invariably ensues. The best way to stop the bleeding without damage to the brain is to grasp the cut vessel with a fine-tip forceps for a period of several min. Of course, this approach requires a steady hand and considerable patience.

With respect to measuring pressure in arterioles with the servo-null system, a number of factors contribute to its successful implementation. Most of these factors are related to the production, filling, and manipulation of the micropipettes. The hardware side of the system is surprisingly straightforward to use, and has provided years of reliable, trouble-free service.

The production of good pipets involves a number of steps. The first step uses a pipet puller (e.g., model 700, David Kopf Instruments) to produce a gradually tapered tip on one end with an inner diameter of less than 3 μm. Because the shape of the tip is not optimal for penetration of a blood vessel, the next step is to bevel the pipet tip. We use a micromanipulator to position the pipet tip on a beveler (e.g., model 1300M, World Precision Instruments). All aspects of the process are monitored at a high level of magnification, using a stereomicroscope. Because optimal beveling requires a thin layer of water on the beveling surface, foreign material mixed into the water is introduced into the micropipet by way of capillary action. To prevent clogging of the tip, we force air through the pipet as the tip is lifted from the beveling surface. As the last step in the process, we examine each pipet under a compound light microscope at moderate levels of magnification (about 100 ×) to ensure that we have achieved an adequate inner diameter (3–5 μm), a smooth beveled end, and an optimal taper.

Once you have created the optimal pipet, the next challenge is to fill it with hypertonic saline (usually 1.5M). One option is to insert the untapered end of the pipet into PE 50 polyethylene tubing that is attached to a syringe filled with hypertonic saline and force-fill the pipet by applying the appropriate amount of pressure to the syringe plunger. This approach is prone to the problem of introducing foreign debris into the tapered end, which often results in trapping of air bubbles in the tip and suboptimal resistance characteristics. We have recently adopted another option that utilizes borosilicate glass capillary tubes with a solid filament attached to the inner wall (catalog # M1B100F-3, World Precision Instruments, Sarasota, FL). Micropipets made from this tubing are filled in two stages. The first stage consists of placing the nontapered end of the pipet into a pool of saline. The saline is drawn into the opposite tapered end by capillary action of the filament. Once the tapered end is filled, the next stage is to back-fill the rest of the pipet using a 34-gauge MicroFil nonmetallic syringe needle (catalog #MF34G World Precision Instruments, Sarasota, FL) designed especially for this purpose. We have found that this method for filling micropipettes greatly reduces problems with foreign debris and air bubbles in the pipet tip.

After filling and calibrating the micropipet, the next challenge is to insert the pipet tip into an arteriole. The key to successful insertion depends primarily on the ability to visualize and control the pipet tip. Visualization is best accomplished using a high-quality stereomicroscope interfaced with a good video imaging system. We have found that it often is easier to visualize the pipet on the video monitor than through the oculars. Success with pipet insertion also is enhanced by a stereomicroscope with a relatively long working distance. For a compound microscope objective, a working distance of 1.5 cm or greater is ideal, whereas a working distance of at least 2.5 cm is required for a stereomicroscope objective. The working distance between the microscope objective, and the craniotomy site determines the insertion angle of the micropipet. If the insertion angle is too shallow, it may not be possible to bring the pipet tip down to the level of the brain surface before hitting the edge of the craniotomy, thus deflecting the pipet and making insertion impossible.

Control of the pipet tip requires a precise, high-quality micromanipulator on a stable, solid working surface. We have always used a Leitz micromanipulator (Type M) with good success. Characteristics that we believe to be desirable in a micromanipulator include precise control in all three primary axes, particularly in the z-axis. Another desirable feature in a micromanipulator is the ability to control the pipet in the x- and y-axes through a joy-stick type of mechanism. Joy-stick control enables precise, rapid positioning of the pipet during pipet insertion and during movements of the brain after the pipet is inserted.

In studies of vascular mechanics, pressure-diameter relationships are obtained during deactivation of smooth muscle with ethylenediaminetetraacetic acid (EDTA). We have shown that suffusion of cerebral arterioles with artificial CSF containing EDTA (25 mg/mL) produces maximal dilatation of cerebral arterioles *(13)*. Arteriolar pressure is reduced in 10-mmHg increments using controlled hemorrhage to reduce arterial pressure. After each pressure step, arteriolar diameter is permitted to achieve a steady state prior to measuring diameter. Circumferential wall stress, strain, and incremental elastic modulus are calculated from measurements of arteriolar pressure, diameter, and cross-sectional area of the vessel wall (measured histologically) *(13)*.

The method we have used to examine mechanical characteristics in cerebral arterioles takes several factors into consideration that may compromise our calculations of stress and strain in the arteriolar wall. These factors include effectiveness of deactivation of vascular smooth muscle, compressibility of the vessel wall during changes in pressure and diameter, and determination of original diameter. Detailed considerations of these factors, published previously, *(13)* will not be discussed here except for the issue of original diameter.

A possible limitation in our calculation of circumferential wall stress is that diameter of cerebral arterioles cannot be measured reliably at 0 mmHg of arteriolar pressure. Circumferential strain (ε) is calculated as $\varepsilon = (D_i - D_o)/D_o$, where D_i is internal diameter and D_o is original diameter. Ideally, original diameter should be measured at 0 mmHg intravascular pressure. Unfortunately, diameter of cerebral arterioles cannot be measured reliably at 0 mmHg under in vivo conditions. If the pressure-diameter relationship of deactivated cerebral arterioles at pressures above 10 mmHg is not representative of the pressure-diameter relationship between 0 and 10 mmHg of pressure, then the stress-strain relationship of cerebral arterioles could be very different, depending on whether original diameter is defined as diameter at 10 or 0 mmHg of pressure. To address this possibility, we have estimated diameter of cerebral arterioles at 0 mmHg of pressure by fitting our measurements of pressure and diameter to a third-order polynomial equation. Substitution of original diameter estimated at 0 mmHg for original diameter measured at 10 mmHg of pressure in the calculation of strain does not significantly alter our findings in normotensive and hypertensive arterioles.

In one of the first studies in which we utilized the servo-null system, we examined the effect of chronic hypertension on mechanical characteristics of cerebral arterioles in vivo *(13)*. Inner diameter of first-order cerebral arterioles before and during maximal dilatation was 23% and 11% smaller in SHRSP than WKY, respectively. Wall thickness and cross-sectional area of maximally dilated arterioles were 53 and 29% greater in SHRSP than in WKY. Thus, there was hypertrophy and a reduction in maximal dilator capacity of cerebral arterioles with chronic hypertension.

Incremental distensibility of cerebral arterioles that were maximally dilated was greater in SHRSP than in WKY for cerebral arteriolar pressures between 30 and 70 mmHg. In addition, the stress-strain curve in SHRSP was shifted to the right of the curve in WKY, which also indicates that distensibility of maximally dilated cerebral arterioles is greater in SHRSP than WKY. Thus, in contrast to large cerebral vessels, which become less distensible in chronic hypertension, (1,15–17) our findings suggest a paradoxical increase in distensibility of cerebral arterioles during chronic hypertension, despite hypertrophy of the arteriolar wall.

It is apparent from our findings that the reduction in maximal dilatation of cerebral arterioles in chronic hypertension cannot be explained by alterations in distensibility. An alternative explanation is that hypertrophy of the arteriolar wall produces enough encroachment on the vascular lumen to counteract the increase in distensibility, thus reducing inner diameter even during maximal dilatation. Based on this hypothesis, the outer diameter of cerebral arterioles would be expected to be similar in SHRSP and WKY, provided that encroachment is the sole cause of impaired maximal dilatation. We therefore calculated the outer diameter of cerebral arterioles from measurements of inner diameter and cross-sectional area, and found that outer diameter of cerebral arterioles was significantly smaller in SHRSP than in WKY. Thus, outer and inner diameter of cerebral arterioles is reduced in chronic hypertension. Therefore, encroachment on the vascular lm does not account entirely for reduced maximal dilator capacity.

We have proposed another alternative to explain the reduction in maximal dilator capacity of cerebral arterioles. During chronic hypertension, cerebral arterioles may undergo structural changes which result in remodeling of the arteriolar wall and a smaller total circumference. Two of the possible mechanisms of remodeling that might lead to a reduction in total circumference of cerebral arterioles in chronic hypertension are a decrease in the length of individual smooth-muscle-cells (SMCs) without an increase in cell number, and/or a decrease in the number of times each SMC wraps around the arteriole.

UNILATERAL CAROTID LIGATION

A major focus of our research has been to define determinants of cerebral vascular hypertrophy. Determinants of vascular hypertrophy during chronic hypertension appear to include increases in pressure, (18,19) neurohumoral fac-

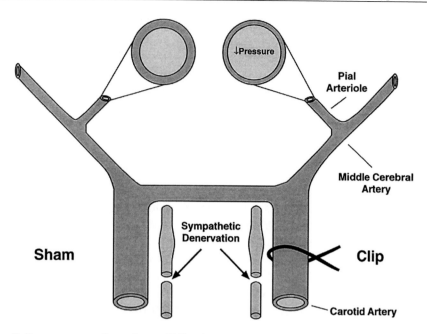

Fig. 3. Response to unilateral carotid ligation. A clip is placed on one carotid to occlude the vascular lumen. To eliminate neural effects, we cut both both sympathetic nerves. We anticipated that pressure in pial arterioles ipsilateral to the clip would be lower than on the sham-operated side. If increases in pressure contribute to hypertrophy, we would expect hypertrophy to be reduced on the clipped side. If, on the other hand, humoral or genetic factors were more important than pressure, hypertrophy might be the same on the two sides.

tors, *(14,20–22)* and genetic factors *(23,24)*. Of these, one might assume that arterial pressure *per se* would play an especially important role in hypertrophy. Despite numerous efforts, however, the role of arterial pressure has been difficult to elucidate. One of the methods that we have found particularly useful in this regard is unilateral carotid ligation.

Inspiration for ligation of the carotid artery came from Bjorn Folkow's work in which ligation was used in a hindlimb preparation. Using this approach in the hindlimb cat, Folkow and Sivertsson *(25)* found that ligation of femoral and epigastric arteries reduced arterial pressure in hindlimb by 30–40 mmHg and resulted in a reduction of both wall-to-lumen ratio and tissue mass in arteries distal to the ligation. This finding suggests that the level of intravascular pressure may be a determinant of mass of the vessel wall during normotension.

The goal of carotid ligation is to lower intravascular pressure in cerebral arterioles of one cerebral hemisphere while maintaining the same conditions in both hemispheres with respect to neural and humoral regulation of cerebral blood vessels (Fig.3). Carotid arteries are exposed through a midline incision in the neck. A clip designed to completely occlude the vascular lm is placed on one common carotid artery. Clips with a gap size of about 0.1 mm are made from 1-mm wide strips of silver sheet. Because sympathetic nerves modulate structure and mechanics of cerebral arterioles, *(14)* and because of the close proximity of the internal carotid artery and sympathetic nerves, one cannot rule out the possibility that the carotid clip, or fibrosis induced by the clip, might damage sympathetic nerves and thus alter structure of cerebral arterioles independently of reductions in cerebral arteriolar pressure. To ensure that cerebral arterioles in both cerebral hemispheres are exposed to the same level of sympathetic input during the interval between placement of the carotid clip and examination of arteriolar mechanics and composition, we remove the superior cervical ganglia on both sides at the time of carotid ligation. To control for the possibility that the clip may influence other neurohumoral factors, such as parasympathetic nerves, a clip adjusted to avoid luminal deformation is placed around the carotid artery on the sham-operated side.

Using this approach, we have found that carotid ligation in SHRSP prevents hypertrophy of cerebral arterioles and normalizes arteriolar pulse pressure, but not mean pressure *(26)*. There also is a strong correlation between cross-sectional area and pulse pressure, but not systolic or mean pressure, in sham and ligated cerebral arterioles of normotensive Wistar Kyoto rats (WKY) and SHRSP *(26)*. These findings suggest that pulse pressure, but *not* mean pressure, is an important determinant of cerebral vascular hypertrophy during chronic hypertension. The findings are not conclusive, because carotid ligation in SHRSP does not fully normalize cerebral arteriolar mean pressure. Another interpretation of the findings is that hypertrophy of cerebral arterioles in SHRSP does not occur until cerebral arteriolar pressure exceeds a critical threshold lower than pressures normally found in SHRSP, but higher than pressures normally found in WKY. Thus, even though cerebral arteriolar mean pressure is not normalized by carotid ligation in SHRSP, it may have been reduced sufficiently to prevent hypertrophy of cerebral arterioles.

In another study in which unilateral carotid ligation proved useful, we have found that treatment of Sprague-Dawley rats with N^G-nitro-L-arginine methyl ester (L-NAME)—an inhibitor of nitric oxide (NO) synthase—results in hypertrophy of cerebral arterioles *(27)*. Unilateral carotid ligation does not attenuate hypertrophy of cerebral arterioles in L-NAME-treated rats, although arteriolar mean pressure is attenuated and pulse pressure is normalized. These findings suggest that NO may be a determinant of cerebral vascular hypertrophy during chronic hypertension. The findings have alternative interpretations, however, because L-NAME may have indirect effects in addition to suppression of NO production, such as altered production of endothelin *(28)* and increased activity of the renin-angiotensin system *(29–31)*.

Before   **After**

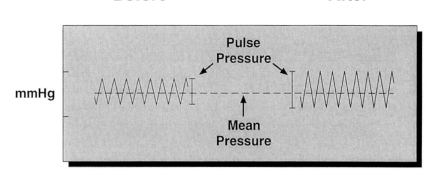

Fig. 4. Response of arterial pressure to A-V fistula. These are hypothetical tracings of arterial pressure before and at some point after the creation of an A–V fistula. We anticipated that that an A-V fistula would lead to an increase in systolic pressure and at the same time a decrease in diastolic pressure. Because pulse pressure is the difference between systolic and diastolic pressure—and because mean pressure is equal to diastolic pressure plus one-third of pulse pressure—it seemed likely that these changes would result in an increase in pulse pressure without an increase in mean pressure.

ARTERIOVENOUS FISTULA

A major conclusion from our unilateral carotid ligation study in SHRSP *(26)* was the possibility that pulse pressure is an important determinant of vascular hypertrophy during chronic hypertension. The findings were not conclusive, because mean pressure was also reduced by ligation. Our goal therefore was to find a method that would allow us to test the hypothesis that increases in pulse pressure, even in the absence of increases in mean pressure, produce hypertrophy of cerebral arterioles.

We adapted the aorto-caval arteriovenous (AV) fistula model *(32)* to accomplish our goal based on the previous finding that aorto-caval fistulae in Sprague-Dawley rats increases pulse pressure in the carotid artery without increasing mean pressure *(33,34)*. The concept of how AV fistulae lead to increases in pulse pressure is shown in Fig. 4. We utilized the unilateral carotid ligation method to address the concern that AV fistulae may activate other trophic factors in addition to pulse pressure, such as neurohumoral factors.

Fig. 5 illustrates the approach to creating an aorto-caval fistula. The abdominal aorta and inferior vena cava are isolated at the level of the right iliolumbar vein through an incision in the right flank. After cross-clamping the aorta and vena cava proximal and distal to their bifurcation, a venotomy is performed through the right lateral aspect of the vena cava. The aorta then is penetrated transcavally with a 25-gauge needle. The transcaval opening is enlarged to 1.0 mm in diameter using microscissors. We have chosen a 1.0-mm opening be-

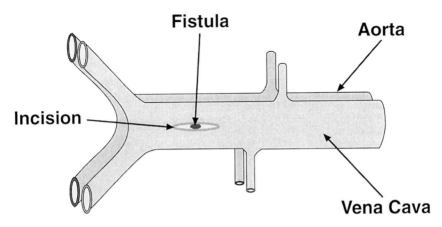

Fig. 5. Aorto-caval A-V fistula. An incision is made in the ventral aspect of the inferior vena cava to expose the common wall between the vena cava and the abdominal aorta. We then create the fistula by making a defect in the common wall between the dorsal aspect of the vena cava and the ventral aspect of aorta. The size of the defect is about 1 mm in diameter.

cause Glassford et al. *(34)* have shown that a 1.0-mm fistula between the abdominal aorta and vena cava results in a large increase in pulse pressure without altering mean arterial pressure in carotid artery. After irrigation of the opened aorta and vena cava to remove thrombogenic material, the venotomy is closed with 10–0 nylon.

AV fistulae resulted in hypertrophy and increases in pulse pressure, but not mean pressure, in cerebral arterioles of Sprague-Dawley rats *(32)*. In addition, both hypertrophy and increases in pulse pressure were prevented by carotid ligation. These findings provide strong evidence, therefore, that increases in pulse pressure—even in the absence of increases in mean pressure—are sufficient to produce hypertrophy of cerebral arterioles.

One consideration with respect to the AV fistula method is the period of time between creation of AV fistulae and examination of cerebral arterioles. Hypertrophy of left ventricle and aorta occurs within 3–9 d following induction of aortic coarctation in rats *(35)*. In our study, effects of AV fistula on structure of cerebral arterioles were not examined until 5 mo after fistulae were created. One might speculate, therefore, that the time between creation of AV fistulae and induction of cerebral arteriolar hypertrophy may be substantially less than the time between fistula creation and examination of cerebral arterioles. If so, one could further speculate that pulse pressure may not be the controlling variable with respect to induction of cerebral arteriolar hypertrophy by AV fistulae. We cannot rule out this possibility, because we have not determined the time required to develop cerebral arteriolar hypertrophy after fistula creation. On the

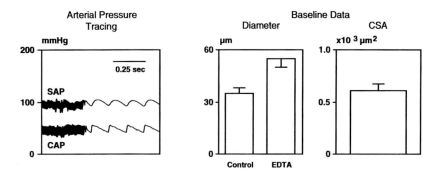

Fig. 6. Pressure, diameter and cross-sectional area of cerebral arterioles in Swiss-Webster mice. A representative tracing of arterial pressure in femoral artery (SAP) and cerebral arteriole (CAP) of a mouse (*left*). Diameter of cerebral arterioles of mice before (control) and during maximal dilatation with EDTA (*middle*). Cross-sectional area of the vessel wall (CSA; measured histologically) of mice cerebral arterioles (*right*).

other hand, it is likely that cerebral arteriolar pulse pressure is increased simultaneously with creation of AV fistulae, or shortly thereafter. It would thus be possible for increases in pulse pressure to induce, as well as maintain, cerebral arteriolar hypertrophy in AV fistulae rats.

FUTURE DIRECTIONS

One of the most promising directions we are pursuing for the future is the use of genetically altered mice to further clarify mechanisms of altered cerebral vascular structure in chronic hypertension. To determine feasibility of adapting in vivo and morphometric methods that were developed originally in rats to examine mechanics and composition of cerebral arterioles in mice, we measured intravascular pressure (servo-null), diameter, and cross-sectional area of the vessel wall (CSA) in fourth-order branches of the anterior cerebral artery (counted from origin) in anesthetized, ventilated Swiss-Webster mice. We have obtained measurements of cerebral arteriolar pressure, including pulse pressure (demonstrated in representative recording in Fig. 6), in 40 mice. Pressure in cerebral arterioles was about 45–50% of systemic arterial pressure (100–110 mmHg). Pulse pressure in cerebral arterioles of mice was about 10–15 mmHg, which is similar to pulse pressure in cerebral arterioles of rats. Suffusion of cerebral arterioles with EDTA (to produce maximal dilatation) resulted in a 70% increase in internal diameter (Fig. 6).

Cross-sectional area of the arteriolar wall in mice was about 50% of cross-sectional area typically found in normotensive rats. These findings indicate that fourth-order cerebral arterioles in normotensive mice are about one-half the size of fourth-order cerebral arterioles in normotensive rats, even though arteriolar mean and pulse pressures are approximately the same in the two groups.

The findings also demonstrate the feasibility of using in vivo and morphometric methods to examine structural characteristics of cerebral arterioles in mice as well as in rats.

ACKNOWLEDGMENT

Original studies by the author described in this chapter were supported by funds from National Institutes of Health Grants HL-22149, NS-24621, and HL94–006. I also wish to acknowledge Jay Siems and Shams Ghoniem for their technical assistance in carrying out many of these studies.

REFERENCES

1. Brayden JE, Halpern W, Brann LR. Biochemical and mechanical properties of resistance arteries from normotensive and hypertensive rats. Hypertension 1983; 5:17–25.
2. Harper SL, Bohlen HG. Microvascular adaptation in the cerebral cortex of adult spontaneously hypertensive rats. Hypertension 1984; 6:408–419.
3. Fujishima M, Sadoshima S, Ogata J, Yoshida F, Shiokawa O, Ibayashi S, et al. Autoregulation of cerebral blood flow in young and aged spontaneously hypertensive rats (SHR). Gerontology 1984; 30:30–36.
4. Jones JV, Fitch W, MacKenzie ET, Strandgaard S, Harper AM. Lower limit of cerebral blood flow autoregulation in experimental renovascular hypertension in the baboon. Circ Res 1976; 39:555–557.
5. Strandgaard S, Jones JV, MacKenzie ET, Harper AM. Upper limit of cerebral blood flow autoregulation in experimental renovascular hypertension in the baboon. Circ Res 1975; 37:164–167.
6. Strandgaard S, Olesen J, Skinhoj E, Lassen NA. Autoregulation of brain circulation in severe arterial hypertension. Br Med J 1973; 1:507–510.
7. Sadoshima S, Busija DW, Heistad DD. Mechanisms of protection against stroke in stroke-prone spontaneously hypertensive rats. Am J Physiol 1983; 244:H406–H412.
8. Werber AH, Heistad DD. Effects of chronic hypertension and sympathetic nerves on the cerebral microvasculature of stroke-prone spontaneously hypertensive rats. Circ Res 1984; 55:286–294.
9. Milnor WR. Hemodynamics. Williams and Wilkins, Baltimore, 1982, pp. 80–84.
10. Wiederhielm CA, Woodbury JW, Kirk S, Rushmer RF. Pulsatile pressures in the microcirculation of frog's mesentery. Am J Physiol 1964; 207:173–176.
11. Intaglietta M, Pawula LRF, Tompkins WR. Pressure measurements in the mammalian microvasculature. Microvasc Res 1970; 2:212–220.
12. Zweifach BW. Quantitative studies of microcirculatory structure and function. I. Analysis of pressure distribution in the terminal vascular bed in cat mesentery. Circ Res 1974; 34:843–857.
13. Baumbach GL, Dobrin PB, Hart MN, Heistad DD. Mechanics of cerebral arterioles in hypertensive rats. Circ Res 1988; 62:56–64.
14. Baumbach GL, Heistad DD, Siems JE. Effect of sympathetic nerves on composition and distensibility of cerebral arterioles in rats. J Physiol (London) 1989; 416:123–140.
15. Toda N, Okunishi H, Miyazaki M. Length-passive tension relationships in cerebral and peripheral arteries isolated from spontaneously hypertensive and normotensive rats. Jpn Circ J 1982; 46:1088–1094.

16. Toda N, Hayashi S, Miyazaki M. Length-tension relationship of cerebral and peripheral arteries isolated from normotensive and spontaneously hypertensive rats. Jpn Heart J 1979; (Suppl 1)20:255–257.

17. Winquist RJ, Bohr DF. Structural and functional changes in cerebral arteries from spontaneously hypertensive rats. Hypertension 1983; 5:292–297.

18. Weiss L, Hallbäck M. Time course and extent of structural vascular adaptation to regional hypotension in adult spontaneously hypertensive rats (SHR). Acta Physiol Scand 1974; 91:365–373.

19. Folkow B, Gurevich M, Hallbäck M, Lundgren Y, Weiss L. The hemodynamic consequences of regional hypotension in spontaneously hypertensive and normotensive rats. Acta Physiol Scand 1971; 83:532–541.

20. Hart MN, Heistad DD, Brody MJ. Effect of chronic hypertension and sympathetic denervation on wall/lumen ratio of cerebral vessels. Hypertension 1980; 2:419–423.

21. Owens GK, Geisterfer AAT, Yang YW-H, Komoriya A. Transforming growth factor-?-induced growth inhibition and cellular hypertrophy in cultured vascular smooth muscle cells. J Cell Biol 1988; 107:771–780.

22. Geisterfer AAT, Peach MJ, Owens GK. Angiotensin II induces hypertrophy, not hyperplasia, of cultured rat aortic smooth muscle cells. Circ Res 1988; 62:749–756.

23. Lee RMKW. Vascular changes at the prehypertensive phase in the mesenteric arteries from spontaneously hypertensive rats. Blood Vessels 1985; 22:105–126.

24. Eccleston-Joyner CA, Gray SD. Arterial hypertrophy in the fetal and neonatal spontaneously hypertensive rat. Hypertension 1988; 12:513–518.

25. Folkow B, Sivertsson R. Adaptive changes in "reactivity" and wall/lumen ratio in cat blood vessels exposed to prolonged transmural pressure difference. Life Sci 1968; 7:1283–1289.

26. Baumbach GL, Siems JE, Heistad DD. Effects of local reduction in pressure on distensibility and composition of cerebral arterioles. Circ Res 1991; 68:338–351.

27. Chillon JM, Ghoneim S, Baumbach GL. Effects of nitric oxide inhibition on mechanics of cerebral arterioles in rats. Hypertension 1997; 30:1097–1104.

28. Sventek P, Li JS, Grove K, Deschepper CF, Schiffrin EL. Vascular structure and expression of endothelin-1 gene in L-NAME-treated spontaneously hypertensive rats. Hypertension 1996; 27:49–55.

29. Kumagai H, Averill DB, Khosla MC, Ferrario CM. Role of nitric oxide and angiotensin II in the regulation of sympathetic nerve activity in spontaneously hypertensive rats. Hypertension 1993; 21:476–484.

30. Jover B, Herizi A, Ventre F, Dupont M, Mimran A. Sodium and angiotensin in hypertension induced by long-term nitric oxide blockade. Hypertension 1993; 21:944–948.

31. Ribeiro MO, Antunes E, de Nucci G, Lovisolo SM, Zatz R. Chronic inhibition of nitric oxide synthesis. A new model of arterial hypertension. Hypertension 1992; 20:298–303.

32. Baumbach GL. Effects of increased pulse pressure on cerebral arterioles. Hypertension 1996; 27:159–167.

33. Mickle J, Menges JT, Day AL, Quisling R, Ballinger W. Experimental aortocaval fistulae in rats. J Microsurg 1981; 2:283–288.

34. Glassford E, D'Silva M, Ghorab H, Bai S, Lee SU, Moossa AR, et al. Arterialization of the liver. II. Systemic pressure gradients in rats following variously sized arteriovenous fisulae. Microsurgery 1990; 11:177–183.

35. MacIver DH, Green NK, Gammage MD, Durkin H, Izzard AS, Franklyn JA. Effect of experimental hypertension on phosphoinositide hydrolysis and proto-oncogene expression in cardiovascular tissues. J Vasc Res 1993; 30:13–22.

19 Monocrotaline-Induced Pulmonary Hypertension in Rats

Marlene Rabinovitch, MD

CONTENTS

INTRODUCTION

Research has shown that certain seeds—the products of pyrolizidine alkaloids—can induce pulmonary vascular disease in animals. Calves that fed on these seeds developed right-sided congestive heart failure. The accumulation of nuchal edema explains the description of this condition as "brisket disease." Efforts have been made to reproduce this phenomenon in a variety of other species so that the evolution of the pulmonary vascular and hemodynamic changes could be studied in a laboratory setting. Of all the species tested, the laboratory rat appeared to be the most reliable, but even in the rat, age- and stain-related differences had to be considered. The male Sprague-Dawley rat, age 6–8 wk—obtained from Charles River supplier—is most commonly used. Our laboratory has unsuccessfully attempted to reproduce monocrotaline-induced pulmonary vascular disease in strains of obese and lean rats (JCR:LA-cp) (1). In this study, female Sprague-Dawley animals appear to be as responsive as males.

While a number of studies have used monocrotaline seeds—relying on the active hepatic metabolite monocrotaline pyrrole to induce the disease in animals—it has been more convenient to obtain the monocrotaline as a powder (Transworld Chemical, Rockville MD), which is dissolved and adminstered in a single 60 mg/kg subcutaneous dose. To prepare monocrotaline, 200 mg of the

From: *Contemporary Cardiology: Vascular Disease and Injury: Preclinical Research*
Edited by: D. I. Simon and C. Rogers © Humana Press Inc., Totowa, NJ

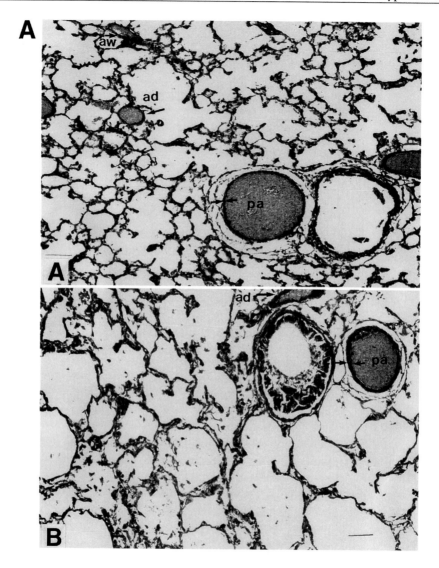

Fig. 1A. (**A**) Photomicrographs of neonatal lung. Photomicrograph of a lung-tissue section in a control neonatal rat 2 wk after saline injection. Observe muscular preacinar (pa) artery of normal wall thickness (arrows) and numerous nonmuscular alveolar duct and wall (ad,aw) arteries. Note normal proportion of alveoli and arteries in the field. (**B**) Photomicrograph of a lung-tissue section in a neonatal rat 2 wk after monocrotaline injection. Observe thick-walled preacinar (pa) artery (arrows) and abnormally muscular alveolar duct (ad) artery. Note few alveoli/mm2 and few arteries. (Bar = 50 μm, elastic Van Gieson stain. Reproduced with permission from ref. *(2)*.

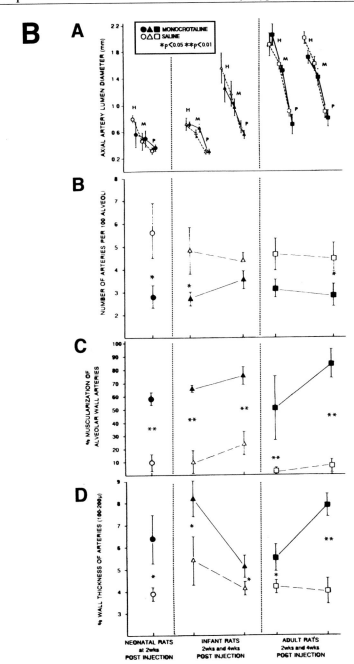

Fig. 1B. (A) Arterial size. Lumen diameter of the axial artery measured on the arteriogram at hilum (**H**), midlung (**M**, 50% from hilum), and periphery (P, 90% from periphery). The lower limit of artery diameter measured is 200M (0.2 mm). Monocrotaline does

crystalline compound is dissolved in 0.6 mL of normal HCl; 5 mL of distilled water are added, and the pH is adjusted to 7 with 0.5 N NaOH and diluted in a final volume of 10 mL. This method is reliable and it is extremely rare to find a nonresponder (less than 1 in 100). The age and weight of the animals, however, appear to be important *(2)*. Neonatal rats injected at 2 d of life develop emphysema and do not live beyond 2 wk of life. The toxin seems to interfere with lung development in this age group (Fig. 1). Curiously, infant rats injected at 2 wk develop disease with the pathologic severity seen in adult rats 2 wk after injection, but 4 wk after injection, the infant rats appear to show spontaneous regression of their lesions, whereas adult rats continue to have progressive disease. Beyond 8 wk of life (or in rats > 350 g), the monocrotaline appears to have less effect. The reasons why young animals regress spontaneously and old animals are relatively resistant to the effects of monocrotaline have not been fully addressed. In our studies, we showed a sustained increase in the activity of a serine elastase enzyme observed in the adult 6–8-wk-old rat, but no sustained increase in enzyme activity in the infant rat. We judge this to be a critical factor in the malignant vs benign pathophysiology *(3)*. The mechanism which leads elastase to induce pulmonary vascular changes of a malignant nature are described later in this chapter. The infant rats showing nonsustained elevation in elastase activity were similar to rats that had been subjected to chronic hypoxia in that all the changes were potentially reversible. In chronically hypoxic rats, increased elastase activity is only apparent at the initiation of the hypoxic exposure, and is not sustained with the development of structural changes.

Although it would be extremely advantageous to study the pathophysiology of monocrotaline-induced pulmonary hypertension in mice—given the opportunities for addressing mechanistic hypotheses through the use of transgenic animals—mice are relatively resistant to the effects of the toxin (M. Botney, personal communication). A diffuse pulmonary infiltrate is observed, but the vascular changes are extremely mild to minimal in nature. Monocrotaline pulmonary vascular disease has been reproduced in a variety of canine species, but not in sheep (H. O'Brodovich, personal communication).

---

not significantly affect artery size. Artery diameter doubles with increasing duration of the experiment in the infant group, but does not change in the adult group. **(B)** Arterial concentration relative to alveoli. A decreased concentration of arteries relative to alveoli is a feature of all monocrotaline-treated rats. In the infant group there is a trend toward a return to normal values 4 wk after the injection. **(C)** Extension of muscle. Extension of muscle into peripheral arteries—judged by an increased percentage of arteries at alveolar wall level—fully and partially muscularized is apparent in all monocrotaline-injected rats. **(D)** Medial hypertrophy. An increase in wall thickness of normally muscularized arteries is evident in all monocrotaline-injected rats. In the infant rats, medial hypertrophy regresses with increasing duration after the injection, whereas in the adult rats it increases. Reproduced with permission from ref. *(2)*.

HEMODYNAMIC ASSESSMENT

The reliability of monocrotaline-induced pulmonary vascular disease in rats has led to the development of a variety of techniques to study the progressive nature of pulmonary hypertension in these animals. We modified a technique to monitor pulmonary-artery pressure when the rats were awake and not under anesthesia *(4–12)*. This involved introducing a blunted 18-gauge needle as a sheath through the jugular vein beyond the right atrium into the right ventricle. The needle was fashioned in such a way that the tip was turned at a $30°$ angle, similar to a hockey stick. Fine Silastic tubing (0.32 mm-inner diameter, 0.65 mm-outer diameter) was fully heparinized, inserted into the introducer, and attached to a transducer (MS20 Electromedics, Englewood, CO) and electrostatic recorder (Gould, Cleveland, OH). Right ventricular pressure was monitored, and as the tip of the introducer was turned upwards towards the pulmonary outflow tract, the catheter was advanced about 1–2 cm. The entry of the catheter into the pulmonary artery was judged by the change in the contour of the pressure wave from right ventricular to a state compatible with the pulmonary artery, with an excellent phasic display of respiratory variation. The sheath could then be withdrawn and the catheter permanently fixed in the pulmonary artery for chronic monitoring. The end of the catheter was stretched, using ether over heavier polyethylene tubing (PE-20) which was then secured with sutures and exteriorized at the back of the neck to about 1–2 cm, heparinized, and plugged with a metal tip. The animals did not interfere with the catheter when it was at the back of their necks, and the procedure enabled us to monitor them daily in the awake condition reliably for 1–2 wk. This catheter also served as a source for drawing blood for a variety of determinations. In clinical use, Swann Ganz catheters will occasionally slip back into the right ventricle, but when the technique was well-practiced in the rats, this occurred in less than 10% of animals. It was most critical to maintain the catheter, flushing every few days with heparinized saline. We have not attempted to monitor animals beyond 2 wk using this technique, but it has nonetheless been helpful in monitoring the later stages of pulmonary hypertension, because the animals at that point are brittle and cannot tolerate the anesthetic procedure. For placement of the catheters, the animals are anesthetized with pentobarbital 33–45 mg/kg, and the anesthesia generally lasts about 2 h. The rats recover from the anesthetic and appear fully active within 24 h. A top up of half a dose of anesthetic is generally all that is necessary if any part of the procedure takes longer than $1^1/_2$ h.

We have monitored systemic-artery pressure in these animals as previously described *(5,12)*. Maintaining an indwelling carotid or descending abdominal aorta line permits easy monitoring of blood gases and pressure through the evolution of pulmonary vascular disease. The abdominal aortic catheter is introduced through a midline incision just above the iliac bifurcation. Polyethylene is used (1.09-mm-outer diameter and 0.32 mm-inner diameter), and the catheter is also exteriorized and tunnelled along the back of the animal to the base of the neck. We have also used left ventricular catheters to measure left ventricular end-disatolic pressures (8). The right carotid artery is isolated and ligated distally with 3–0 silk. A preformed polyenthelene catheter consisting of a 3.5-cm length of PE-10 melded to PE-20 is exteriorized, and the PE-10 part is introduced into the carotid artery and advanced until a left ventricular pressure tracing is obtained.

We have found that it is also possible to introduce a pulmonary-artery catheter through the right jugular vein, and another catheter through the left jugular vein for continuous infusion of a variety of different agents with a mini osmotic pump (11). It is advisable to wait a day between procedures, because we have found that the head of the animal can become suffused when both external jugular veins are simultaneously tied off. Thus, in response to monocrotaline, one can assess the effects of continuous infusion of iv medications by continuous measurement of pulmonary-artery pressures and saturations, cardiac output, and pulmonary vascular resistance, as well as the systemic arterial pressure and resistance. All these measurements can be made in the awake and unanesthetized animal.

For calculation of the cardiac output, we have also constructed chambers that have allowed us to measure oxygen consumption in rats using the Fick principle (7). The measurement of oxygen is done in a closed plexiglass chamber similar to a "space capsule." The catheters are exteriorized and air is circulated through the closed chamber at a flow rate of 2 L/min. Consumed oxygen is replaced from a Krogh spirometer filled with 100% oxygen saturated with water. The movement of the spirometer is recorded with a Sanborn carrier amplifier (350–2700) and a Mosely autograph recorder (680 M). The system is run, refilling the spirometer until a stable linear utilization of O_2 is achieved (about 5–10 min). The time required to consume 50 mL of O_2 is determined, and the rate of consumption is calculated, correcting the vol removed to STP. Cardiac index (CI) may be calculated as normalized per body wt according to the formula: $VO2/(SAO2–SVO2) \times Hg$ capacity. VO_2 = oxygen consumption, and $SAO_2\_SVO_2$ = difference between systemic arterial and venous saturations. The measurement of oxygen consumption permits better estimates of pulmonary vascular resistance (Rp): $Rp = (Ppa–Ppv)/CI$.

Animals usually begin to die 5–6 wk following injection of monocrotaline, or it becomes necessary to sacrifice them in accordance with recommendations of Animal Care Committees. The presumed etiology of their demise is right-sided congestive heart failure, as the animals at this point have ascites and hepatomegaly, more marked elevation in pulmonary-artery pressure, and increased pulmonary vascular resistance. Pulmonary-artery pressure values can be at systemic or near systemic levels, but are generally of the order of one-half

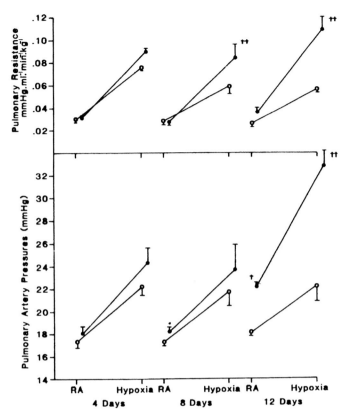

Fig. 2. Pulmonary artery pressure (P_{pa}) and pulmonary resistance (R_p) in room air (RA) and hypoxia ($10\%FIO_2 \times 10$ min) in groups studied 4, 8, and 12 d postinjection with monocrotaline (MC, l, $n = 6$) or normal saline (S, m, $n = 6$). Greater increase in R_p is seen in MC-injected animals at 8 and 12 d postinjection. A similar, greater increase in P_{pa} is seen only in 12–d group, a point at which RA pressure is also elevated. † Significantly different from S control at $p<0.05$.‡ Significantly different from S control at $p<0.01$. Reproduced with permission from ref. *(8)*.

to two-thirds systemic. The development of right heart failure in response to one-half or two-thirds systemic pulmonary-artery pressure may be related to the relative rapidity with which pulmonary hypertension develops. This may result in profound tricuspid-valve regurgitation. Although echocardiographic monitoring of parameters of ventricular function is possible, studies have not been conducted to assess these features.

In the hemodynamic evaluation of pulmonary hypertension following monocrotaline injection there is no evidence of heightened pulmonary vascular reactivity preceding the evolution of structural changes (Fig. 2). We have shown

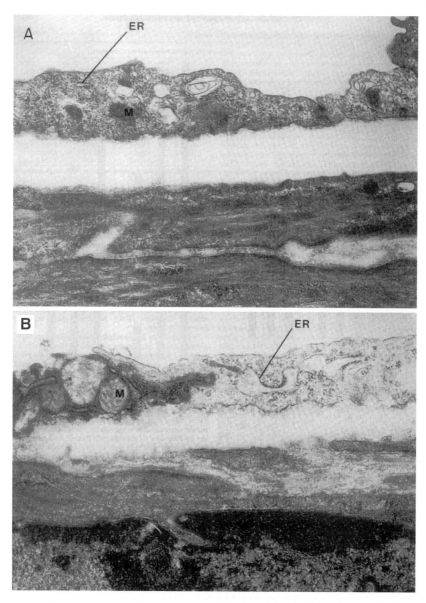

Fig. 3. Photomicrographs of small preacinar artery 4 d after injection with monocrotaline (**B**) or normal saline (**A**). Endothelium from monocrotaline-injected animals appears swollen and less dense. Note swollen mitochondria (M) and dilated endoplasmic reticulum (ER). Reproduced with permission from ref. *(8)*.

that pulmonary-artery pressure and resistance values are normal for the first wk after injection of the toxin monocrotaline. At the same time, reactivity to hypoxia or to norephinephrine does not differ from that in saline-injected (control) animals. We have shown endothelial injury as early as 4d after injection of the toxin, marked by cytoplasmic swelling and a decrease in the surface area of myofilaments (Fig. 3). Later evolution of muscularization of distal vessels occurs at about 8 d, and medial hypertrophy of muscular arteries at 12 d when pulmonary-artery pressure begins to rise. Elevation in pulmonary vascular resistance is a relatively late feature, suggesting that an increase in cardiac output accompanies the early elevation in pulmonary-artery pressure. Beginning from a mean pulmonary-artery pressure of 18–20 mmHg, by 2 wk after injection of the toxin, mean pulmonary-artery pressures are elevated to about 22 mmHg, and after 3 wk to about 35 mmHg. Mean pressures as high as 50 mmHg are seen at 4 wk after injection of the toxin. Mean systemic arterial pressures are generally unchanged—approx 90 mmHg.

STRUCTURAL AND BIOCHEMICAL CHANGES

We have developed a technique that allows us to study both the structure and ultrastructure of pulmonary arteries in the same animal. The rats are anesthetized with pentobarbital (33 mg/kg), and then intubated and ventilated at a stroke vol of 3.5 mL and a rate of 75 ventillations/min (Harvard Rodent Ventilator Model 683, South Natik, MA) *(13)*. A midline sternotomy is performed to expose the heart and lungs, and heparin 1000 USP U/mL is injected (0.5 mL) into the venous circulation. The pulmonary artery is subsequently cannulated via the right ventricle. The left atrium is vented and the lungs are cleared of blood by perfusing preheated (37°C) heparin (0.5% v/v PBS) at 20 cm water pressure for 5 min. The left lung is temporarily isolated by occluding the left pulmonary artery and bronchus, and the right lung is perfused with fixative for electron microscopy (1% glytaraldehyde in 4% formaldehyde) at 20 cm water pressure for 10 min and then clamped. The left pulmonary artery is then unclamped, perfused with PBS for 1 min and injected with a hot 60°C radiopaque barium gelatin mixture at 100 mmHg pressure for 5 min. The lung is inflated with fixative for light microscopy (10% formalehhyde) at 36 cm water pressure and perfused continuously at that pressure for 3 d.

The barium-gelatin injection prevents contrast from entering vessels <15 mm, so arteries that fill can be landmarked according to their accompanying airway. This technique also ensures even filling and distension, making measurements of wall thickness less variable. The mechanism of extension of muscle into peripheral arteries is thought to be related to differentiation of pericytes or intermediate cells into mature smooth-muscle-cells (SMCs). Hypertrophy of muscular pulmonary arteries measured as 2x wall thickness/exter-

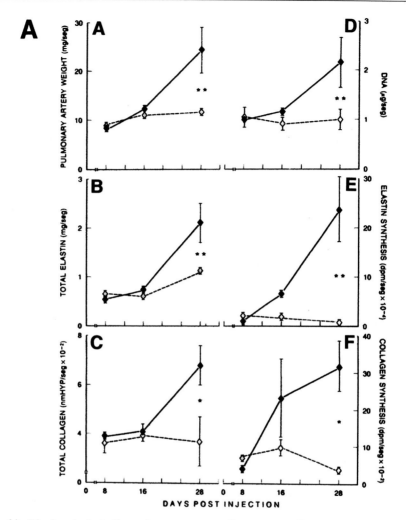

Fig. 4A. Biochemical studies-pulmonary artery. In monocrotaline-treated rats (♦), compared with control (◊), the following were increased significantly by 28 d after injection; **(A)**, vessel segment weight; **(B)** total insoluble elastin content; **(C)** total collagen content, **(D)** DNA; **(E)** insoluble elastin synthesis, and **(F)** collagen synthesis. Insoluble elastin synthesis increased progressively compared with controls over the duration of the experiment ($p<0.01$, 2–way ANOVA). $*p<0.05$, $**p<0.01$ assessed by Tukey analysis. Reproduced with permission from ref. *(8)*.

nal diameter is related to an increase in both the size and number of underlying SMCs, and loss of arteries may be the by-product of the severe narrowing of the proximal vessels.

In our initial ultrastructural studies, we observed features that were compatible with heightened turnover of elastin in the vessel wall *(13)* (Fig. 4). We

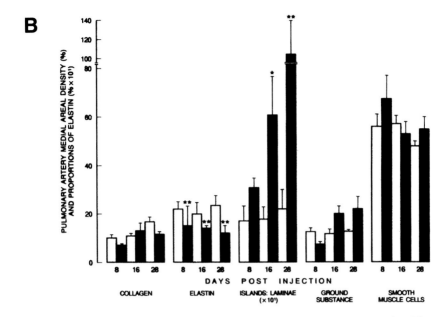

Fig. 4B. Morphometric assessment of medial features of hilar pulmonary arteries. The control vessels (open bars) were similar at all time points. In monocrotaline-treated rats (closed bars) there was a significantly decreased percentage proportion of amorphous elastin in the wall at all time points. There was also a progressive increase in the proportion of amorphous elastin organized as islands relative to lamina. $*p < 0.05$; $**p < 0.01$, assessed by Tukey analysis. Reproduced with permission from ref. *(8)*.

identified a 20-fold increase in elastin synthesis that was associated with a two-fold increase in elastin accumulation. Rather than an increased number of elastic laminae, the newly synthesized elastin appeared to be deposited as interlamellar islands. As an early feature, there also appeared to be initial fragmentation of the elastic laminae associated with the endothelial changes.

Based on these observations—not seen in infant rats which show the potential for regression—we began to investigate whether heightened elastase activity was responsible for the structural and hemodynamic abnormalities associated with progressive pulmonary hypertension *(3)* (Fig. 5). We documented increased elastase activity as early as 2 d after injection of monocrotaline, and showed that it was also prevalent with sustained and progressive pulmonary vascular disease at 28 d. The elastase was a serine elastase in nature, as judged by its inhibitor profile. It was measured by extracting pulmonary-artery hemogenates and incubating them with [³H]-elastin. We made the assumption that the changes in the central pulmonary arteries reflected similar abnormalities in the distal pulmonary arteries that were responsible for the ultimate hy-

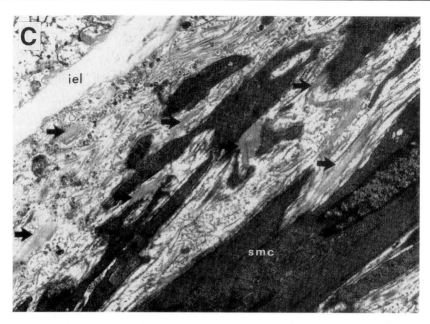

Fig. 4C. Electron photomicrograph of amorphous elastin islands in the media of the hilar pulmonary artery. In monocrotaline-treated rats 28 d after injection, the amorphous elastin islands (arrows) were found predominantly in the media between elastic lamina. Internal elastic lamina = iel; smooth muscle = smc. cell. × 17,500. Reproduced with permission from ref. *(8)*.

pertrophy of the vessel wall and the increase in resistance. We were able to show that increased elastase activity was associated with both an increase in size and number of SMCs in the central pulmonary arteries. A cause-and-effect relationship was later shown in studies in which we inhibited elastase activity with a variety of serine elastase inhibitors, including SC-37698, *(9,10)* and showed that this reduced the severity or prevented the development of pulmonary vascular disease in distal vessels. We also showed that even when the inhibitor was given later in the course of the disease, we could prevent the progression of pulmonary hypertension and associated vascular abnormalities (Fig. 6).

A variety of biochemical features, in addition to elastase activity, have been shown to accompany the evolution of pulmonary vascular disease after monocrotaline. These include an increase in polyamine synthesis *(14)* as well as increased production of growth factors, such as epidermal growth factor and fibroblast growth factor *(15)*. In our studies, we have shown increased accumulation of the glycoprotein tenascin C in the pulmonary-artery wall *(16)*. This is apparent in the lung as early as 7 d after injection of monocrotaline, and in the

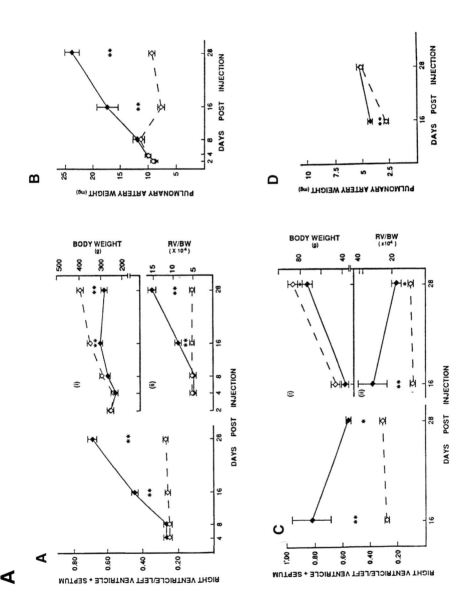

273

B

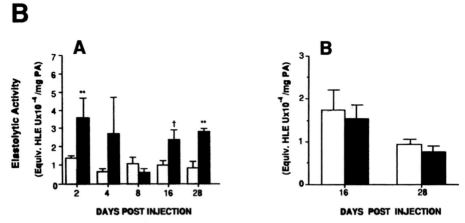

Fig. 5B. Central pulmonary-artery elastolytic activity in adult and infant rats. Elastolytic activity was observed in all rats and normalized per mg PA. In all control rats, the amount of elastolytic activity remained low throughout the experiment (open bars). **(A)** Monocrotaline-treated adult rats (closed bars) had greater elastolytic activity compared with control rats at 2 and 28 d post-injection. **(B)** Values for elastolytic activity expressed per mg PA in infant rats seemed to decrease between 16 and 28 d, but the differences were not significant. There was no difference in elastolytic activity comparing saline-and monocrotaline-injected rats. In these assays, pulmonary-artery weights varied slightly but insignificantly from those reported in Fig. 1. equiv. = equivalents; HLE = human leukocyte elastase; mg = milligram vessel weight; PA = central pulmonary artery. Mean values ± standard error; $n = 3$, each representing a mean of triplicate determinations from eight pooled adult rat or 12 pooled infant rat central pulmonary arteries (trunk and right and left mainstream branches); $**p < 0.01$; $†p = 0.054$. Reproduced with permission from ref. *(3)*.

Fig. 5A. *(previous page)* Right ventricular hypertrophy and pulmonary-artery weights in adult and infant rats. **(A)** In adult monocrotaline-treated rats (closed symbols), the ratios of right ventricular weight relative to the weight of left ventricle plus septum and (ii) relative to body wt (RV/BW) were increased significantly at both 16 and 28 d compared with saline-injected adult rat controls (open symbols). (i) An increase in body wt measured in g was impaired in monocrotaline-treated adult animals at both 16 and 28 d after injection. **(B)** An increase in pulmonary-artery weight measured in mg was observed at both 16 and 28 d after infection in monocrotaline-treated compared with control rats. (A and B) Mean values are given ± standard error. For time points 2 and 4, $n = 3$; for time points 8, 16, and 28, $n = 8$; $**p < 0.01$. **(C)** In infant rats, the ratios of right ventricular weight relative to the weight of the left ventricle plus septum and (ii) relative to body wt (RV/BW) were increased significantly at 16 d after injection, but showed lack of progression by 28 d in monocrotaline-treated infant rats compared with saline-injected infant control rats. **(D)** Mean pulmonary-artery weights in infant monocrotaline-treated rats were significantly greater than those of control rats at 16 d after injection ($p < 0.01$), but were similar at 28 d. In C and D, mean values are given ± standard errors; $n = 3$ for both time points; $*p < 0.05$; $**p < 0.01$. Reproduced with permission from ref. *(3)*.

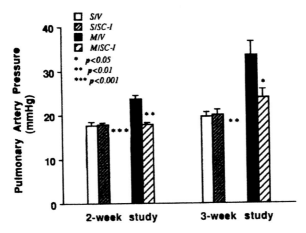

Fig. 6. Mean pulmonary-artery pressures. S-saline; V-vehicle; SC-I, SC-37698 elastase inhibitor (2 mg/d in 2-wk study and 3 mg/d in 3-wk study); M-monocrotaline. For 2-wk study: S/V ($n = 6$), S/SC-I ($n = 6$), M/V ($n = 7$), M/SC-I ($n = 6$). 3-wk study: S/V ($n = 3$), S/SC-I ($n = 3$), M/V ($n = 6$), M/SC-I ($n = 6$). Values are means ± SE. Reproduced with permission from ref. *(10)*.

central vessel at 14 d by an increase in immunodetectable tenascin on lung-tissue sections (Fig. 7) as well as by western immunoblot. It is also associated with an increase in mRNA levels for tenascin. Tenascin is first seen at the adventitial medial border (d 14), and then throughout the media (d 21), but with more advanced disease (d 28) it appears in the newly evolving inner media and neointima (Fig. 7). This heightened tenascin expression is also seen in patients with progressive pulmonary vascular disease *(17)*. The mechanistic significance was elucidated in cell-culture studies showing that tenascin is critical for EGF-induced SMC proliferation *(18)*. It appears that the increased production of tenascin is related to proteolytic activity which unravels collagen in the extracellular matrix and allows for the engagement of cryptic RDG sites by β3 integrins. The αvβ3 integrin appears to be responsible, and signals the increased transcriptional activity of the tenascin promoter via a MAP kinase pathway *(19)*. A region in the tenascin promoter of approx 122 base pairs has been identified as incorporating the critical elements of induction of gene expression *(19)*.

Once increased tenascin is produced, it appears to codistribute with proteolyzed collagen and cluster β3 integrin receptors. The clustering of β3 integrins leads to focal adhesion contact formation and subsequent clustering of EGF receptors, which phosphorylate promptly upon ligation and signal cell growth *(18)*. Tenascin is important to cell survival. We have also shown that withdrawal of tenascin either directly by antisense technology or by suppression of proteases, either serine elastases or matrix metalloproteinases, results in

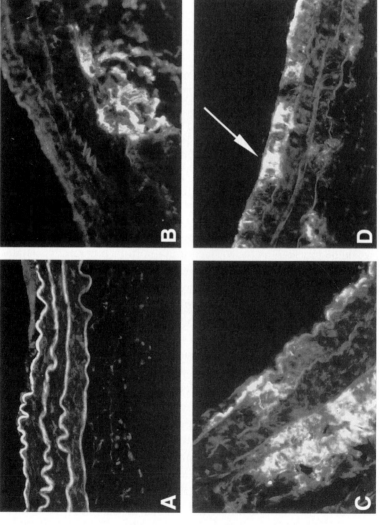

Fig. 7. Representative photomicrographs of immunofluorescent staining for TN-C in PAs of saline (**A**) and monocrotaline-treated (**B** through **D**) adult rats. Negative staining for TN-C was seen in PA tissue isolated from saline-treated animals (**A**). The elastic laminae show intense autofluorescence. In contrast, by d 14, focal deposition of TN-C was observed in the outer medial and adventitial layers of monocrotaline-treated rats (**B**). By d 21, TN-C was seen throughout the media (**C**), and by d 28, it was also apparent in close proximity to the developing neointima (arrow, **D**). Bar = 35 µm (n = 3 per time point). Reproduced with permission from ref. (16).

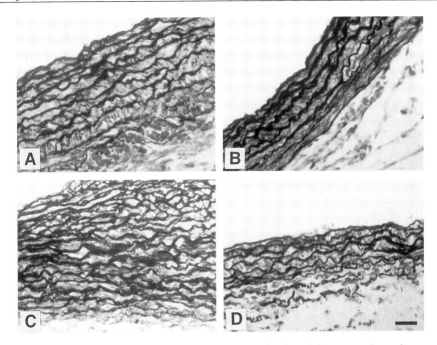

Fig. 8. Representative photomicrographs of Movat-stained rat PA organ-culture tissue collected from attached and floating cultures at 0 d and 8 d. Rat PAs taken at 21 d—the point at which they would be placed into culture—show medial hypertrophy (**A**) in contrast to PAs from saline-injected rats (**B**). On attached collagen gels, these vessels continue to thicken over the 8 d (**C, E**). Vessels on floating gels, however, show a progressive regression of medial thickness over the 8 d (**D, E**). Bar = 25 μm. Measurements of medial hypertrophy (**E**) showed significant corresponding differences and are associated with modulation of matrix, represented as increases in elastin on attached cultures and decreases in floating cultures. This is assessed by the number of elastic laminae (**F**) and by relative densitometric units of elastin in the vessel wall (data not shown). Bars = mean + SEM of $n = 3$ vessels at each timepoint ($n = 8$ for graph of medial thickness), * = $p<0.05$ comparing attached and floating conditions, and † = $p<0.05$ compared to d 0. Reproduced with permission from ref. *(20)*.

apoptosis of SMCs *(18)*. More recently, these observations in cell culture have been adapted to organ culture.

It is possible to grow pulmonary arteries from monocrotaline-injected rats in organ culture, and to follow the evolution of cellular and molecular changes. We have observed that the monocrotaline vessels continue to hypertrophy in organ culture, whereas incubation with proteinase inhibitors or stress unloading of these vessels by floating the collagen gels results in SMC apoptosis *(20)*. The SMC apoptosis is accompanied by loss of extracellular matrix (elastin and collagen), and by regression of the hypertrophy (Fig. 8). In more recent studies, we have shown that inhibiting tenascin induces apoptosis and does not induce regression, but prevents progression of hypertrophy in organ culture. This was attributed to the induction of an alternative β3 ligand in the presence of a proteolytic environment namely, osteopontin *(21)*. In our more recent studies, we have shown that rats fed serine elastase inhibitors orally, beginning at 21 d after injection of monocrotaline, show regression of pulmonary hypertension to normal values within 2 wk. The survival of the treated animals is 85%, compared to 0 in the untreated and regression of the structural changes is virtually complete *(22)*.

Studies have also shown that L-arginine might protect against the development of monocrotaline-induced pulmonary hypertension *(23)*. We have pursued studies in cultured cells, and have recently shown that nitric oxide, a product of L-arginine inhibits the intracellular signalling pathway necessary for the induction of SMC elastase activity *(24)*.

CONCLUSION

The monocrotaline model of pulmonary vascular disease has proven to be highly effective in studying regression and progression of pulmonary hypertension. It can be induced in the rat, allowing for hemodynamic monitoring and correlative biochemistry, cell, and molecular biology. However, there are several drawbacks when comparing the monocrotaline model to the human disease. The plexiform lesion is not evident and the levels of pulmonary hypertension are subsystemic. Recent studies by Okada et al. *(25)* have shown that the concomitant pneumonectomy at the time of monocrotaline injection results in more severe vascular changes and some neointimal lesions. Alternative approaches to induce more slowly progressive lesions might be effective. In comparison to hypoxia-induced pulmonary vascular disease, monocrotaline does produce a more malignant form of pulmonary hypertension, which is relevant to resolving questions related to advanced primary or secondary pulmonary hypertension in human patients.

REFERENCES

1. Mitani Y, Russell J, Brindley D, Rabinovitch M. Dexfenfluramine in obese and lean JCR:LA-corpulent and Sprague Dawley rats and pulmonary hypertension. Circulation 1997; 96:1–244.
2. Todd L, Mullen M, Olley P, Rabinovitch M. Pulmonary toxicity of monocrotaline differs at critical periods of lung development. Pediatr Res 1985; 19:731–737.
3. Todorovich-Hunter L, Dodo H, Ye C, McCready L, Keeley F, Rabinovitch M. Increased pulmonary artery elastolytic activity in adult rats with monocrotaline-induced progressive hypertensive pulmonary vascular disease compared with infant rats with nonprogressive disease. Am. Rev Respir Dis 1992; 146:213–223.
4. Herget J, Palecek F. Pulmonary arterial blood pressure in closed chest rats. Changes after catecholamines, histamine and serotonin. Arch Int Pharmacodyn 1972; 198:107–117.

5. Weeks J, Jones J. Routine direct measurement of arterial pressure in unanesthetized rats. Proc Soc Exp Biol Med 1960; 104:646–648.

6. Rabinovitch M, Konstam M, Gamble W, Papanicolaou N, Aronovitz M, Treves S, et al. Changes in pulmonary blood flow affect vascular response to chronic hypoxia in rats. Circ Res 1983; 52: 432–441.

7. Fried R, Meyrick B, Rabinovitch M, Reid L. Polycythemia and the acute hypoxia response in awake rats following chronic hypoxia. J Appl Physiol: Respir Environ Exerc Physiol 1983; 55:1167–1172.

8. Rosenberg H, Rabinovitch M. Endothelial injury and vascular reactivity in monocrotaline pulmonary hypertension. Am J Physiol 1988; 255:H1484–H1491.

9. Ilkiw R, Todorovich L, Maruyama K, Shin J, Rabinovitch M. SC-39026 (Searle), a serine elastase inhibitor, prevents muscularization of peripheral arteries suggesting a mechanism of monocrotaline-induced pulmonary hypertension in rats. Circ Res 1989; 64:814–825.

10. Ye C, Rabinovitch M. Inhibition of elatolysis by SC-37698 reduces development and progression of monocrotaline pulmonary hypertension. Am J Physiol 1991; 261:H1255–H1267.

11. Rabinovitch M, Mullen M, Rosenberg H, Maruyama K, O'Brodovich H, Olley P. Angiotensin II prevents hypoxic pulmonary hypertension and vascular changes in rats. Am J Physiol 1988; 254:H500–H508.

12. Rabinovitch M, Gamble W, Miettinen O, Reid L. Age and sex influence on pulmonary hypertension of chronic hypoxia and in recovery. Am J Physiol 1981; 240:H62–H72.

13. Todorovich-Hunter L, Ranger P, Johnson D, Keeley F, Rabinovitch M. Altered elastin and collagen synthesis associated with progressive pulmonary hypertension induced by monocrotaline. A biochemical and ultrastructural study. Lab Investig 1988; 58:184–195.

14. Gillespie M, Rippetow P, Haven C, Shiao R, Orlinska U, Maley B, et al. Polyamines and epidermal growth factor in monocrotaline-induced pulmonary hypertension. Am Rev Respir Dis 1989; 140:1463–1466.

15. Arcot S, Lipke D, Gillespie M, Olson J. Alterations of growth factor transcripts in rat lungs during development of monocrotaline-induced pulmonary hypertension. Biochem Pharmacol 1993; 14:1086–1091.

16. Jones P, Rabinovitch M. Tenascin-C is induced with progressive pulmonary vascular disease in rats is functionally related to increased smooth muscle cell proliferation. Circ Res 1996; 79:1131–1142.

17. Jones P, Cowan K, Rabinovitch M. Progressive pulmonary vascular disease is characterized by a proliferative response related to deposition of tenascin-C and is preceded by subendothelial accumulation of fibronectin. Am J Pathol 1997; 150:1349–1360.

18. Jones P, Crack J, Rabinovitch M. Regulation of tenascin-C, a vascular smooth muscle cell survival factor that interacts with the $\alpha v \beta 3$ integrin to promote epidermal growth factor receptor phosphorylation and growth. J Cell Biol 1997; 139:279–293.

19. Jones P, Jones F, Zhou B, Rabinovitch M. Denatured type I collagen induction of vascular smooth muscle cell tenascin-C gene expression is dependent upon a $\beta 3$ integrin-mediated mitogen-activated protein kinase pathway and a 122 bp promotor element. J Cell Science 1999; 112:435–445.

20. Cowan K, Jones P, Rabinovitch M. Regression of hypertrophied rat pulmonary arteries in organ culture is associated with suppression of proteolytic activity, inhibition of tenascin-C and smooth muscle cell apoptosis. Cir Res 1999; 84:1223–1233.

21. Cowan K, Jones P, Rabinovitch M. Tenascin-C antisense induces apoptosis of smooth muscle cells and expansion of a resistant population. Mol Biol Cell 1998; (Suppl)9:303a.

22. Cowan KN, Heilbut A, Lam C, Ito S, Rabinovich M. Reversal of severe pulmonary hypertension by a serine elastase inhibitor. Nat Med. 2000; 6:698–702.

23. Mitani Y, Maruyama K, Minoru S. Prolonged administration of L-arginine ameliorates chonic pulmonary hypertension and pulmonary vascular remodeling in rats. Circulation 1997; 96:689–697.

24. Mitani Y, Zaidi SHE, Dufourcq P, Thompson K, Rabinovich M. Nitric oxide reduces vascular smooth muscle cell elastase activity through cGMP-mediated suppression of ERK phosphorylation and AML1B nuclear partitioning. FASEB J. 2000; 14:805–814.

25. Okada K, Tanaka Y, Bernstein M, Zhang W, Patterson G, Botney M. Pulmonary hemodynamics modify the rat pulmonary artery response to injury. A neointimal model of pulmonary hypertension. Am J Pathol 1997; 151:1019–1025.

20 Chronic Pulmonary Hypertension in the Hypoxic Rat and in the Sheep Following Continuous Air Embolization

Barbara Meyrick, PhD
and Elena Tchekneva, MD

CONTENTS

INTRODUCTION

Chronic pulmonary hypertension (CPH) is a common complication of many chronic lung diseases, such as chronic bronchitis and emphysema, pulmonary fibrosis, AIDS, and scleroderma. The onset of CPH is accompanied by several characteristic structural changes in the pulmonary arteries, including increased thickness of the media, adventitia, and intima of normally muscular arteries, appearance of muscle in smaller, more peripheral arteries than normal, and a decrease in peripheral vascular volume *(1)*. Since it is not possible to follow the pathogenesis of this disease in human patients, our current knowledge is based largely on the use of animal models. This chapter outlines currently available techniques for two of the models of CPH. The huge literature base precludes a detailed inclusion of all models and authors.

From: *Contemporary Cardiology: Vascular Disease and Injury: Preclinical Research*
Edited by: D. I. Simon and C. Rogers © Humana Press Inc., Totowa, NJ

The most commonly used experimental models of CPH are the rat which has been exposed to chronic hypoxia or has received monocrotaline (*see* Chapter 19). Exposure to high oxygen tension also leads to the onset of CPH in rats *(2)*. Larger animal models of CPH are also available, such as the dog administered monocrotaline *(3)* and the sheep receiving continuous air embolization (CAE) into the pulmonary artery *(4)*. Neonatal models of pulmonary hypertension are also available, such as the neonatal cow and pig exposed to hypoxia *(5,6)* and aorto-pulmonary shunts in the fetal sheep *(7)*. Several recent studies have utilized knockout mice to examine the pathogenesis of hypoxia-induced CPH *(8–10)*.

Primary pulmonary hypertension (PPH), the idiopathic form of the disease, occurs much less frequently than CPH, and in familial cases it is probably linked to an aberration in the genetic code on chromosome 2q31–32 *(11)*. To date, no good animal model of PPH exists—e.g., neither the hypoxia nor monocrotaline-induced models of CPH show increased intimal thickness and plexiform lesions. However, the fawn hooded rat, *(12)* a spontaneous model of CPH, has been suggested to best mimic PPH, although whether its genotype is similar to that of patients with PPH is unknown.

THE RAT AS A MODEL OF CHRONIC PULMONARY HYPERTENSION

Basic assessment of the development of—and recovery from—CPH usually entails measurement of pulmonary hemodynamics, demonstration of the characteristic structural changes in the pulmonary vasculature, and assessment of right ventricular hypertrophy.

Hemodynamic Measurements

Measurements of pulmonary-artery pressure (P_{PA}) and pulmonary vascular resistance (PVR) are possible, and in some laboratories routine, in the normal and hypertensive rat. In the hypoxic rat, the hemodynamic measurements are usually made in room air. This obviates any rise in pressure caused by hypoxic vasoconstriction. Under anesthesia (e.g., ketamine HCL; 50–100 mg/kg, im and rompun; 15 mg/kg, im), a catheter is placed into the pulmonary artery via the jugular vein, and another into the aorta *(13)*. A PE-50 catheter is placed into the aorta and a polyvinyl catheter (inner diameter, 0.028, outer diameter, 0.061 mm) into the pulmonary artery. The pulmonary-artery catheter is introduced through the jugular vein and gently passed into the pulmonary artery through the right ventricle. This catheter has a small curve at its distal end to facilitate entry into the pulmonary artery from the heart. A P_{PA} trace is used to document passage of the catheter into the pulmonary artery. The catheters are tunneled subcutaneously and secured at the base of the skull. Catheterized rats are housed in individual cages to prevent other animals from chewing the catheters. Animals are allowed to recover from surgery for a period of approx 3 d prior to initiation of an experiment. The catheters allow measurements to be made in conscious animals, and enable a single animal to be monitored over a period of time—i.e., during the development of CPH—in a consistent and reproducible manner. Several detailed descriptions of this methodology are published (13,14). Cardiac output may also be assessed using the indocyanine green-dye technique. Blood is pumped by way of a shunt from the carotid artery to a jugular-vein catheter at a rate of 3 mL/min through a cuvette (Waters Associates, Milford, MA) and densitometer, and the cardiogreen dye (0.05 mL containing 1 mg/mL) is detected after injection into the pulmonary artery (13). Calculation of cardiac output may be monitored by a Nova computer using an algorithm based on the Stewart-Hamilton method (15). Small aliquots of blood may be drawn from the catheters for measurement of blood gases and hematocrit, considering that a 200-g rat has a total blood vol of only 5–6 mL.

Measurements of right ventricular pressure may also be made in the anesthetized animal immediately prior to death. Right ventricular pressure has been used to monitor the development of CPH in place of direct measurements of P_{PA}. The major drawbacks to this technique are that it does not allow measurements over time and the measurements are only possible in the anesthetized animal.

CHRONIC HYPOXIA

Exposure to hypobaric or normobaric hypoxia leads to the development of CPH. A simple hypobaric chamber may be constructed from a heavy metal container such as an old autoclave (16). Decompression is achieved by a rotary pump. Most experiments to date have used a pressure of one-half an atmosphere (380 mmHg), equivalent to approx 5,500 m above sea level or 10% oxygen. It is customary to acclimatize the rat by exposing the animals to 500 mmHg pressure on the first day of exposure and then to 380 mmHg on the second. To maintain a CO_2 level within the chamber of less than 0.4% and to remove excess humidity, air flow through the chamber should be approx 30 L/min.

Normobaric hypoxia causes changes similar to those of hypobaric hypoxia. The apparatus used for normobaric hypoxia usually consists of a plexiglass isolation chamber flushed with 10% oxygen. Hypoxia may be maintained in a number of ways—e.g., using a Pro:ox model 350 unit (Reming Bioinstruments, Redfield, NY). Fractional concentrations of inspired oxygen are controlled by this unit by solenoid infusion of nitrogen (Roberts Oxygen, Rockville, MD) vs inward leak of air through holes in the chamber. Humidity, ammonia, and CO_2 are removed by pumping the chamber through Bara Lyme (barium hydroxide

Table 1
Hemodynamic and Structural Data from Control and Hypoxic Rats

	Controls	Hypoxia (14 d)
P_{PA} (mmHg)	20.8 ± 1.4	44.6 ± 4.0[a]
P_{SA} (mmHg)	110.0 ± 2.4	108.8 ± 8.5[a]
Hematocrit (%)	45 ± 1	60 ± 1[a]
SvO_2 (%)	56 ± 4	32 ± 2[a]
LV±S/RV	3.4 ± 0.1	1.9 ± 0.1[a]
Alv:Art	24.5 ± 1.4	30.8 ± 2.2[a]
% Musc. Art	0	44.8 ± 6.0[a]
% Advent. Thick	18.2 ± 2.2	39.0 ± 4.3[a]

P_{PA} = pulmonary-artery pressure; P_{SA} = systemic artery pressure; SvO_2 = systemic venous oxygen saturation; Alv:Art = # alveolar to one artery; % Musc. Art = % fully muscular arteries at alveolar duct level; % Advent. Thick = % adventitial thickness;[a] p <0.05 . Data collected from ref. *(14,21,27,31)*.

lime, USP, Chemetron Medical Division, Allied Health Care Products, St Louis, MO), Drierite (anhydrous calcium sulfate, Fisher Scientific, Atlanta, GA), and activated carbon (Fisher Scientific) *(17)*. The animals are on a 12:12 h light:dark cycle. For both exposure techniques, the chamber is usually returned to normal atmosphere once a day for a period of approx 15 min to allow bedding and food to be replenished. At the end of this time, the animals are returned directly to 10% oxygen (380 mmHg).

Hemodynamic Measurements

Rats are the animals most frequently used for long-term hypoxic experiments. Hemodynamic measurements in the rat reveal a significant increase in P_{PA} by 3 d of hypoxia and a doubling by 14 d (Table 1) *(14)*. A cautionary note for long-term measurements is that maintenance of patent catheters necessarily involves the use of heparin, an agent that is linked to amelioration of CPH in hypoxic guinea-pigs and mice *(18,19)*. However, even with heparin, P_{PA} has been shown to increase significantly in the hypoxic rat and the rat following administration of monocrotaline *(14,20)*. Systemic venous O_2 levels are significantly reduced and hematocrit is strikingly increased (Table 1). Upon return to room air, these hypoxia-induced changes are reversed *(21)*. Most species of rats may be used, although not all types of rats are equally susceptible to hypoxia, as shown by a more modest increase in P_{PA} and less severe alterations in pulmonary-artery structure *(22)*. Specific pathogen-free male Sprague-Dawley rats respond well to hypoxia. Occasionally, rats are encountered that are nonresponsive to hypoxia, but this is not limited to one particular line. Other animals may also be successfully exposed to hypoxic environments—e.g., guinea pigs for long-term exposure (18). Mice have also been used, but their size makes the endpoints more difficult to assess (19). The structural response in the mouse is strikingly less pronounced than in the rat. However, it is now possible to monitor pulmonary vascular pressures in the open-chest mouse (10).

Structural Studies

The structural changes in the pulmonary artery are an important marker of CPH, and are usually part of studies to examine the effect of agonists, antagonists, or other agents, on the development of CPH. The best approach to the structural studies is morphometrics. The pulmonary artery is of several types as assessed by structure—muscular, partially muscular, and nonmuscular (1). The arteries that run and divide are termed conventional arteries, and those that divide without an accompanying airway are termed supernumerary arteries (1). A special muscular artery—the thick-walled oblique muscle artery—has also been described in the rat, and may complicate assessment of medial thickness (23). This type of artery is also present in many other species, e.g., rabbit and sheep (Meyrick, B., unpublished observation). Several techniques have been used to examine the structural changes of CPH. For example, in uninjected material, increased medial and adventitial thickness and appearance of muscle into smaller arteries than normal may be determined (e.g., 18,24). Calculation of the volume of the intima, media, and adventitia of the larger arteries has also been applied (25). However, use of nondistended arteries may not always detect the more subtle changes produced by antagonists and other agents. It is impossible to easily assess whether a reduction in peripheral vascular volume has occurred. Distending the pulmonary artery with a contrast medium—e.g., barium-sulfate/gelatin mixture—provides a more complete picture and assessment of the more minimal changes of CPH (1,2,21). For this technique, the lungs and heart are removed at death and the pulmonary artery is cannulated by way of the right ventricle. The artery is injected with a barium/gelatin mixture at a temperature of 60°C and a pressure of 75 mm Hg over a period of 3 min. The cannula is occluded and the lung is inflated with 10% formol-saline at a pressure of 23 cm H_2O and kept at this pressure in a bath of formol-saline for 24 h. The use of a constant pressure to fill the pulmonary artery ensures that all arteries—control and hypertensive—are fully distended, and allows comparison between the two groups. Fixation under a constant airway pressure fully dilates the alveoli in control and hypertensive lungs, and allows numbers of alveoli to be counted and compared. Arteriograms can be made of the injected lungs as a first assessment of the number of peripheral arteries (assessment of background haze) and of any dilation or constriction of the larger arteries (1,7,14,20,21). These techniques allow measurements of intimal, medial, and adventitial thickness related

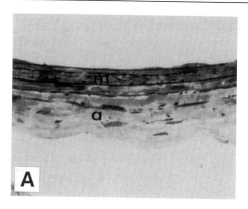

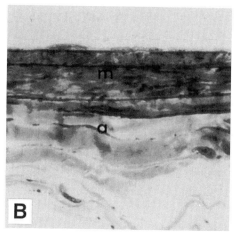

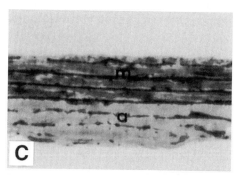

Fig. 1. Micrographs of 1-μm sections showing the hilar pulmonary artery from a control rat (**A**) (m, media and a, adventitia), an animal after 10 d of hypoxia (**B**) (the media and adventitia are thickened), and an animal after 70 d recovery from 10 d hypoxia (**C**) (media and adventitia are returned to the normal range, although there is marked fibrosis of the adventitia. ×50. Reprinted with permission from ref. *(28)*.

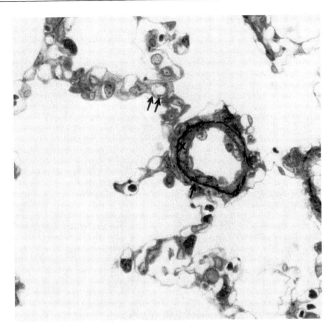

Fig. 2. Micrograph of a 1-μm section showing a newly muscularized artery, approx 30-μm in external diameter, at alveolar wall level after 10 d hypoxia. Intermediate cells (x) are situated beneath plump endothelial cells and internal to a single elastic lamina (single arrow). The endothelial cells of many of the alveolar capillaries appear thicker than normal (double arrow). Toluidine blue ×500. Reprinted with permission from ref. *(31)*.

to external diameter to determine increases in their thickness; assessment of external diameter and medial thickness in relation to accompanying airway level (e.g., terminal or respiratory bronchiolus, alveolar duct, or alveolar wall) to determine appearance of muscle into the wall of smaller arteries than normal; measurement of internal diameter of artery related to external diameter to show alterations in lumen diameter; and counts of the number of alveoli related to the number of arteries in the same fields to determine reduction of peripheral arterial volume. The fixed heart is used for assessment of right ventricular hypertrophy, which is usually assessed as the weight of the left ventricle plus septum/ the weight of the right ventricle *(26)*.

Such structural studies have revealed, in the rat, a doubling in medial thickness in the smallest arteries (50–100 μm) by 3 d of hypoxia and a significant increase in the larger arteries (500–1000 μm) by 5 d *(27;* Fig. 1). Adventitial thickness was also significantly increased by 3 d and doubled by 14 d *(28)* (Table 1). Appearance of muscle into smaller and more peripheral arteries than normal (Table 1 and Fig. 2) was significantly increased from 3 d of hypoxia, and reduction in number of peripheral vessels was significant from d 14 (Table 1).

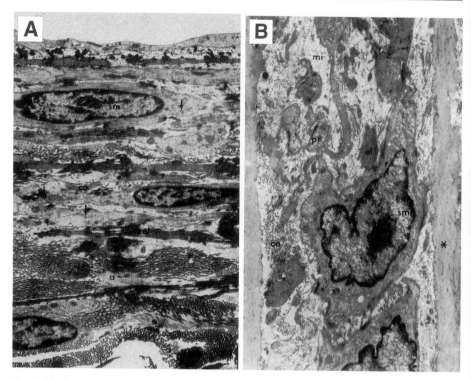

Fig. 3. Electron micrographs of the hilar pulmonary artery from a control rat **(A)** and after 10 d hypoxia **(B)**. Following hypoxia, the SMCs (sm) are hypertrophied and show cytoplasmic processes (pr), the elastic laminae (*) are thickened, and the extracellular connective tissue (mi-microfibrils; co-collagen fibers; el-elastin) is increased compared to control. In **(A)** smooth muscle dense bodies at arrow; internal elastic lamina-iel; external elastic lamina-eel; ×10,500. Reprinted with permission from ref. *(28).*

Each of the structural changes are partially reversible upon return to room air *(28,29).* Increased medial thickness, appearance of muscle into normally nonmuscular arteries, and reduction in peripheral vascular volume have been shown to correlate with the increase in P_{PA} *(14).* The increase in adventitial thickness was shown to be caused by early and marked proliferation of fibroblasts and an accompanying increase in connective tissue, particularly collagen *(28,30).* A similar response has also been shown in the hypoxic neonatal cow *(25).* Endothelial hypertrophy is also apparent in both small and large arteries *(31,32).* In the media, electron microscopic and cell proliferation studies revealed striking hypertrophy of the smooth muscle cells (SMCs) with an early but modest proliferative response, increased deposition of connective tissue and increased thickness of the elastic laminae *(28,30)* (Fig. 3). Appearance of muscle into the wall of smaller arteries than normal was shown to be due to hypertrophy and proliferation of precursor SMCs—e.g., pericytes and intermediate cells—normally present in the walls of nonmuscular arteries *(23,30)* (Fig. 1). The reduction in peripheral arterial volume is probably the result of a narrowing of lumen diameter caused at least in part by the extension of muscle to the periphery. Obliteration of arteries is not a feature of this form of CPH.

These studies have provided insight into the pathogenesis of CPH, although the mechanism underlying the development of the structural changes is not fully understood. Remodeling of the elastic laminae—both through increased connective tissue deposition *(33)* and breakdown by an elastase *(34)* have been shown to play a role, and the increase in vascular collagen has been linked to the rise in intravascular pressure *(33)*. Other mediators—e.g., angiotensin-converting enzyme inhibitor, *(36)* atrial natriuretic factor, *(36)* nitric-oxide synthase, *(37)* endothelin-1, *(38)* 5-lipoxygenase-activating protein, *(8)* cyclooxygenase products, *(39)* angiotensin II, *(40)* platelet-derived growth factor, and vascular endothelial growth factor *(41)* have also been implicated, but whether the alterations in these putative mediators reflect a trigger event or occur as a result of the structural remodeling is still undetermined. The agents with the greatest effect on the development, prevention, and reversal of hypoxic CPH at this time are the endothelin-1 (ET-1) receptor, ET_A, antagonists *(38,42)*. Studies with knockout mice have shown that 5-lipoxygenase may at least contribute to the onset of right ventricular hypertrophy, and that disruption of the endothelial nitric-oxide synthase gene is associated with a loss of vasodilation that may contribute to the development of CPH *(8–10)*. The reason for the increase in P_{PA} is not well-defined, although in the hypoxic model, vasoconstriction is likely to contribute to the onset of the structural changes as well as to the pressure rise. Increased hematocrit is another factor that contributes to the rise in P_{PA}, *(43)* as is the reduction in peripheral vascular volume. Appearance of muscle in smaller arteries than normal is also likely to contribute to the rise in pressure. Medial thickening is secondary to the CPH. Whether hypoxia is a good model for all forms of CPH, such as those associated with inflammation, is uncertain. Future studies will probably detect differences between the various models and better define triggers to the hypertension.

THE SHEEP AS A MODEL OF CPH

Large animal models have generally been used to examine neonatal CPH, including the neonatal cow and pig exposed to hypoxia, and the neonatal lamb with increased intrauterine pulmonary blood flow *(5–7)*. Use of such large animal models allows catheter insertion to be more easily performed than in the rat and mouse, and pulmonary hemodynamic measurements to be taken on a daily basis in an accurate and reproducible manner. Our laboratory has used the chronically catheterized sheep to develop models of CPH. The advantage of the sheep for such studies is that the caudal-mediastinal lymph node can be cannulated, allowing collection of lymph samples that are derived mainly from the lung. Comparison of measurements of proteins and other putative mediators of CPH in lung lymph with those of plasma samples allows assessment of changes that occur in the lung during the pathogenesis of CPH.

Surgical Preparation of Sheep

A detailed description of the surgical preparation of the chronically catheterized awake sheep has been provided in ref. *44*. Yearling sheep (from a local farmer in our case) are fasted for 24 h prior to surgery. Anesthesia is induced initially by an iv injection of barbiturates (thiopental), and the sheep is intubated. Anesthesia is maintained with halothane and nitrous oxide. The left and right areas of the chest are shaved and washed with Betadyne solution. An incision is made in the fifth intercostal space of the right side. The rib space is widened initially with the fingers, and then with retractors, with care taken to avoid fracturing the ribs. A malleable retractor is used to retract the lungs ventrally. The lymph node is located under the pleura between the aorta and the esophagus. The efferent lymph duct is marked by injecting indocyanine green dye (Hyson, Westcott, and Dunning, Baltimore, MD) into the head of the node using a 25-gauge needle. The pleura overlying the duct is torn, and the distal portion of the duct is ligated with a 5-0 silk suture. Special care should be taken to prevent ligation of the small veins and arteries that may supply the lymph node. Any additional ducts from the node should be ligated. After removing any adherent tissue from the surface of the duct, a second silk suture is placed 1 cm from the site of ligation, and a heparin-filled sialastic cannula (0.025 in id, 0.047 in od) with a beveled end approx 2 cm from a silicone glue bead is inserted into the lymph duct. The cut for insertion of the catheter is made with iridectomy scissors, and, because of the friability of the duct, should not be more than one-third of its diameter. The catheter is placed into the duct bevel down, and advanced with bayonet forceps until maximal flow is achieved, and the 5–0 silk suture is tied and then tied again around the glue bead. The catheter is exteriorized by way of a stab wound at the interspace caudal to the thoracotomy and secured with silicone glue. The chest is closed by loosely closing the rib space with a double loop of stainless steel wire, closing the muscle layers with 0 chronic gut sutures, and closing the skin with 2-0 cuticular silk sutures. The lungs should be hyperinflated several times before closing the chest. The animals are allowed to recover for a minimum of 7 d prior to initiation of the experiment. During this time all catheters must be flushed with saline and refilled with heparin and an antibiotic on a daily basis. The lymph cannula should be checked and stripped to remove any fibrin clots.

The animal is turned, and an incision is made in the left fifth intercostal space to allow placement of catheters in the left ventricle and pulmonary artery. A retractor is used to open the ribs. The lungs are retracted dorsally with a malleable retractor, and the pericardium is punctured and pulled dorsally to expose the main pulmonary artery. A small portion of the main pulmonary artery is lifted and clamped with a curved Kapp-Beck clamp and a 2-0 silk suture, and two teflon felt pledgets are placed in a purse-string configuration around the clamped portion of the pulmonary artery. A small incision is made between the suture loop, a saline-filled silicone catheter (0.062 inner diameter, 0.125 outer diameter) is inserted into the incision, and the catheter is inserted and advanced 4.5. cm in an antegrade direction. After removing the Kapp-Beck clamp, the suture is tightened with a friction knot and a second suture is used to boot-lace the catheter in position. The chest is closed. Using the same technique, a second catheter is placed in the right atrium, but with a 2-cm insertion. Catheters are also placed in the jugular vein and carotid artery at the neck. In addition, an 8-French Cordis introducer is placed in the other jugular vein to allow later placement of a Swan-Ganz thermistor-tipped catheter for measurements of body temperature and cardiac output.

CONTINUOUS AIR EMBOLIZATION

We have used the chronically catheterized sheep with a lung lymph fistula to develop several models of CPH. For example, CPH has been induced following repeated administration of endotoxin, *(45)* following thoracic irradiation, *(46)* and following repeated sc injection of the cyclooxygenase inhibitor indomethacin *(47)*. The following account is of our CAE model of CPH, a model which is currently used in our laboratory.

Administration of Continuous Air Emboli

The machine shop at Vanderbilt University constructed stainless-steel metabolic cages to house the sheep according to our specifications. The cages have an area of 15 sq ft (2'8" by 6'2") with one side and a back panel that can be moved inward to limit movement of the sheep during hemodynamic monitoring. Water and food are freely available to the sheep at all times. A stainless-steel lead and catheter trolley is included on the top of the cage to which is fitted a standard size three-channel swivel (Harvard Apparatus Bioscience) through which filtered air (Acrodisc filters 0.2 μm, Gelman Sciences, Ann Arbor, MI) passes en route to the sheep. The swivel and trolley allow the sheep to move freely about the cage when it is not constrained for monitoring. Air is delivered to the sheep using a Masterflex pump. The filtered air passes through Masterflex tubing to the top of the cage and into the three-channel swivel. From here, air is delivered through more tubing which is encased in a flexible metal cylinder

Table 2
Hemodynamic (Off Air) and Structural Changes Following 12 Days
of Continuous Air Embolization Into Sheep

	Control	Air embolization
PVR (U)	3.7 ± 0.2	7.0 ± 0.7[a]
P_{PA} (mmHg)	19 ± 1	31 ± 3[a]
P_{LA} (mmHg)	-1 ± 1	-3 ± 1
CO (L/min)	5.4 ± 0.3	4.3 ± 0.4
SaO_2 (Torr)	93 ± 2	65 ± 1[a]
Alv:Art	3.3 ± 0.2	1.8 ± 0.2[a]
% Musc Art	1.2 ± 1.2	37.3 ± 8.2[a]
% MT (51–100)	3.7 ± 0.9	9.1 ± 1.1[a]
(501–1000)	1.0 ± 0.1	4.1 ± 0.4[a]

PVR = pulmonary vascular resistance; P_{PA} = pulmonary-artery pressure; P_{LA} = left atrial pressure; CO = cardiac output; SaO_2 = systemic artery oxygen saturation; Alv:Art = # alveoli to one artery; % Musc Art = % fully muscular arteries; % MT = medial thickness related to external diameter. [a] p <0.05. (Data collected from ref. *4,49*).

into the proximal port of the Swan-Ganz catheter. The Swan-Ganz catheter is housed in a side-pocket of a sheep jacket (Alice King Chatham Medical Arts, Hawthorne, CA). The sheep end of the flexible tubing is tied onto the jacket. A continuous flow of air (CAE) is initiated after several reproducible baseline measurements. The initial rate of flow is approx 0.04 mL/kg/h, which is achieved in a stepwise manner over a period of 4 h. The exact rate of air flow is dependent on the response of each sheep. Our endpoint is an increase in PVR that is greater than 2, but less than three times the sheep's baseline value. Air flow is adjusted on a daily basis to maintain PVR at this level. The rate of air flow generally decreases with the development of CPH *(4,55)*. Following monitoring, the catheters are flushed and filled with heparin and antibiotic.

Hemodynamic Measurements

We have followed the onset of CPH over a period of 12 d of CAE and shown a significant increase in PVR by 4 d, increasing in severity to 12 d (*4*; Table 2). The measurements are made after turning the air flow off and allowing the animal to equilibrate for a period of 1–2 h. A doubling in P_{PA} was also apparent by 8 d. Left atrial pressure and cardiac output showed modest, but insignificant, reductions (Table 2). The pulmonary pressor response to a bolus injection of the thromboxane mimic, PGH_2–analog, was significantly elevated above baseline by 4 d of CAE. Hypoxemia is modest in the CAE animals, and is not sufficient to cause hypoxic vasoconstriction (Table 2).

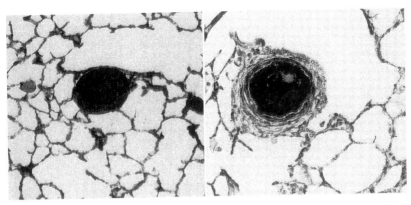

Fig. 4. Light micrographs showing a barium-filled artery running at respiratory bronchiolar level from a control sheep (*left*) and from a sheep following continuous air embolization for 12 d (*right*). Following air embolization, the wall is thickened showing appearance of new muscle and increased thickness of the adventitia. Verhoeff's elastin stain followed by Van Gieson, × 230. Reprinted with permission from ref. *(49)*.

Structural Studies

Examination of the structure of barium-filled pulmonary arteries demonstrated an increase in percent medial thickness in arteries of all sizes by d 12 and as early as 4 d in those between 50 and 200 μm (Table 2). Appearance of muscle into smaller and more peripheral arteries than normal (Fig. 4) and reduction in peripheral arterial volume both by direct counts and by arteriograms showed a similar time course *(49)* (Table 2). One of the striking features of the air embolization model is the development of intimal thickening, particularly in arteries less than 500 μm in external diameter (Fig. 5). This is one of the characteristic pulmonary-artery changes seen in CPH in humans. Intimal thickening is not a feature in the rat models of CPH, but has been shown to occur in monocrotaline-induced CPH with increased flow *(50)*. With cessation of CAE, these changes are reversible over a period of 7 d (Meyrick, B. unpublished findings). Structural changes in the pulmonary veins have also been identified, as well as an increase in the volume of bronchial vessels *(51)*. Early, transient sequestration of granulocytes in the peripheral vasculature is part of the response to CAE *(49)*. Using granulocyte-depleted sheep, we have shown inhibition of the CAE-induced onset of sustained pulmonary hypertension and of the reduction in pulmonary vascular volume *(52)*. However, the increased medial thickness and appearance of muscle into smaller arteries than normal was not attenuated *(52)*. These studies demonstrate that granulocytes contribute to the functional changes of CAE-induced CPH and to the reduction in peripheral

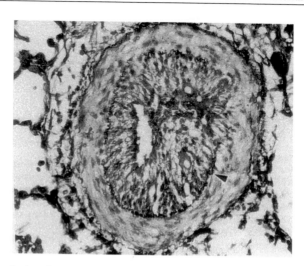

Fig. 5. Micrograph showing an artery (500 μm in external diameter) from lung biopsy tissue from a sheep following 12 d of air embolization. The media is thickened, and there is a striking increase in the intima. The internal elastic lamina is noted by the arrow. Verhoeff's elastin stain followed by Van Gieson, × 100. Reprinted with permission from ref. *(54)*.

vascular volume, suggesting a link between these two changes; the smooth-muscle changes are independent of granulocytes and are probably secondary to the rise in P_{PA}. Use of an elastase inhibitor—recombinant secretory leukocyte protease inhibitor (rSLPI)—slowed, but did not inhibit, the onset of CAE-induced CPH *(48)*.

Measurements of lung lymph revealed an increase in lung lymph flow, an indicator of increased permeability *(4)*; an increase in elastin peptide release from the lung *(49)*; an increase in thromboxane release and a transient increase in prostacyclin *(4)*; and an increase in release of transforming growth factor-β (TGF-β) *(53)* and insulin-like growth factor-1 *(54)*. *In situ* hybridization studies demonstrate an increase in the TGF-β mRNAs and protein in the SMCs around normally muscular arteries and in the walls of the newly muscularized arteries; the hybridization signal was most pronounced for TGF-β_1 and β_3 *(55)*. Using immunocytochemical techniques, IGF-1 has been shown in the thickened intima of CAE-induced CPH *(54)*. These findings demonstrate the complex response of the lung during the development of CPH.

Recently, we have shown an increase in ET-1 exiting the lung, *(56)* and our current studies are focused on the cellular source of ET-1 and its local synthesis in the pulmonary vascular wall. We have shown, by semiquantitative RT-PCR, regional variation in preproET-1 (ppET-1) transcripts in the main and midregion pulmonary artery of control sheep. The hilar artery shows more ppET-1 tran-

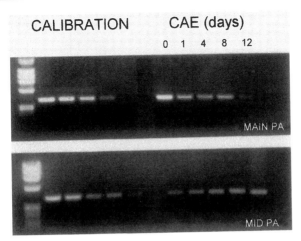

Fig. 6. Representative data showing that the ppET-1 gene is differentially expressed in main and midregion pulmonary artery (PA) of control (0) sheep, and is altered during continuous air embolization (CAE). *(left)* PCR images of the ppET-1 cDNA after serial dilutions of the RT products from control main and midregion PA. *(right)* PCR images of ppET-1 cDNA from sheep receiving 0, 1, 4, 8, 12 d CAE. Reprinted with permission from ref. *(56)*.

scripts than the midregion (9–10th generation) artery *(56)*. Further, we have shown that, with the development of CAE-induced CPH, the regional variability remained but was reversed—ppET-1 transcripts were reduced in the main pulmonary artery but increased in the midregion *(56)* (Fig. 6). To understand the cell types responsible for these differences in ET-1 mRNA, we have isolated and cultured SMCs from the intimal and inner medial layer (L1 and L2 layers, respectively; *57*) of the main and midregion pulmonary artery of control and hypertensive sheep. In control sheep, we found phenotypic differences in L2 cells from the two levels of pulmonary artery, as well as in the two cell types from adjacent layers of the hilar artery *(56,58)*. The L2 cells of the main pulmonary artery exhibit higher expression of the ppET-1 gene and higher intracellular levels of big-ET-1 and mature ET-1 than those of the midregion *(59)*. The L1 cells of the main pulmonary artery synthesize and release larger amounts of ET-1 than the L2 cells and have higher levels of intracellular endothelin-converting enzyme—the enzyme responsible for the metabolizing proET-1 to mature ET-1 *(58)*. The L2, but not the L1, cells increase their intracellular levels of ET-1 in the presence of the exogenous peptide. These findings demonstrate that SMCs from adjacent layers of the pulmonary artery are phenotypically different. The L1 cells are a more synthetic cell type than the L2 cells (like the adjacent endothelial cells) and the L2 cells are more responsive to local ET-1 levels than L1 cells.

The CAE model of CPH differs in many respects to the hypoxic rat. While both show similarities in many of the structural features, the CAE model does not include hypoxic vasoconstriction, but does exhibit robust intimal proliferation and intimal thickening and obliteration of small arteries—features of many forms of CPH in humans. The larger animal models also allow changes in larger arteries to be examined than is possible in the rat. Our data demonstrate that CAE induces an inflammatory form of CPH and is more like the monocrotaline model of CPH than that observed following exposure to high oxygen concentrations *(60,61)*. Our data demonstrate that the structural remodeling of CPH may be a case of dysregulated repair. For example, in CAE-induced CPH there is early granulocyte sequestration in the lung, an increase in pulmonary vascular permeability, and accumulation of edema followed by increases in growth factors—e.g. TGF-β, IGF-1 and ET-1. Whether this model mimics CPH in patients with inflammatory disorders—e.g., the adult respiratory distress syndrome, cystic fibrosis, and AIDS—is uncertain but similarities in the structural changes suggests that this is likely.

REFERENCES

1. Meyrick B, Reid L. Pulmonary hypertension: anatomic and physiologic correlates. Clin Chest Med 1983; 4:199–217.
2. Hu LM, Jones R. Injury and remodelling of pulmonary veins by high oxygen: a morphometric study. Am J Pathol 1989; 134:253–262.
3. Okada M, Yamashita C, Okada M, Nohara H, Yamagishi H, Wakiyama H, et al. Single lung transplantation of canine pulmonary hypertension. J Heart Lung Transplant 1997; 16:532–537.
4. Perkett EA, Brigham KL, Meyrick B. Continuous air embolization into sheep causes sustained pulmonary hypertension and increased pulmonary vasoreactivity. Am J Pathol 1988; 132:444–454.
5. Orton EC, LaRue SM, Ensley B, Stenmark K. Bromodeoxyuridine labeling and DNA content of pulmonary artery medial cells from hypoxia-exposed and nonexposed healthy calves. Am J Vet Res 1992; 53:1925–1930.
6. Haworth SG, Hislop AA. Effect of hypoxia on adaptation of the pulmonary circulation to extra-uterine life in the pig. Cardiovasc Res 1982; 16:293–303.
7. Reddy MV, Meyrick B, Wong J, Khoor A, Liddicoat JR, Hanley F, et al. In utero placement of aortopulmonary shunts. A model of postnatal pulmonary hypertension with increased pulmonary blood flow in lambs. Circulation 1995; 92:606–613.
8. Voelkel NF, Tuder RM, Wade K, Hoper M, Lepley RA, Goulet JL, et al. Inhibition of 5-lipoxygenase-activating protein (FLAP) reduces pulmonary vascular reactivity and pulmonary hypertension in hypoxic rats. J Clin Invest 1996; 97:2491–2498.
9. Steudel W, Scherrer-Crosbie M, Block KD, Weimann J, Huang PL, Jones RC, et al. Sustained pulmonary hypertension and right ventricular hypertrophy after chronic hypoxia in mice with congenital deficiency of nitric oxide synthase 3. J Clin Investig 1998; 101:2468–2477.
10. Steudel W, Ichinose F, Huang PL, Hurford WE, Jones RC, Bevan JA, et al. Pulmonary vasoconstriction and hypertension in mice with targeted disruption of the endothelial nitric oxide synthase (NOS3) gene. Circ Res 1997; 81:34–41.

11. Nichols WC, Koller DL, Slovis B, Foroud T, Terry VH, Siemieniak DR, et al. Localization of the gene for familial primary pulmonary hypertension to chromosome 2q31–32. Nat Genet 1997; 15:277–280.

12. Sato K, Webb S, Tucker A, Rabinovitch M, O'Brien RF, McMurtry IF, et al. Factors influencing the idiopathic development of pulmonary hypertension in the fawn hooded rat. Am Rev Respir Dis 1992; 145:793–797.

13. Haynes J, Chang SW, Morris KG, Voelkel NF. Platelet-activating factor antagonists increase vascular reactivity in perfused rat lungs. J Appl Physiol 1988; 65:1921–1928.

14. Rabinovitch M, Gamble W, Nadas A, Miettinen OS, Reid L. Rat pulmonary circulation after chronic hypoxia: hemodynamic and structural features. Am J Physiol 1979; 236:H818–H827.

15. Huber F, Sodal IE, Weil JV. On-line cardiac output by digital computer. J Appl Physiol 1976; 40:266–268.

16. Wright BM. Apparatus for exposing animals to reduced atmospheric pressure for long periods. Br J Haematol 1964; 10:75–79.

17. Palmer LA, Semenza GL, Stohler MH, Johns, RA. Hypoxia induced type II NOS gene expression in pulmonary artery endothelial cells via HIF-1. Am J Physiol 1998; 274:L212–L219.

18. Spence CR, Thompson BT, Janssens SP, Steigman DM, Hales CA. Effect of aerosol heparin on the development of hypoxic pulmonary hypertension in the guinea-pig. Am Rev Respir Dis 1993; 148:241–244.

19. Hales CA, Kradin RL, Brandstetter RD, Zhu YJ. Impairment of hypoxic pulmonary artery remodelling by heparin in mice. Am Rev Respir Dis 1983; 128:747–751.

20. Meyrick B, Gamble W, Reid L. Development of Crotalaria pulmonary hypertension: hemodynamic and structural study. Am J Physiol 1980; 239:H692–H702.

21. Rabinovitch M, Gamble WJ, Miettinen OS, Reid L. Age and sex influence on pulmonary hypertension of chronic hypoxia and on recovery. Am J Physiol 1981; 240:H62–H72.

22. Hill NS, Thron CD, Smith RP. Time course of cardiopulmonary responses to high altitude in susceptible and resistant rat strains. Respir Physiol 1987; 70:241–249.

23. Meyrick B, Hislop A, Reid L. Pulmonary vasculature of the normal rat—the oblique muscle segment. J Anat 1978; 125:209–221.

24. Poiani GJ, Tozzi CA, Yohn SE, Pierce A, Belsky SA, Berg RA, et al. Collagen and elastin metabolism in hypertensive pulmonary arteries of rats. Circ Res 1990; 66:968–978.

25. Durmowicz AG, Parks WC, Hyde DM, Mecham RP, Stenmark KR. Persistence, re-expression, and induction of pulmonary arterial fibronectin, tropoelastin, and type I collagen mRNA expression, neonatal hypoxic pulmonary hypertension. Am J Pathol 1994; 145:1411–1420.

26. Fulton RM, Hutchinson EC, Jones AM. Ventricular weight in cardiac hypertrophy. Brit Heart J 1952; 14:413–420.

27. Hislop A, Reid L. New findings in pulmonary arteries of rats with hypoxia-induced pulmonary hypertension. Br J Exp Pathol 1976; 57:542–554.

28. Meyrick B, Reid L. Hypoxia-induced structural changes in the media and adventitia of rat hilar pulmonary artery, and their regression. Am J Pathol 1980; 100:151–178.

29. Hislop A, Reid L. Changes in the pulmonary arteries of rat during recovery from hypoxia-induced pulmonary hypertension. Br J Exp Pathol 1977; 58:653–662.

30. Meyrick B, Reid, L. Hypoxia and incorporation of ^{3}H-thymidine by cells of rat pulmonary arteries and alveolar wall. Am J Pathol 1979; 96:51–70.

31. Meyrick B, Reid L. The effect of continued hypoxia on rat pulmonary artery circulation: an ultrastructural study. Lab Invest 1978; 38:188–200.

32. Meyrick B, Reid L. Endothelial and subintimal changes in rat pulmonary artery during recovery from hypoxia. Lab Invest 1980; 42:603–615.

33. Tozzi CA, Christiansen DL, Poiani GJ, Riley DJ. Excess collagen in hypertensive pulmonary arteries decreases vascular distensibility. Am J Respir Crit Care Med 1994; 149:1317–1326.

34. Maruyama K, Ye CL, Vankatacharya H, Lines LD, Silver MM, Rabinovitch M. Chronic hypoxic pulmonary hypertension in rats with increased elastolytic activity. Am J Physiol 1991; 261:H1716–H1726.

35. Morrell NW, Atochina EN, Morris KG, Danilov SM, Stenmark KR. Angiotensin converting enzyme expression is increased in small pulmonary arteries of rats with hypoxia-induced pulmonary hypertension. J Clin Invest 1995; 96:1823–1833.

36. Klinger JR, Wrenn DS, Warburton RR, Pietras L, Ou LC, Hill NS. Atrial natriuretic peptide expression in rate with different pulmonary hypertensive responses to hypoxia. Am J Physiol 1997; 273:H411–H417.

37. La Cras TD, Tyler RC, Horan MP, Morris KG, Tuder RM, McMurtry IF, et al. Effects of chronic hypoxia and altered hemodynamics on endothelial nitric oxide synthase expression in the adult rat lung. J Clin Invest 1998; 101:795–801.

38. DeCarlo VS, Chen SJ, Meng QC, Durand J, Yano M, Chen YF, et al. ET-A receptor antagonist prevents and reverses chronic hypoxia-induced pulmonary hypertension in rat. Am J Physiol 1995; 269:L690–L697.

39. Russell P, Wright C, Kapeller K, Barer G, Howard P. Attenuation of chronic hypoxic pulmonary hypertension in rats by cyclooxygenase products and by nitric oxide. Eur Respir J 1993; 6:1501–1506.

40. Zhao L, al-Tuberly R, Sebkhi A, Owji AA, Nunez DJ, Wilkins MR. Angiotensin II receptor expression and inhibition in the chronically hypoxic rat lung. Br J Pharmacol 1996; 119:1217–1222.

41. Pfeifer M, Blumberg FC, Wolf K, Sandner P, Elsner D, Riegger GA, et al. Vascular remodeling and growth factor gene expression in the rat lung during hypoxia. Respir Physiol 1998; 111:210–212.

42. Chen SJ, Chen YF, Opgenoth TJ, Meng QC, Durand J, DiCarlo VS, et al. The orally active nonpeptide endothelin A-receptor antagonist A-127722 prevents and reverses hypoxia-induced pulmonary hypertension and pulmonary vascular remodeling in Sprague-Dawley rats. J Cardiovasc Pharmacol 1997; 29:713–725.

43. Fried R, Meyrick B, Rabinovitch M, Reid L. Polycythemia and the acute hypoxic response in awake rats following chronic hypoxia. J Appl Physiol 1983; 55:1167–1172.

44. Parker RE. Sheep as an animal model of endotoxemia-induced diffuse lung injury. In: Cantor J, ed. Handbook of Animal Models of Pulmonary Disease, Vol 1. CRC Handbooks, 1989 31–45.

45. Meyrick B, Brigham KL. Repeated E. coli endotoxin induced pulmonary inflammation causes chronic pulmonary hypertension in sheep: structural and functional changes. Lab Invest 1986; 55:164–176.

46. Perkett EA, Brigham KL, Meyrick B. Increased vasoreactivity and chronic pulmonary hypertension following thoracic irradiaton in sheep. J Appl Physiol 1986; 61:1875–1881.

47. Meyrick B, Niedermeyer ME, Ogletree ML, Brigham KL. Pulmonary hypertension and increased vasoreactivity caused by repeated indomethacin treatment in sheep. J Appl Physiol 1985; 59:443–452.

48. Gossage JR, Perkett EA, Davidson JM, Starcher BC, Carmichael D, Brigham KL, et al. Secretory leukoprotease inhibitor attenuates lung injury induced by continuous air embolization in sheep. J Appl Physiol 1995; 79:1163–1172.

49. Perkett EA, Davidson JM, Meyrick B. Sequence of structural changes and elastin peptide release during vascular remodeling in sheep with chronic pulmonary hypertension induced by air embolization. Am J Pathol 1991; 139:1319–1332.

50. Okada K, Tanaka Y, Bernstein M, Zhang W, Patterson GA, Botney MD. Pulmonary hemodynamics modify the rat pulmonary artery response to injury. A neointimal model of pulmonary hypertension. Am J Pathol 1997; 151:1019–1025.

51. Johnson JE, Perkett EA, Meyrick B. Pulmonary veins and bronchial vessels undergo remodeling in sustained pulmonary hypertension induced by continuous air embolization into sheep. Exp Lung Res 1997; 23:459–473.

52. Perkett EA, Brigham KL, Meyrick B. Granulocyte depletion attenuates sustained pulmonary hypertension and increased pulmonary vasoreactivity caused by continuous air embolization in sheep. Am Rev Respir Dis 1990; 141:456–465.

53. Perkett EA, Lyons RM, Moses HL, Brigham KL, Meyrick B. Transforming growth factor-β activity in sheep lung lymph during the development of pulmonary hypertension. J Clin Invest 1990; 86:1459–1464.

54. Perkett EA, Badesch DB, Roessler MK, Stenmark KR, Meyrick B. Insulin-like growth factor-I and pulmonary hypertension induced by continuous air embolization in sheep. Am J Respir Cell Molec Biol 1992; 7:81–89.

55. Perkett EA, Pelton RW, Meyrick B, Gold I, Miller DA. Expression of transforming growth factor-β mRNAs and proteins in pulmonary vascular remodeling in the sheep air embolization model of pulmonary hypertension. Am J Respir Cell Molec Biol 1994; 11:16–24.

56. Tchekneva E, Quertermous T, Christman BW, Lawrence M, Meyrick B. Regional variability in preproEndothelin-1 gene expression in sheep pulmonary artery and lung during the onset of air-induced chronic pulmonary hypertension. Participation of arterial smooth muscle cells. J Clin Invest 1998; 101:1389–1397.

57. Frid MG, Aldashev AA, Dempsey EC, Stenmark KR. Smooth muscle cells isolated from discrete compartments of the mature vascular media exhibit unique phenotypes and distinct growth capabilities. Circ Res 1997; 81:940–952.

58. Tchekneva E, Dikov M, Meyrick B. ppET-1 and ECE gene expression in pulmonary vascular smooth muscle cells (PVSMC): effect of hypertension associated factors. Am J Respir Crit Care Med 1997; 155:A784.

59. Tchekneva E, Lawrence M, Meyrick B. Cell-specific differences in ET-1 system in adjacent layers of main pulmonary artery. A new source of ET-1. Am J Physiol Lung Cell Mol Physiol 2000; 278:L813–822.

60. Jones R, Zapol WM, Reid L. Pulmonary artery remodeling and pulmonary hypertension after exposure to hyperoxia for 7 d. Am J Pathol 1984; 117:273–285.

61. Jones R, Zapol WM, Reid L. Pulmonary arterial wall injury and remodeling by hyperoxia. Chest 1983; 83:S40–S42.

VI ANIMAL CARE AND TISSUE PROCESSING

21 Veterinary Issues and Anesthesia Options

Robert P. Marini, DVM

CONTENTS

VETERINARY ISSUES

Biomedical research is highly regulated by a number of federal, state, and local statutes. The application of these statutes may depend upon the species of animal used, the funding source, the location of the facility, and the status of the facility as a component of the US government. The most important of these regulations are summarized below.

Regulations

THE LABORATORY ANIMAL WELFARE ACT (PL 89–544; THE ACT) (1)

This legislation was enacted by Congress in 1966 as a response to public concern that pets might be used in animal research. It has been amended many times since its promulgation and is published in Title 9, Code of Federal Regulations (CFR), Chapter 1, Subchapter A, Parts 1–3. It defines animals as *"any live or dead dog, cat, non-human primate, guinea pig, hamster, rabbit, or any other warm blooded animal, which is being used, or is intended for use in research, testing, experimentation, or exhibition purposes, or as a pet."(1)* Those animals which fit the definition are covered by the Act regardless of the funding source for research in which these animals are used. Specifically excluded

From: *Contemporary Cardiology: Vascular Disease and Injury: Preclinical Research*
Edited by: D. I. Simon and C. Rogers © Humana Press Inc., Totowa, NJ

by the Act are *"birds, rats of the genus Rattus and mice of the genus Mus bred for use in research,"* as well as horses not used in research or poultry and livestock used for food and fiber or food and fiber research. Some of these exemptions are currently being challenged *(2)*. The Act requires licensure of animal dealers, exhibitors, and operators of auctions, and also requires registration of carriers, intermediate handlers, exhibitors, and institutions using regulated species.

The Act contains standards for handling, housing, husbandry, shelter, veterinary care, and separation of species. Among the most important and substantive amendments are provisions for exercise requirements of dogs, an environment to promote the psychological well being of primates, consideration of strategies to minimize pain and distress, the search for painless alternatives, and the proper use of anesthetics, analgesics, and tranquilizers.

The Act is administered by Animal Care, the Animal Plant Health Inspection Service (APHIS), US Department of Agriculture (USDA). The USDA now also regulates horses and livestock used in biomedical or nonagricultural research.

Health Research Extension Act of 1985 (PL99–158) *(3)*

The Health Research Extension Act of 1985 establishes guidelines for the care and treatment of animals in biomedical and behavioral research conducted with funds provided by the Extension Act. The Public Health Service (PHS) Policy on Humane Care and Use of Laboratory Animals (the Policy) *(4)* serves to implement the Health Research Extension Act of 1985. Institutions that are awarded funds by the PHS are required to operate in accordance with the provisions published in the Guide for the Care and Use of Laboratory Animals (The Guide) *(5)*. The Guide was first published in 1963 by the Institute of Laboratory Animal Resources (ILAR), National Academy of Sciences, and was revised most recently in 1997. It is divided into five sections: Introduction; Institutional Policies and Responsibilities; Animal Environment, Housing and Management; Veterinary Medical Care; and Physical Plant. In contrast to the Act, the PHS Policy defines animals as *"any live, vertebrate animal used or intended for use in research, research training, experimentation, or biological testing or for related purposes"* thereby encompassing poikilotherms (fish, amphibians, reptiles) as well as mice, rats, and birds. Housing, husbandry, and veterinary care agree in general with the standards found in the Act.

US Government Principles for the Care and Utilization of Vertebrate Animals in Testing, Research, and Training (the Principles; Appendix A) *(6)*

These guidelines were developed by the Interagency Research Animal Committee, whose purposes include education, program coordination, and policy issues. The Principles are endorsed by the PHS Policy which both implements and supplements the Principles.

Additional regulations and licensure requirements may exist in the form of state or local statutes. Such regulations may include pound seizure laws, inspection, and oversight provisions by state or local agencies, and the existence of local commissioners who are empowered to oversee animal research. The IACUC, in coordination with the program veterinarian, maintains compliance with these various organizations and agencies.

Institutional Animal Care and Use Committee (IACUC)

In both the Act and the Policy, the Chief Executive Officer of the research facility is responsible for appointing an IACUC. The composition of the IACUC differs between these two documents in number (three in the Act vs five in the Policy) but not in the requirements for a veterinarian with specialty training or experience in laboratory animal medicine and a member without any other affiliation with the research facility. The IACUC has many key responsibilities in the oversight of research involving animals, but the responsibility that accounts for most of the interaction between principal investigators and the IACUC is protocol review. The IACUC must confirm, through review of protocols describing proposed research projects, that components of the protocol that involve animals are planned in accordance with the Act and the PHS Policy. The general areas evaluated by the IACUC are those enumerated in the Principles. The following areas require special attention by investigators submitting proposals to the IACUC.

ALTERNATIVES SEARCH

Investigators must provide assurance that the activities planned do not unnecessarily duplicate previous experiments. They must also assure that alternatives to procedures that cause more than slight or momentary pain or distress to experimental animals have been evaluated and considered. If alternatives do not exist or are inadequate for the subject under study, a written narrative must be provided that includes the databases, sources, and methods of the search for alternatives.

PROCEDURES CAUSING PAIN OR DISTRESS

Procedures with the potential for causing more than momentary pain or distress must be performed with appropriate sedatives, analgesics, or anesthetics, and must be planned in consultation with the attending veterinarian. Scientific justification must be provided in writing if these agents must be withheld. Each proposal must include a description of procedures and stratagems to minimize pain and discomfort. Techniques for euthanasia must also be included and should be in accordance with veterinary consultation and the AVMA Panel on Euthanasia *(7)*.

INVESTIGATOR TRAINING

The IACUC must determine that investigators are adequately trained to conduct planned procedures using animals. The IACUC may require attendance at training courses, seminars, and wet labs, or require oversight by veterinary technicians, other investigators, or the program veterinarian.

CHOICE OF SPECIES AND NUMBER OF ANIMALS

Investigators must provide a rationale for using animals, for the choice of the animal species used and for the proposed number of animals. Some IACUCs may require that appropriate numbers be determined by application of statistical principles while others may be less formal. Common rationales for the choice of species include the existence of historical data, special anatomic or physiologic features, and the requirement for multiple samples or samples of a particular weight or volume.

Requirements for Surgery

ASEPTIC TECHNIQUE

Aseptic technique is required for all species, including rodents, which are to be used in procedures from which the animal is expected to recover. Aseptic technique must be applied to the surgical subject, instruments, the surgeon, and other relevant members of the surgical team.

SURGICAL FACILITY

For survival procedures in nonrodent mammalian species, a dedicated surgical facility is required. This facility should contain the following areas: a surgical support area, an area for preparation of the animal, a surgeon preparation area, operating room or rooms, and an area for intensive and postoperative care of the animal *(5)*. Aseptic procedures in rodents may be performed in any clean laboratory space that may be isolated from normal traffic flow and which is easily sanitized. A recent review provides more detailed information *(8)*.

ANESTHESIA OPTIONS

The choice of anesthetic is determined by degree of invasiveness, duration of the procedure, age and condition of the surgical subject, and species-specific considerations. Only animal species included in this text will be considered in the following section. Details on handling these species and preferred anesthetic regimens should be sought in primary references and from veterinarians at your institution. Table 1 and Table 2 provide information on anesthetic agents and equipment mentioned in this chapter.

Table 1
Sources of Anesthetic Agents

Agent	Trade name	Concentration	Manufacturer (see Appendix B)
Acepromazine maleate	Promace	10 mg/mL	Fort Dodge Laboratories, Inc.
	Acepromazine	10 mg/mL	Fermenta Animal Health Co.
Atropine sulfate	Atropine sulfate	0.04 mg/mL	Elkins-Sinn Inc.
Buprenorphine	Buprenex	0.3 mg/mL	Reckitt & Colman Pharmaceuticals, Inc.
Butorphanol	Torbutrol	0.5 mg/mL	Fort Dodge Laboratories, Inc.
Diazepam	Valium	5 mg/mL	Roche Products Inc.
Fentanyl/fluanisone	Hypnorm		Janssen Pharmaceutica, Inc.
Glycopyrrolate	Robinul-V injectable	0.2 mg/mL	A. H. Robins Co, Inc.
Isoflurane	Aerrane		Anaquest
Ketamine	Ketaset	100 mg/mL	Bristol Laboratories
Lidocaine	Lidocaine hydrochloride oral topical solution	20 mg/mL	Barre-National Inc.
Methoxyflurane	Metofane		Schering-Plough Animal Health
Midazolam	Versed	1 mg/mL	Roche Laboratories
Pentobarbital	Nembutal	50 mg/mL	Abbott Laboratories
Propofol	Diprivan	10 mg/mL	Zeneca Pharmaceuticals
Thiopental	Pentothal		Abbott Laboratories
Tiletamine/zolazepam	Telazol	100 mg/mL	AH Robins
Tribromoethanol		100 g	Aldrich (SIGMA-ALDRICH Fine Chemicals)
Amylene hydrate			Aldrich
Xylazine	Rompun	20 mg/mL	Bayer Corp.Co
		100 mg/mL	

Table 2
Sources of Anesthetic Equipment (Selected Manufacturers and Distributors)

Hallowell Engineering & Manufacturing Corp.
74 North Street
Pittsfield, MA 0120
413–945–4263

North American Drager
148 B Quarry Road
Telford, PA 18969
215–723–9824

Columbus Instruments
9150 N. Hague
Columbus, OH 43204
614–276–0861; 800–669–5011

Harvard Apparatus, Inc.
22 Pleasant Street
South Natick, MA 01760
800–272–2775; 508–655–7000

Braintree Scientific, Inc.
P.O. Box 850929
Braintree, MA 02185–0929
718–843–2202

Sensor Devices, Inc.
407 Pilot Court, #400A
Waukesha, WI 53188
414–524–1000

ANESCO
115 Etter Lane
Georgetown, KY 40324
502–867–0784

Viking Medical
P.O. Box 2142
Medford Lakes, NJ 08055
800–920–1033; 609–953–0138

Ohmeda
Ohmeda Drive
PO Box 7550
Madison, WI 53707–7550
608–221–1551

TW Medical Veterinary Supply
P.O. Box 1745
Cedar Park, TX 78630–1745 (US)
512–258–6604; 888–787–4483

Vet Equip Inc.
P.O. Box 10785
Pleasanton, CA 94588–0785
925–463–1828

Equipment Sources Compendia

Marketplace for New and Used Medical Equipment
Annual Buyer's Guide And Monthly Catalog
   Medical Equipment
   Publishing Office
   1 Penn Plaza
   New York, NY 10119
   (212) 615–3058

Compendium of Vendors for Animal Research
Annual Buyers Guide
   Lab Animal
   Nature America Inc.
   Editorial and Executive Offices
   345 Park Avenue South, 10th Floor
   New York, NY 10010
   (212) 726–9200

Mice and Rats

Among the challenges of anesthetizing rats and mice are their small size, a small and inaccessible larynx that makes endotracheal intubation difficult, size and accessibility of peripheral vessels, and difficulties in physiologic monitoring and determining anesthetic depth (9,10). Strain differences in response to anesthesia complicate adoption of general recommendations (e.g., the inhalant anesthetic methoxyflurane may produce a diabetes insipidus-like syndrome in F344 rats). A large surface area-to-body wt ratio makes hypothermia in the anesthetized animal particularly common.

PREOPERATIVE CONSIDERATIONS

Mice and rats should be purchased from quality vendors and be free of murine adventitial viruses and other agents that may compromise health and impact tolerance of and recovery from anesthesia. They should be allowed 3 d to acclimate to their new environment. It is generally considered unimportant to withhold food from rats and mice prior to surgery. If food restriction is employed, the duration should be limited to less than 12 h (more typically 2–4 h) (10). Atropine (0.05 mg/kg SQ, ip) may be used as an anticholinergic, but is often omitted in practice. Similarly, pre-anesthetic agents (e.g., tranquilizers) that are commonly used in larger species are seldom used in rodents, in which the induction agent may also be used for maintenance throughout the procedure.

ANESTHESIA

Injectable techniques are very commonly used in rodents (9,10). Several combinations are listed below:

Mice

1. Tribromoethanol (250 mg/kg ip equivalent to approx 0.2 mL/10 g of a 1.2% w/v solution): this agent is prepared from stock solutions of 3,3,3 tribromoethanol and amylene hydrate. It produces approx 20 min of surgical anesthesia and is commonly used in procedures involved in the production of transgenic mice. Anesthesia may be prolonged with incremental doses of one-quarter to one-third the induction dose. Tribromoethanol should be made fresh from stock solutions or, if preprepared, should be stored at 4°C in brown bottles (Table 3; ref. 4). Improper storage (exposure to heat and light) leads to decomposition into toxic products that cause gastrointestinal irritation. While this agent is certainly efficacious and is widely used, a recent study reports the production of peritonitis at 24 h postadministration (12).
2. Ketamine/xylazine: Ketamine (120 mg/kg ip) and xylazine (16 mg/kg ip) diluted with 0.9% NaCl to concentrations of 1.2% and 0.16% respectively, produces 25–35 min of surgical anesthesia in mice (12). The agents may be mixed in the same syringe.

Table 3
Formula for Tribromoethanol Anesthesia[a]

Ingredients

2.5 g	2,2,2–tribromoethanol (Aldrich)
5 m	2–methyl-2–butanol (tertiary amyl alcohol; Aldrich)
200 m	distilled water

Method

1. Add tribromoethanol to butanol and dissolve by heating (approx 50°C) and stirring.
2. Add distilled water and continue to stir until butanol is totally dispersed.
3. Aliquot and store in the dark at 4°C.
4. Warm to 37°C and shake well before use.
5. Decomposition can result from improper storage. Provided the pH of the original soln was >5. This can be tested by adding 1 drop of Congo red (0.1% w/v) to 5 mL anesthetic. Purple color developing at pH <5 indicates decomposition to dibromoacetic aldehyde and hydrobromic acid. If this occurs, the anesthetic should be discarded, as it is toxic and can cause death within 24 h of injection.

[a]Adapted with permission from ref. *11*.

3. Fentanyl/fluanisone with midazolam or diazepam: Fentanyl/fluanisone (0.4 mL/ kg ip) and diazepam (5.0 mg/kg ip) produces 30–40 min of surgical anesthesia in mice *(9)*. The fentanyl/fluanisone combination is not available in the US.
4. Inhalant anesthesia: Anesthesia induction may be achieved in mice via bell-jar or other chamber induction techniques. The agent traditionally used for this purpose is methoxyflurane. Methoxyflurane induction via bell jar is safe and effective, because the low vapor pressure (tendency to volatilize) of the agent and its high solubility in blood makes anesthetic overdose unlikely provided attention to loss of movement is monitored in animals placed in the jar. An aliquot of inhalant is added to gauze or cotton balls at the bottom of a chamber (bell jar), the inhalant–impregnated gauze is covered with a woven wire mesh to avoid contact of the animal with the gauze, and then the animal is placed within the jar. If isoflurane is used in a bell jar, a measured amount must be used and animals must be evaluated continuously. Goldenthal (1992) used a 2.5-L jar in conjunction with a lid altered to serve as an isoflurane reservoir *(13)*. Five mL of isoflurane added to the cotton contained within the lid was sufficient to anes-thetize mice within 2 min of exposure. Animals recovered within 2 min of exposure *(9)*. The vapor pressure of isoflurane is high and its blood solubility is low compared with methoxyflurane, making anesthetic overdose an important risk. Whenever chamber induction of this type is used, the entire apparatus must be subject to adequate local scavenging or be placed in an appropriate fume

hood. Protection of personnel from exposure to waste concentrations of anesthetic gases should be addressed in facility guidelines and respected by investigators.

An anesthetic chamber connected via appropriate hosing to a precision vaporizer for methoxyflurane or isoflurane may also be used for anesthetic induction. Animals are then maintained using the same inhalant via face mask. Circuits, face masks, and vaporizers for use in rodents are commercially available (Table 2).

Rats

1. Ketamine/xylazine: ketamine (40–80 mg/kg ip) and xylazine (3–10 mg/kg ip) produce 20–30 min of anesthesia in the rat. Both agents may be mixed in the same syringe. A variation of this regimen involves the following cocktail:

   25% ketamine (v/v) 100 mg/mL;

   2.5% xylazine (v/v) 100 mg/mL;

   14.2% absolute ethanol; and

   58.3% 0.9% saline.

   A 250-g rat may be administered 0.3–0.6 mL/ip depending upon stock or strain *(14)*.

2. Fentanyl/fluanisone with midazolam or diazepam: fentanyl/fluanisone (0.6 mL/ kg ip) and diazepam (2.5 mg/kg ip) may be used initially and increments of 0.1mL/kg im may be used every 30–40 min to prolong anesthesia. Flecknell describes a premixed dilution consisting of 2 parts water for injection, 1 part Hypnorm, and 1 part midazolam, which is stable for at least 2 mo *(9,10)*. The dosage for rats is 2.7–4.0 mL/kg.

3. Pentobarbital: pentobarbital (30–60 mg/kg ip) continues to be used for anesthesia in rats despite variability in effect associated with strain or stock of rat, poor analgesic properties independent of its ability to cause loss of consciousness, and poor margin of safety. Consistency and efficacy may be improved by withdrawing food from rats for 1 h prior to surgery and by allowing rats 1–3 h to acclimate to the area in which the injection will be given *(8)*. One major supplier of surgically modified rats uses pentobarbital in procedures on Sprague–Dawley rats (TAC: N[SD]) and has developed a dose/weight chart from many years' experience using this agent (Personal Communication: Eric Arlund, Taconic, (518)537–6208; e-mail: taconicser@aol.com). Pentobarbital is diluted with sterile saline to a C of 13 mg/mL. Dosage varies by stock or strain, and gender, and is not linearly related to body wt. This supplier uses methoxyflurane by nose cone to adjust anesthetic plane, if necessary, after pentobarbital administration.

4. Inhalant anesthesia: inhalants may be used in rats in much the same fashion as that described for mice. Rats may be intubated using 14- to 20-gauge, over the needle Teflon catheters with the stylets filed down. Catheters may also be adapted with Silastic tubing to reduce mucosal injury *(15)*. Intubation is facilitated by customized laryngoscopes or by use of a mouth speculum and transillumination. In the latter technique, the rat is maintained in dorsal recumbency (supine), or is restrained on customized restraining boards and a powerful light source is shone on the ventral neck to illuminate the pharyngeal tissues *(16)*.

Rabbits

Rabbits may be safely and reliably anesthetized. Their past reputation as anesthetic risks has been largely influenced by the prevalence of underlying respiratory disease prior to the wide adoption of *Pasteurella*-free animals. Investigators in today's biomedical research environment should purchase rabbits from vendors with animals of high quality that are specific pathogen free for *Pasteurella*. Healthy, *Pasteurella*-free rabbits are more tolerant of anesthesia and have fewer postprocedural complications that may compromise results and lead to loss of data.

Rabbits are coprophagic, and as a consequence their stomachs are never empty. The inability to vomit precludes aspiration during anesthetic induction as a potential hazard. The withdrawal of food from rabbits prior to anesthesia is motivated by the purported advantage of improving diaphragmatic excursions against an emptier gastrointestinal tract. Overnight food withdrawal is sufficient, but is not uniformly practiced. Atropine (0.05 mg/kg) may be administered to rabbits prior to anesthesia, but the existence in some individuals of many strains of rabbits of the enzyme atropinesterase may obviate the effectiveness of the agent. Glycopyrrolate (0.01 mg/kg iv, 0.1 mg/kg im or sc) is an effective alternative and should be considered in inhalant procedures and when xylazine is used. The use of a good quality, mixed-grass hay postprocedurally helps promote the restoration of gastrointestinal function in rabbits.

Anesthetics are administered most frequently to rabbits by im injection into either the antero-lateral thigh or the lumbar epaxial musculature. Thigh injections should be given at right angles to the femur, and should avoid infiltration adjacent to the sciatic nerve (Fig. 1). Perineural injection of anesthetics may cause autotomy and self-amputation of digits. Common anesthetic regimens are listed below *(9,17)*:

1. Ketamine/xylazine: ketamine 35–50 mg/kg im and xylazine 5–10 mg/kg im produce approx 30 min of pedal withdrawal reflex loss. Procedures of moderate invasiveness may be performed with this combination alone. Anesthesia may be incremented by administration of one-half the original dose of ketamine. The addition of 0.75 mg/kg acepromazine or of 0.1 mg/kg butorphanol to ketamine/xylazine may prolong anesthesia and provide enhanced anesthetic depth.

2. Fentanyl/fluanisone and midazolam: fentanyl/fluanisone (0.3 mL/kg im) followed by midazolam (0.5–2 mg/kg iv, to effect) provides 20–40 min of surgical anesthesia. Increments of 0.1 mL/kg fentanyl/fluanisone iv every 30–40 min may be used to prolong anesthesia. The respiratory depressant effects of fentanyl may be reversed with naloxone (0.1 mg/kg iv) or buprenorphine (0.001 mg/kg iv). Use of the latter drug—a partial agonist opioid—effects reversal of respiratory depression with preservation of post-operative analgesia.

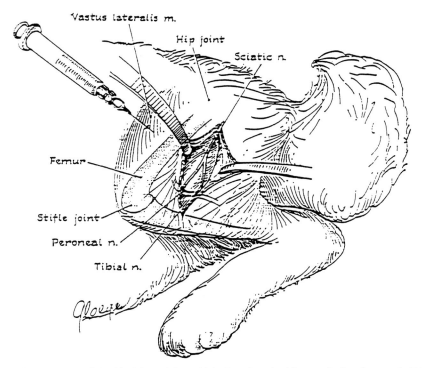

Fig. 1. Anatomy of the hind leg of the rabbit. Reprinted with permission from ref. *(20)*.

3. Inhalant anesthesia: isoflurane is currently the agent most commonly used in the rabbit. Isoflurane may be administered via tight-fitting face mask or via endotracheal tube. The latter is preferred to minimize operating-theater pollution and to allow for more efficient assisted ventilation. Isoflurane is used to effect, from 1–4%, in balance oxygen administered via coaxial (Bain) circuit in nonrebreathing fashion. Twice the min respiratory vol (the product of tidal volume and respiratory rate) is used as a fresh gas-flow rate; for most rabbits this is approx 4 L/min (Table 4) *(9)*. Face-mask and endotracheal-tube administration may be used after induction with ketamine/xylazine or fentanyl/fluanisone/midazolam, or after sedation with diazepam (1 mg/kg iv). Rabbits frequently hold their breath when first administered isoflurane. Gradual increase in isoflurane concentration may minimize this effect.

Endotracheal intubation may be achieved by visualization of the *aditus laryngicus* using a laryngoscope handle and a 1 Wisconsin or 1 Miller blade. Lidocaine oral topical solution should be used to lubricate the endotracheal tube and to reduce laryngeal irritability. Benzocaine-containing solns should not be used to spray the larynx, as methemoglobinemia may result. An assistant should restrain the anesthetized rabbit in sternal recumbency, with the head and neck extended in extreme dorsiflexion and with the tongue under manual traction

Table 4
Recommended Fresh Gas Flow Rates for Different Anesthetic Circuits[a]

Body weight (kg)	Estimated tidal vol (mL)	Minute vol (L)	Flow rate, open system (L min^{-1})	Flow rate, T-piece or Bain circuit (L min^{-1})	Flow rate, Magill circuit (L min^{-1})	Flow rate closed circuit L/min
0.5	5–7.5	0.4–0.6	1–2	1–1.5	–	–
1	10–15	0.5–1	1.5–3	1.5–2.5	–	–
3	30–45	1–1.5	3–4.5	2.5–3.5	–	–
6	60–90	1.5–3	4.5–9	3.5–7.5	–	–
10	100–150	3–6	9–18	6–12	3–6	0.3
20	200–300	5–9	15–27	10–18	5–9	0.5

[a]Adapted with permission from ref. (9).

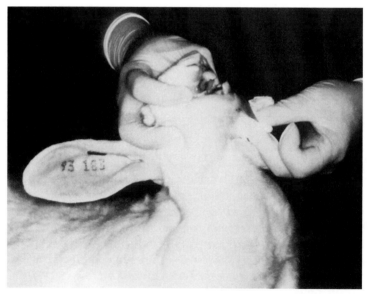

Fig. 2. Restraint of the rabbit for endotracheal intubation.

through one or the other diastema (Fig. 2). Endotracheal tubes may be 2.5–4.0-internal-diameter tubes, and may be cuffed or uncuffed.

Intubation may also be achieved blindly by placing the tube (preferably transparent) into the supraglottic area, and subsequently advancing the tube into the trachea as the animal inhales. Restraint as described above or with less dorsiflexion and more neutral extension of the head facilitates this procedure. Condensation on the transparent tube allows the operator to time insertion so that it corresponds to the disappearance of condensation, which occurs at approx the start of inspiration.

Swine

Swine are monogastric animals which are capable of vomiting, and should therefore have food withdrawn 12 h prior to anesthesia *(9,18)*. Water should remain *ad libitum*. Restraint of swine can be challenging, as they may object loudly and struggle vigorously. Pigs under 10 kg may be restrained manually; in larger pigs a useful technique is to force the animal into a corner or against the sides of its primary enclosure with a panel. Restraint slings in which swine may be suspended comfortably are commercially available. The dorsolateral neck and the thigh muscles are commonly used injection sites in pigs. Slapping the neck several times prior to insertion of a 20-gauge needle or 20-gauge butterfly catheter with 12" extension tubing often distracts the animal enough for a relatively uneventful needle stick. The needle may then be attached to an iv extension set or—in the case of the butterfly—to a syringe, and the injection may be made while following the pig about the enclosure. The use of tranquilizers may reduce stress and allow smoother induction. Atropine (0.04 mg/kg im) should be used to eliminate vagal reflexes and control bronchial and salivary secretions. Some investigators prefer glycopyrrolate (0.004–0.01 mg/kg im) in procedures involving manipulation of the heart. Typically, swine are administered agents that result in deep sedation or light anesthesia, and—if anesthetic depth is inadequate for intubation—are administered an injectable induction agent by ear vein (Table 5) or inhalant by face mask, and are then maintained with inhalant anesthetics delivered by mask or endotracheal tube.

Investigators should be aware of the genetic susceptibility of certain breeds of swine to malignant hyperthermia. Malignant hyperthermia is not a genetic condition of miniature swine. Susceptible breeds include Landrace, Pietrain, and Poland China; use of these breeds should be avoided in surgical protocols. All modern inhalants, stress, exercise, and succinylcholine are known to trigger malignant hyperthermia. This condition results from a defect in the ryanodine receptor gene that results in excessive liberation of Ca^{2+} from the sarcoplasmic reticulum and subsequent Ca^{2+} accumulation within the cytoplasm of myocytes. Signs include elevated end-tidal CO_2, hypercarbemia ($P_aCO_2 > 45$–50 mmHg), acidosis (pH <7.25), hyperthermia, and rhabdomyolysis with hyperkalemia, myoglobinemia, and myoglobinuria. Dantrolene (dose for prophylaxis 3.5–5 mg/kg iv, 1 h prior to the procedure) may be used prophylactically or for treatment of malignant hyperthermia *(18)*. Injectable agents are listed below:

1. Ketamine/acepromazine: ketamine (22 mg/kg im) and acepromazine (1.1 mg/kg im) produce approx 20–30 min of light anesthesia. This allows insertion of a catheter into the marginal ear vein, but is often inadequate for endotracheal intubation. Intubation may be achieved with mask induction using an inhalant or by iv administration of a barbiturate.

Table 5
Sites for Venous Access

Species	Vessel		
Mouse	Retro-orbital sinus	Tail vein	Medial saphenous vein
Rat	Retro-orbital plexus	Tail vein	
Rabbit	Marginal ear vein	Jugular vein	
Pig	Marginal ear vein	Cephalic vein	
Nonhuman primate	Saphenous vein	Cephalic vein	Femoral vein

2. Tiletamine/zolazepam: tiletamine/zolazepam (6–8 mg/kg im) produces approx 20–30 min of light anesthesia. Tiletamine/zolazepam (2–7 mg/kg im) and xylazine (0.2–1.0 mg/kg im) produce light to medium anesthesia of 30–40-min duration. The latter combination is adequate for endotracheal intubation.
3. Thiopental: This agent is administered in dilute soln (6–9 mg/kg of a 1–2.5% iv soln) to effect an anesthetic plane adequate for short procedures or endotracheal intubation in the preanesthetized pig.
4. Propofol: propofol (2.5–3.5 mg/kg iv) may be used for induction of anesthesia in preanesthetized swine, and has been used as a sole agent for anesthesia at rates of 8–12 mg/kg/h. It may cause apnea immediately after injection. Investigators should be prepared to assist ventilation when propofol is used in this fashion.
5. Isoflurane (1–4% in balance oxygen) is the most commonly used inhalant anesthetic for swine anesthesia. It may be administered by tight-fitting face mask or by endotracheal tube. Swine over 10 kg should have anesthetic delivery via circle circuit with CO_2 absorption while swine under that weight may be maintained using a coaxial (Bain) circuit. Gas flows with the Bain circuit are quite high and may exceed achievable flow rates in some anesthetic machines.

Endotracheal intubation of swine may be accomplished with the animal in ventral (sternal) or dorsal recumbency. With the animal in sternal recumbency, an assistant lifts the upper jaw and maintains traction on the tongue. The operator uses a larygoscope handle and blade (195 mm; Wisconsin 1–4 depending on the animal) to visualize and depress the epiglottis. An endotracheal tube (5–8 mm-internal-diameter for most swine), with or without stylet, is passed over the epiglottis and then rotated 90 degrees to avoid the laryngeal diverticulum. Tubes should be lubricated with Lidocaine oral topical solution. If resistance is met, the tube is withdrawn and the procedure is repeated using this same corkscrew motion. For intubation of animals in dorsal recumbency, it is imperative that the jaw is not held open, as this practice creates an unfavorable geometry for intubation. The operator uses the laryngoscope blade to visualize the epig-

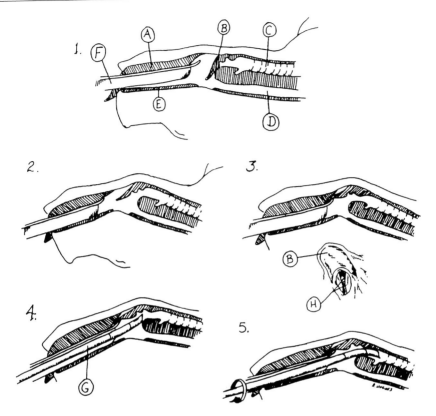

Fig. 3. Method for intubation of the pig. Reprinted with permission from ref. *(18)*.

lottis and forces the maxilla into the table by elevating the tip of the blade as it depresses the epiglottis. The blade should be at a 45-degree angle to permit visualization of the larynx (Fig. 3). The tube may then be advanced as described above. Swine are prone to laryngospasm and should therefore have their larynx sprayed with topical anesthetic as soon as adequate visualization has been achieved.

Nonhuman Primates

The primate order is very diverse, with species differing in habitat, social organization, size, and many other characteristics. The recommendations in this section are specific to the genus Papio, consisting of the baboons and the genus Macaca, which includes the rhesus (*Macaca mulatta*) and the cynomolgus monkey (*Macaca fascicularis*). These three species comprise the most widely used nonhuman primates in cardiovascular research *(9,19)*.

Macaques and baboons are safely anesthetized using a variety of techniques; by far the most widely practiced is the use of a dissociative followed by endotracheal intubation and maintenance with an inhalant. A common alternative for procedures of moderate invasiveness is the use of a premixed soln of ketamine/xylazine. Anticholinergics (atropine 0.04 mg/kg im) should always be used in primates to control the copious salivation that occurs with the use of dissociatives in these species. Another important consideration is the presence of zoonotic agents in macaques and baboons that require strict adherence to standard operating procedures for the use of personal protective equipment. The most important of these is *Herpesvirus simiae*, or B virus of macaques. This agent is shed in bodily secretions, especially saliva, and is potentially fatal if contracted by humans. Techniques must be employed by operators to avoid the placement of hands within the mouth of a macaque during the procedure of endotracheal intubation. Macaques and baboons should always be anesthetized for handling, a procedure that is facilitated by the widespread use of squeeze-back cages. Nonhuman primates should have food withdrawn overnight, or at least 12 h prior to anesthesia. Feeding within 8 h of anesthesia may result in gastric dilation in the dissociative-anesthetized nonhuman primate.

1. Ketamine: ketamine (10 mg/kg im) is adequate for chemical restraint of approx 15–20 min duration and allows investigators to perform minor procedures such as percutaneous catheterization and venipuncture. Experienced operators may perform endotracheal intubation under ketamine alone, but investigators with limited experience should use agents that result in more profound anesthesia. The latter precaution will preclude injury to the operator while performing this technique. Higher doses (up to 20 mg/kg) may promote light anesthesia. Nonhuman primates administered ketamine retain the laryngeal, pharyngeal, and palpebral reflexes.

2. Ketamine/xylazine: ketamine (7–10 mg/kg im) and xylazine (0.5–0.6 mg/kg im) produces 30 min of anesthesia of moderate depth. A common method of ketamine/xylazine anesthesia involves the use of a cocktail consisting of 7 mL of ketamine (100 mg/mL) and 3 mL of xylazine (20 mg/mL). The resulting soln is used at 0.1 mL/kg. This dose corresponds to 7 mg/kg ketamine and 0.6 mg/kg xylazine.

3. Tiletamine/zolazapam: the tiletamine/zolazepam (5 mg/kg) combination provides approx 45 min of chemical restraint or light anesthesia. Recovery is subjectively more placid than that of ketamine, and muscle relaxation is greater than with ketamine alone.

4. Anesthetic induction: both thiopental (3–5 mg/kg iv) and propofol (2–5 mg/kg iv) may be used for induction prior to endotracheal intubation.

5. Pentobarbital: pentobarbital is a useful agent in the nonhuman primate, but must be used with caution because of its powerful respiratory depressant effects. It is

typically used intravenously after ketamine or tiletamine/zolazepam induction. Dilution of the 50 mg/mL stock soln 1:1 with saline allows better control over administration. The dose administered to unanesthetized animals is 20–30 mg/kg, but prior administration of a dissociative necessitates reduction of the dose by at least one-third. One-half of this calculated dose may be administered by bolus, with smaller increments administered to effect. Pentobarbital provides 30–60 min of surgical anesthesia, and recovery is slow.

6. Inhalants: as in other species, isoflurane is currently the inhalant agent of choice. Isoflurane is used to effect (1–4% in balance oxygen) and should be administered via endotracheal tube. Depending on the size of the animal, a coaxial (Bain) circuit (fresh gas-flow of twice the min respiratory vol) or a circle circuit (fresh gas-flow of 1–2 L/min) with CO_2 absorption may be used.

Endotracheal intubation is best achieved with the animal in sternal recumbency. An assistant uses a length of roll gauze placed behind the superior (maxillary) canines to suspend the head of the animal. The operator uses a curved laryngoscope blade (Macintosh 1–3) to advance the tongue from the mouth. The assistant may exert traction on the tongue using a piece of gauze to help the operator visualize the *aditus laryngicus*. At no time should the assistant's hand enter the mouth of the nonhuman primate. The larynx should be sprayed with lidocaine prior to intubation to preclude laryngospasm. Endotracheal tubes (2–8-mm outer diameter, depending on the animal) should be lubricated with lidocaine oral topical solution prior to intubation.

POSTSURGICAL CARE AND ANALGESIA

Programs for postsurgical care and strategies to deal with unexpected events should be detailed in the Animal Care and Use Protocol. Criteria for evaluation include overall demeanor, level of activity, appearance of incision, appetite, hydration state, the presence of urine and stool, and condition of the haircoat. Observations then determine the collection of objective data for animals that are not recovering fully and may include blood work, rectal temperature, radiographs, angiography, and cardiovascular evaluation. Animals should be administered analgesics if they are showing signs of pain or if procedures to which they will be subjected are likely to cause postsurgical pain in humans. Many institutions recommend preoperative use of analgesics with continued administration postoperatively. Institutional guidelines and attending veterinarians should be consulted for preferred techniques of provision of analgesia. If euthanasia is required, techniques used should be in accordance with institutional guidelines and the AVMA Panel on Euthanasia (Table 6).

Table 6
Recommended Techniques for Euthanasia

Species	Method of euthanasia
Mouse	CO_2 asphyxiation
Rat	CO_2 asphyxiation OR pentobarbital IP (120 mg/kg)
Rabbit	Pentobarbital (120 mg/kg iv), preferably after ketamine/xylazine anesthesia (35/5 mg/kg im)
Nonhuman primate	Pentobarbital (120 mg/kg iv) after ketamine anesthesia (10 mg/kg im)
Pig	Pentobarbital (120 mg/kg iv) after tiletamine/zolazepam anesthesia (5 mg/kg im)

APPENDIX A

The Principles: U.S. Government Principles for the Utilization and Care of Vertebrate Animals Used in Testing, Research, and Training

The development of knowledge necessary for the improvement of the health and well-being of humans as well as other animals requires in vivo experimentation with a wide variety of animal species. Whenever U.S. government agencies develop requirements for testing, research, or training procedures involving the use of vertebrate animals, the following principles shall be considered; and whenever these agencies actually perform or sponsor such procedures, the responsible Institutional Official shall ensure that these principles are adhered to:

I. The transportation, care and use of animals should be in accordance with the Animal Welfare Act (7 U.S.C. 2131 et. seq.) and other applicable Federal laws, guidelines, and policies.*

II. Procedures involving animals should be designed and performed with due consideration of their relevance to human or animal health, the advancement of knowledge, or the good of society.

III. The animals selected for a procedure should be of an appropriate species and quality and the minimum number required to obtain valid results. Methods such as mathematical models, computer simulation, and in vitro biological systems should be considered.

IV. Proper use of animals, including the avoidance or minimization of discomfort, distress, and pain when consistent with sound scientific practices, is imperative. Unless the contrary is established, investigators should consider that procedures that cause pain or distress in human beings may cause pain or distress in other animals.

V. Procedures with animals that may cause more than momentary or slight pain or distress should be performed with appropriate sedation, analgesia, or anesthesia. Surgical or other painful procedures should not be performed on unanesthetized animals paralyzed by chemical agents.

VI. Animals that would otherwise suffer severe or chronic pain or distress that cannot be relieved should be painlessly killed at the end of the procedure or, if appropriate, during the procedure.

VII. The living conditions of animals should be appropriate for their species and contribute to their health and comfort. Normally, the housing, feeding, and care of all animals used for biomedical purposes must be directed by a veterinarian or other scientist trained and experienced in the proper care, handling, and use of the species being maintained or studied. In any case, veterinary care shall be provided as indicated.

VIII. Investigators and other personnel shall be appropriately qualified and experienced for conducting procedures on living animals. Adequate arrangements shall be made for their in-service training, including the proper and humane care and use of laboratory animals.

IX. Where exceptions are required in relation to the provisions of these Principles, the decisions should not rest with the investigators directly concerned but should be made, with due regard to Principle II, by an appropriate review group such as an institutional animal care and use committee. Such exceptions should not be made solely for the purposes of teaching or demonstration.

*For guidance throughout these Principles, the reader is referred to the *Guide for the Care and Use of Laboratory Animals* prepared by the Institute of Laboratory Animal Resources, National Academy of Sciences (5).

APPENDIX B
Sources of Anesthetic Agents

Fort Dodge Laboratories, Inc.
800 Fifth St. N.W.
Fort Dodge, IA 50501
(515) 955–4600

Fermenta Animal Health Co.
10150 North Executive Hills Blvd.
Kansas City, MO 64153
(816) 891–5500

Elkins-Sinn Inc.
2 Esterbrook Lane
Cherry Hill, NJ 08003–4099
(610) 688–4400

Reckitt and Colman Pharmaceuticals, Inc.
1909 Huguenot Road
Richmond, VA 23235
(804) 379–1090

Roche Products, Inc.
Manati, Puerto Rico
(for medical information, contact Roche Laboratories)
(800) 526–6367

Janssen Pharmaceutica, Inc.
1125 Trenton-Harbourton Rd.
P.O. Box 200
Titusville, NJ 08560–0200
(800) 526–7736

A. H. Robins Co., Inc.
1407 Cummings Drive
Richmond, VA 23220
(610) 688–4400

Aldrich (SIGMA-ALDRICH Fine
Chemicals)
P.O. Box 355
Milwaukee, WI 53201
(800) 771–6737

Bristol Laboratories (BRISTOL-
MYERS SQUIBB CO.)
P.O. Box 4500
Princeton, NJ 08543–4500
(609) 897–2000

Barre-National Inc. (ALPHARMA)
U.S. Pharmaceuticals Division
7205 Windsor Blvd.
Baltimore, MD 21244
(800) 638–9096

Schering-Plough Animal Health
1095 Morris Avenue
P.O. Box 3182
Union, NJ 07083–1982
(908) 298–4000

Roche Pharmaceuticals Roche Laboratories Inc.
340 Kingsland Street
Nutley, NJ 07110–1199
(800) 526–6367

Abbott Laboratories
100 Abbott Park Rd.
Abbott Park, IL 60064
(800) 633–9110

Bayer Corporation Pharmaceutical
Division
400 Morgan Lane
West Haven, CT 06516
(800) 288–8371

Anaquest (Ohmeda Pharmaceutical
Products Division Inc.)
110 Allen Road, Box 804
Liberty Corner, NJ 07938–0804
(908) 322–8272

Zeneca Pharmaceuticals
Wilmington, Delaware 19850–5437
(302) 886–3000

REFERENCES

1. U.S. Department of Agriculture Animal Welfare Act, Subchapter A, part 1, 3, USDA, Washington, DC, (7 U.S.C. 2131 et seq.) 1993.
2. McArdle J. Reassessing Rodents: animals outside the AWA. Lab Anim 1999; 28:2, 22–25.
3. National Institutes of Health. Health Research Extension Act of 1985, Animals in Research. NIH, OPRR (Office for Protection from Research Risks), Rockville, MD, 1996.
4. National Institutes of Health. Public Health Service Policy on Humane Care and Use of Laboratory Animals. NIH, OPRR (Office for Protection from Research Risks), Rockville, MD, 1986.

5. Institute of Laboratory Animal Resources, Commission on Life Sciences, National Research Council. Guide for the Care and Use of Laboratory Animals. National Academy Press, Washington, DC, 1996.

6. US Government Principles for the Utilization and Care of Vertebrate Animals Used in Testing, Research, and Training. Appendix D. In: Guide for the Care and Use of Laboratory Animals. National Academy Press, Washington DC, 1996 116–118.

7. Report of the AVMA Panel on Euthanasia. JAVMA 1993; 202:229–249.

8. White WJ, Blum JR. Design of Surgical Suites and Postsurgical Care Units. In: Kohn DF, Wixson SK, White WJ, Benson GJ, eds. Anesthesia and Analgesia in Laboratory Animals. Academic Press, San Diego,1997, 149–162.

9. Flecknell, PA. Laboratory Animal Anaesthesia, 2nd ed. Academic Press, London, 1987, 26(3).

10. Kohn DF, Wixson SK, White WJ, Benson JG. Anesthesia and Analgesia in Rodents. In: Kohn DF, Wixson SK, White WJ, Benson GJ, eds. Anesthesia and Analgesia in Laboratory Animals. Academic Press, San Diego, 1997; 165–200.

11. Papaioannou VE, Fox JG. Efficacy of tribromoethanol anesthesia in mice. Lab Anim Sci 1993; 43(2):189–192.

12. Zeller W, Meier G, Burki K, Panoussis B. Adverse effects of tribromoethanol as used in the production of transgenic mice. Lab Anim 1998; 32:407–413.

13. Goldenthal A. Use of isoflurane in a drop system. Lab Anim 1992; 21(5):47–48.

14. Wu MP, Tamada JA, Brem H, Langer R. In vivo versus in vitro degradation of controlled release polymers for intracranial surgical therapy. J Biomed Mat Res 1994; 28:387–395.

15. De Leonardis JR, Clevenger R, Hoyt RF. Approaches to rodent intubation and endotracheal tube design. Contemp Top Lab Anim Sci 1995; 34(4):60.

16. Cambron H, Latulippe JF, Nguyen T, Cartier R. Orotracheal intubation of rats by transillumination. Lab Anim Sci 1995; 45(3):303–304.

17. Lipman NS, Marini RP, Flecknell PA. Anesthesia and Analgesia in Rabbits. In: Kohn DF, Wixson SK, White WJ, Benson GJ, eds. Anesthesia and Analgesia in Laboratory Animals. Academic Press, San Diego, 1997; (10)205–228.

18. Smith AC, Ehler WJ, Swindle MM. Anesthesia and Analgesia in Swine. In: Kohn DF, Wixson SK, White WJ, Benson GJ, eds. Anesthesia and Analgesia in Laboratory Animals. Academic Press, San Diego, 1997; (14), 315.

19. Popilskis SJ, Kohn DF. Anesthesia and Analgesia in Nonhuman Primates. In: Kohn DF, Wixson SK, White WJ, Benson GJ, eds. Anesthesia and Analgesia in Laboratory Animals. Academic Press, San Diego, 1997; 233–254.

20. Hodesson S et al. Anesthesia of the Rabbit with Equi-Thesin following the administration of preanesthetics. Lab Anim Care 1965; 115, 336–337.

22 Histological and Immunohistochemical Methods for Vascular Animal Model Studies

Philip Seifert, MS, HTL(ASCP),
Campbell Rogers, MD, FACC
and Elazer R. Edelman, MD, PhD, FACC

Contents

INTRODUCTION

The compound microscope was probably invented in the late sixteenth century, and by the eighteenth century, physiologists were using the microscope to define anatomical structures. However, it was not until dyes, developed by the textile industry in the nineteenth century, were applied to tissue sections that the full potential of histology could be realized. Monochromatic images could now be transformed, allowing the user to easily distinguish between adjacent microscopic structures. Recent advances in biomedical technology have stimulated ever more sophisticated viewing, analysis, and measurement of the tissue reaction to implanted devices and administered drugs. As a result, histotechnology is in the midst of a renaissance in the development of new

From: *Contemporary Cardiology: Vascular Disease and Injury: Preclinical Research*
Edited by: D. I. Simon and C. Rogers © Humana Press Inc., Totowa, NJ

Table 1
Steps in Histological Preparation

1. Fixation

2. Processing

3. Embedding

4. Microtomy

5. Staining

6. Analysis

techniques and incorporation of innovations in monoclonal antibody science
with automated equipment that produce images never before imagined.

This chapter provides references and an overview of various histopathological techniques and methods for studying vascular biology in animal models.
Six fundamental steps must be addressed in dealing with tissue specimens
(Table 1). These include techniques to preserve tissue integrity, from orientation to ultrastructure, as well as the choice of specific stains to highlight elements of interest. No one technique can be applied to every tissue and
indication. Indeed, methods for microscopic examination of vascular tissues
vary from whole-mount preparations to routine frozen and paraffin procedures
to the recent use and adaptation of specialized bone methacrylate methods for
histologic examination of stent-implanted vessels. Numerous manuals and texts
are available which expound on theory, practice, and methods, with detailed
instructions for the performance of histological and immunohistochemical
preparations on various tissues (1–3). There are a large number of schemes and
strategies to keep in mind when designing animal experiments that involve histology. To adequately determine what is needed, the desired current or future
evaluation must be decided. This in turn dictates fixation and preparation procedures. Preparation procedures that allow serial sectioning and extended
archiving (paraffin and methacrylate) are preferred. Most histology labs are
equipped to process and stain tissues routinely using automated techniques, but
specialized stains may need to be performed manually. In the following sections, we discuss the various steps involved in tissue fixation, processing, embedding, microtomy, staining, and analysis.

FIXATION

Pioneering microscopists were plagued by the natural decay of tissues with
time, and needed to view their specimens within moments of harvest or risk

tissue distortion. Excised tissues undergo autolytic, putrefaction, and environmental degradation. Fixation preserves morphological structure for subsequent chemical processing, microtomy and staining at any time. A range of fixatives is available to account for differences in tissue dimensions, tissue composition, and stains that will be used. Equally important is the matter of time. Occasionally tissues will undergo structural changes such as shrinkage faster than the penetration time for many fixatives. Fixatives can serve as mordants, or simply make tissue chemically receptive to specific stains.

To examine these types of tissue, and materials containing fats and lipids (Table 3) or to use immunohistochemical staining with antigens sensitive to environmental conditions (Table 5) frozen preparation should be performed. Tissues may be fixed in formaldehyde-based fixatives or snap frozen in liquid-nitrogen cooled isopentane *(1,3)*. In either case, they must be infused with specialized embedding media which will serve as scaffolding for microtomy. Frozen processing retains much of the tissue antigenicity, but creates artifacts and morphological alterations. To fully preserve tissue architecture, more stringent fixatives are used.

Vascular structures have a resting tone, and are distended by physiological pressures. When removed from the body, they collapse. Routine histology for imaging of *in situ* morphology often utilizes pressure-perfusion fixation to prevent collapse and shrinkage of vessels from muscle contraction and elastic recoil. Pressure-perfusion fixation is accomplished by rinsing clear the whole heart or peripheral vascular tissue with physiological solutions, such as Ringer's lactate, followed by perfusion at 100 mmHg pressure with a formaldehyde-based fixative should be at least longer than 15 min. After perfusion, tissues can be dissected free with some assurance that their architecture and orientation will remain intact. To ensure full fixation, these excised specimens should then be immersed in fixative for at least 24 h in a 20:1 of fixative to tissue-volume ratio *(1,3)*.

Fixatives can usually be classified as *coagulative* or *crosslinking*. Coagulative fixatives establish a network in tissues that enables solutions to readily penetrate to the tissue interior. These include reagents such as mercuric chloride and picric acid. The last of these is an essential element in a number of well-known fixatives. In contrast, noncoagulative or crosslinking fixatives link and stabilize tissue proteins, creating a gel that limits denaturation as well as fluid and reagent penetration. Such crosslinking fixatives include formaldehyde, glutaraldehyde, osmium tetroxide, acetic acid, and potassium dichromate.

A fixative used for routine and specialized staining is 10% neutral buffered formalin or phosphate-buffered 4% paraformaldehyde fixative. The 4% paraformaldehyde fixative is composed of pure formaldehyde from a paraformaldehyde stock solution, depolymerized under heat and a high pH, and prepared in a phosphate buffer *(1,3)*. Formaldehyde is a crosslinking fixative that reacts

Table 2
Fixatives for Vascular Animal Model Studies

Fixatives	Applications	References
10% Neutral buffered formalin	General-purpose fixative, H and E, special stains, immunohistochemistry	(1–16)
4% Paraformaldehyde (0.1 M phosphate-buffered)		
Methanol-Carnoy's	An alcohol-based coagulative fixative useful for PCNA and BrDU immunostaining	(5,9,17–19)
Karnovsky's fixative	Scanning and transmission electron microscopy	(1–3)
Osmium tetroxide	Scanning and transmission electron microscopy, lipid fixative for embedding	(1–3)

on the side chains of amino acids. There are numerous special fixatives (Orth's solution, Zenker's, Bouin's, B-5, and Carnoy's), yet none is more readily utilized and commercially available than 10% neutral buffered formalin (1,3). Table 2 lists fixatives that are used in a variety of vascular animal models.

PROCESSING, EMBEDDING AND STAINING

All tissues need to be embedded with some support media before microtome sectioning (Table 3). The harder the tissue, the stronger the support material must be. Only this material prevents the microtome blade from distorting the tissue specimen as the cross-section is cut. Frozen materials may be *fixed* and then *embedded* with media. Nonfrozen materials are fixed first and must be embedded later. As most embedding materials are hydrophobic, the specimens must be chemically dehydrated and cleared of lipids to allow penetration of the media. The processing schedule is dependent upon the size and type of tissue involved; small mouse vessels may be run for 3–5 h or less, while larger arteries may require an extended run of 6–14 h. The use of automated equipment has increased the efficiency and decreased the time required for embedding and processing, but some procedures, such as those that use methacrylate, require manual infiltration and polymerization (4,9–11,16–20).

An important issue in histopathological investigations using polymers and vascular devices is the potential artifactual alteration from histological process-

Table 3
Processing Procedures For Animal Studies

Embedding procedure	Use	References
Frozen	Lipid stains (Oil red-O, Sudan IV)	(1–3)
Paraffin	Routine and special stains	(1–3)
Methacrylate resin	Metallic implants (e.g., stents)	(4,6,9–11,16–20)
Glycol methacrylate	Polymers (susceptible to alteration from processing reagents)	(21,22)
Epoxy resin	Transmission electron microscopy for ultrastructural studies	(1–3)

ing and embedding reagents *(21)*. A test specimen should be processed through-out the entire procedure and examined for potential artifacts. Some inert poly-mers are resistant to alteration, yet others (i.e., polyurethane-based or PLA/PCL) are susceptible to alteration during paraffin- and methacrylate-embedding. Table 4 lists various histological stains that are utilized in vascular animal model studies to identify various tissue components.

PROCEDURES FOR STENT-IMPLANTED TISSUE

The harder the material, the harder the media must be. The use of metallic implants has raised the standard for tissue-processing requirements. Standard techniques in vascular tissue histology will not suffice when vessels are *stented*. Methods modified from the histopathology of orthopedic tissues and implants have enabled examination of stented arteries, particularly those that employ methacrylate embedding *(4,9–11,16–20)*. Yet, conventional methacrylate for-mulations are still too soft for stent pathology, and they must be modified with substantial reduction of the plasticizer to harden the resin *(4,9,10,17–19)*. More-over, the polymerization techniques employed involve environmental exposures that can destroy antibody-antigen recognition. We have developed a modified bone methacrylate method *(20)* that allows histological and immunohistochemi-cal staining on intact stent-implanted vessels via cold–temperature resin em-bedding, sawing, and microtomy (MWM resin; *4,9,10,17–19*; Fig. 1). This allows the generation of a panel of stains on serial sections from the same speci-men block and quantification of the localization via computer-assisted image analysis. We have applied these techniques in several animal studies *(4,9,17–19)* and in human autopsy stent-implanted vessels *(10)*.

Table 4
Histological Stains

Stain	Preparation	Staining characteristics	References
Hematoxylin and Eosin stain	Frozen, paraffin and methacrylate	Classic general-purpose stain, Nuclei = blue, cytoplasm, and extracellular matrix = pinkish red	(1–3)
Verhoeff's elastin	Frozen, paraffin and methacrylate	Elastic fibers and nuclei = blue-black, collagen = red, cellular cytoplasm, and extracellular matrix components = yellow, platelets = yellow-gray	(1–3)
Elastic-Gomori's trichrome	Paraffin and methacrylate	Elastic fibers and nuclei = blue-black, collagen (sulfated mucosubstances) = greenish blue, cellular cytoplasm, and extracellular matrix components = red	(3)
Masson's trichrome	Paraffin and methacrylate	Nuclei = blue-black, collagen (sulfated mucosubstances) = blue, cellular cytoplasm, and extracellular matrix components = red	(1–3)
Mod. Russell-Movat Pentachrome	Paraffin and methacrylate	Elastic fibers and nuclei = blue-black, collagen = yellow, mucosubstances = blue, cellular cytoplasm, and extracellular matrix components = reddish-orange	(2)
Oil red-O	Frozen	Neutral lipids = red, nuclei = blue	(1–3)

330

Table 4 (*Continued*)

Stain	Preparation	Staining characteristics	References
Sudan IV	Whole-mount	Neutral lipids = black	(3)
Evans blue	Whole-mount	Denuded regions of lumen = blue, nondenuded = unstained	(3)
Silver	Whole-mount	Used to visualize endothelial cells by staining intercellular junctions brown-black	(18)
Carstairs fibrin	Paraffin and methacrylate	Fibrin = deep orange, nuclei = blue, cytoplasm = blue, collagen = red	(3)
Picrosirius red	Paraffin and methacrylate	Collagen = red (under brightfield illumination), yellow and greenish-blue (under cross-polarization illumination)	(7)

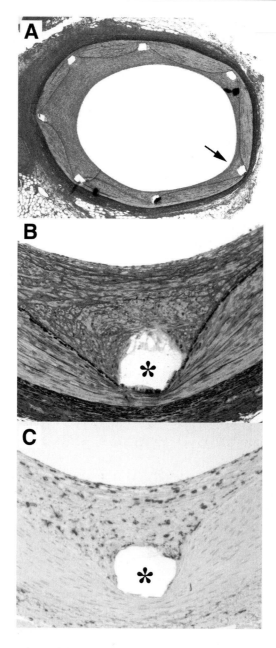

Fig. 1. (A) Endovascular stainless-steel stent-implanted Pig coronary artery, 28 d post implantation, MWM resin-embedded, 5-μm section, Verhoeff's elastin stain, original magnification = 25×. **(B)** High magnification of stent strut (*) region denoted in Fig. A (arrow), 5-μm section, Verhoeff's elastin stain, original magnification = 160×. **(C)** Serial section immunostained for porcine-CD45 (MAC323) using antigen retrieval and a tyramide signal

For large implants (>200-mm wire thickness) or hard metallic compositions (e.g., Nitinol) a sawing/grinding/polishing procedure *(6,11)* should be used after embedding in a methacrylate (nonglycol methacrylate-based) resin. With this technique, the desired planes are sawed out, mounted onto slides, and ground and polished down to approx 20–50 μm in thickness, using a series of grit materials and compounds. This technique retains the entire implant within the specimen, but suffers from a number of drawbacks. These disadvantages include loss of material through sawing and grinding, limitation of step sectioning every 0.5–1.0 mm throughout the specimen, obscuration of adherent cell layers surrounding the implant by a ledging effect at the tissue-implant interface, and inadequate microscopic resolution imposed by the 20–50 μm-section thickness.

IMMUNOHISTOCHEMISTRY

Immunohistochemical staining is an effective means of identifying and localizing specific antigens related to cell and tissue proliferation, specificity, phenotype, and cell types (Table 5). However, antigenicity may be lost in routinely processed tissues with alteration, depletion, or masking effects derived from a crosslinking fixative and solvent processing during paraffin- or methacrylate-embedding. Antigen retrieval (e.g., heat-induced epitope retrieval, antigen unmasking, antigen recovery) arose from the need to immunostain routinely processed tissues. Numerous antigen retrieval methods have been developed throughout the past decade since Shi's groundbreaking publication *(13)*. The use of a pH specific buffer and heat in combination from microwave, steam heat, autoclave, or a water bath unmasks epitopes for greater immunoreactivity, thus intensifying and increasing the number of positive cells in formalin-fixed paraffin-embedded tissues *(12–14)*. This has expanded the possibilities and range of tissues for immunohistochemistry that were previously possible only with frozen tissues or specially fixed tissues.

The use of antigen retrieval techniques is not restricted to paraffin-embedded tissues and can be adapted and utilized in resin embedded tissues *(23)*. Hand et al. *(23)* adapted a methyl methacrylate procedure and utilized antigen retrieval to enhance immunoreactivity for a diverse panel of antigens. We have observed immunostaining intensity loss in methacrylate-embedded vessels and other tissues compared to paraffin-embedded tissues *(4)*. We further investigated the combination of antigen retrieval with tyramide signal amplification *(24)* to increase immunoreactivity in our methacrylate-embedded tissues. This

amplification detection system (Dako Co.), brown cytoplasmic staining leukocytes are localized within the neointima, original magnification = 160 ×. (See color plate 9 appearing in the insert following p. 236).

Table 5
Immunostains used in Vascular Animal Model Studies

Antigen	Clone	Cell or Antigen specificity	Host/isotype	Preparation[a]	Mouse	Rat	Rabbit	Pig	Monkey
BrDU (bromodeoxyuridine)	Bu20a	S-phase cells	Mouse IgG	F, P, M	x	x	x	x	x
Ki-67	MIB-1	G1–M phase	Mouse IgG	F, P, M		x	x	x	x
PCNA (proliferating cell nuclear antigen)	PC10	G0–M phases	Mouse IgG	F, P, M	x	x	x	x	x
SMC α-actin	1A4	Smooth muscle cells and fibroblasts	Mouse IgG	F, P, M	x	x	x	x	x
von Willebrand factor (factor VIII related antigen)		Endothelium, platelets, and plasma	Rabbit/polyclonal	F, P, M	x	x		x	x
			Goat/polyclonal	F, P, M		x			
Rabbit macrophage	RAM-11	Macrophages	Mouse IgG	F, P, M			x		
Human macrophage	HAM56	Monocytes and macrophages	Mouse IgM	F, P, M					x
Mouse F4/80 antigen	Cl:A3–1	Monocyte/ macrophages	Rat IgG	F, P	x				

334

Table 5 (Continued)

Antigen	Clone	Cell or Antigen specificity	Host/isotype	Preparation[a]	Mouse	Rat	Rabbit	Pig	Monkey
Mouse macrophages/ monocytes (intracellular antigen)	MOMA-2	Monocyte/ Macrophages	Rat IgG	F	x				
Mouse Mac-3	M3/84	Macrophages	Rat IgG	F, P	x				
CD3 (pan T-cells)		Pan T-cells	Polyclonal	F, P, M				x	x
Mouse neutrophils	7/4	Neutrophils	Rat IgG	F,P	x				
Porcine CD45 (allotypic variant)	MAC323	Pan leukocytes	Mouse IgG	F, P, M				x	
Mouse CD45 (LCA, Ly-5)	30–F11	Pan leukocytes	Rat IgG	F, P	x				
VCAM-1		Endothelial and leukocytes	Polyclonal	F			x		
ICAM-1		Endothelial and leukocytes	Polyclonal	F			x		

[a]Abbreviations: F = frozen, P = paraffin, M = MWM resin

335

combination has given us excellent results that are comparable to paraffin-embedded tissues for several antigens to identify smooth muscle cells (SMCs), leukocytes, and proliferating cells *(4)*. We have performed novel studies using immunomarkers for smooth-muscle α-actin, von Willebrand factor, macrophages, andseveral proliferation markers (BrDU, PCNA, Ki-67[MIB-1]), CD3 (pan T-cell), CD45(LCA).

IMAGE ANALYSIS AND MORPHOMETRIC QUANTIFICATION

There are numerous computer-aided methods to quantitatively analyze histological *(see* Table 4) and immunostained tissues. For certain vascular studies layers of the vessel must be measured histomorphometrically using an elastin stain as described in Table 4 (Verhoeff's, Movat, Elastic Trichrome) *(1,5,8–10,17–19)*. Color segmentation analysis is utilized to discriminate the area of chromagen distributed and cell density/area in histochemically and immunohistochemically stained tissues *(7,25)*.

HISTOLOGY COMPANIES AND SOCIETIES

The following is a partial list of companies and societies that carry equipment, supplies, reagents, and instructional texts for histology specimen preparation, staining, and immunohistochemical staining:

American Society of Clinical Pathologists.
Dako Co.
Delaware Diamond Knives, Inc.
Fisher Healthcare.
Leica Microsystems Inc.
National Society for Histotechnology.
Polysciences, Inc.
Pharmingen.
Richard-Allen Scientific.
Sakura-Finetek USA, Inc.
Serotec Inc.
Shandon, Inc.
Sigma Diagnostics.
Vector Laboratories.
Carl Zeiss, Inc.
Zymed Laboratories, Inc.

CONCLUSION

Histological analysis for vascular animal models should be planned according to the research goals in mind. Maximal use of experimentally derived tissues that can utilize a variety of stains should allow routine histological staining and immunohistochemical staining. Frozen sections are utilized when lipid stains are to be employed, and for preservation of sensitive antigens. Paraffin-embedding should be employed for studies involving histomorphometry and pathological analysis. The use of a modified bone methacrylate-embedding procedure must be employed when metallic implants (stents) are used for adequate preservation of the tissue-implant interface. Microtomy is the ideal sectioning technique to use for stainless-steel stent-implanted vessels. If any hard metals (i.e., Nitinol) stent–implants are used, a cutting/grinding/polishing methods should be used. Immunohistochemistry is possible with the use of antigen retrieval and tyramide signal amplification methods in both paraffin- and MWM resin-embedded tissues.

REFERENCES

1. Carson FL. Histotechnology: A Self Instructional Text, 2nd ed. ASCP Press, Chicago, 1997.
2. Prophet EB, Mills B, Arrington JB, Sobin LH. Laboratory Methods in Histotechnology Washington, DC, American Registry of Pathology, 1992.
3. Sheehan DC, Hrapchak BB. Theory and Practice of Histotechnology, 2nd ed. Battelle Press, Columbus, OH, 1980.
4. Seifert P, Rogers C, and Edelman ER. Comparison of immunohistochemical staining for porcine CD45, smooth muscle cell αactin, and Ki-67 (MIB-1) in tissues embedded in paraffin and methacrylate. National Society for Histotechnology Annual Symposium/Convention (poster presentation), 1999.
5. Carter AJ, Laird JR, Farb A, Kufs W, Wortham DC, Virmani R. Morphologic characteristics of lesion formation and time course of smooth muscle cell proliferation in a porcine proliferative restenosis model. J Am Coll Cardiol 1994; 24:1398–1405
6. Hehrlein C, Gollan C, Donges, K, Metz J, Riessen R, Fehsenfeld P, et al. Low-dose radioactive endovascular stents prevent smooth muscle cell proliferation and neointimal hyperplasia in rabbits. Circulation 1995; 92:1570–1575.
7. Kratky RG, Ivey J, Roach MR. Collagen quantitation by video-microdensitometry in rabbit atherosclerosis. Matrix Biology 1996; 15:141–144.
8. Nugent HM, Rogers C, Edelman ER. Endothelial implants inhibit intimal hyperplasia after porcine angioplasty. Circ Res. 1999; 84:384–391.
9. Rogers C, Edelman ER. Endovascular stent design dictates experimental restenosis. Circulation 1995; 91:2995–3001.
10. Rogers C, Seifert P, Edelman ER. The neointima provoked by human coronary stenting: contributions of smooth muscle and inflammatory cells and extracellular matrix in autopsy specimens over time Circulation 1998; 98:I-182.
11. Sanderson C. Entering the realm of mineralized bone processing: a review of the literature and techniques. J Histotechnol 1997; 20:259–266.
12. Shetye JD, Scheynius A, Mellstedt HT, Biberfeld P. Retrieval of leukocyte antigens in paraffin-embedded rat tissues. J Histochem Cytochem 1996; 44:767–776.
13. Shi S-R, Key ME, Kalra KL. Antigen Retrieval in formalin-fixed, paraffin-embedded tissues:An enhancement method for immunohistochemical staining based on microwave oven heating of tissue sections. J Histochem Cytochem 1991; 39:741–748.

14. Shi S-R, Cote RJ, Taylor CR. Standardization and further development of antigen retrieval immunohistochemistry: strategies and future goals. J Histochen Cytochem 1999; 22:177–192.

15. Simon DI, Chen Z, Seifert P, Edelman ER, Ballantyne CM, Rogers C. Decreased neointimal formation in *Mac-1$^{-/-}$* mice reveals a role for inflammation in vascular repair after angioplasty J Clin Invest 2000; 105:293–300.

16. Van Beusekom HMM., Whelan DM, van de Plas M, van der Giessen WJ. A practical and rapid method of histological processing for examination of coronary arteries containing metallic stents. Cardiovasc Pathol 1996; 5:69–76.

17. Kjelsberg MA, Seifert P, Edelman ER, Rogers C. Design-dependent variations in coronary stent stenosis measured as precisely by angiography as by histology. J Inv Card 1998; 10:142–147.

18. Rogers C, Parikh S, Seifert P, Edelman ER. Endogenous cell seeding: remnant endothelium after stenting enhances vascular repair. Circulation 1996; 94:2909–2914.

19. Rogers C, Welt FGP, Karnovsky MJ, Edelman ER. Monocyte recruitment and neointimal hyperplasia in rabbits: coupled inhibitory effects of heparin. Arterioscler Thromb Vasc Biol 1996; 16:1312–1318.

20. Wolf E, Roser K, Hahn M, Welkerling H, Delling G. Enzyme and immunohistochemistry on undecalcified bone and bone marrow biopsies after embedding in plastic:a new method for routine application. Virchows Arch A Pathol Anat Histopathol 1992; 420:17–24.

21. Emmanual J, Emmanual JG, Koeneman JB. Alteration of retrieved implants in vitro by processing and infiltrating fluids. Biomed Mater Res: Applied Biomaterials 1989; 23:337–347.

22. Gerrits PO, Eppinger B, van Goor H, Horobin RW. A versatile, low toxicity glycol methacrylate embedding medium for use in biological research, and for recovered biomaterials prostheses. Cells Mater 1991; 1:189–198.

23. Hand NM, Blythe D, Jackson P. Antigen unmasking using microwave heating on formalin fixed tissue embedded in methyl methacrylate. J Cellullar Pathol 1996; 1:31–37.

24. Bobrow MN, Harris TD, Shaughnessy KJ, Litt GJ. Catalyzed reporter deposition, a novel method of signal amplification. Application to immunoassays. J Immunol Methods 1989; 125:279–85.

25. Hunt, JA, McLaughlin PJ, Flanagan BF. Techniques to investigate cellular and molecular interactions in the host response to implanted biomaterials. Biomaterials 1997; 18:1449–1459.

26. Hsu SM, Raine L, Fanger HU. Use of avidin-biotin-peroxidase (ABC) in immunoperoxidase techniques: a comparison between ABC and unlabelled antibody (PAP) procedures. J Histochem Cytochem 1981; 28:577

Index

A

ACE inhibitors, *see* Angiotensin-converting enzyme inhibitors

Anesthesia, *see also* specific models, agents and sources, 307, 321, 322

equipment sources, 308
euthanasia guidelines, 319, 320
mice, 309–311
monkeys, 317–319
pigs, 315–317
rabbits, 312–314
rats, 309, 311

Angiotensin-converting enzyme (ACE) inhibitors, neointimal formation prevention in animals versus humans, 30–32

Apolipoprotein E, knockout mice, 150, 151, 161, 162

Arterial thrombosis,
cyclic flow model, *see* Folts cyclic flow model
historical perspective of models, 127
ideal model criteria, 128
mouse models, *see* Carotid thrombosis

Arteriovenous fistula model,
cerebral arteriolar hypertrophy, 257, 258
pulse pressure response, 256, 257
surgery, 256, 257

Arteriovenous grafting models,
baboon ex vivo chronic arterio-venous shunt, 73–75
canine models,
carotid interposition vein graft, 70, 71

ex vivo arteriovenous series shunts, 69, 70
femoral artery interposition vein graft, 70, 71
femoral artery to femoral vein end-to-side loop artiovenous graft, 68, 69
large animal models,
access sites, 67
surgical considerations, 66, 68
mouse carotid interposition vein graft, 62, 63
porcine carotid interposition vein graft, 73
prospects for development, 75, 76
prosthetic conduits, 61, 62, 75, 76
rabbit models,
carotid interposition vein graft, 66
femoral artery interposition vein graft, 66
surgical considerations, 65, 66
rat models,
aortic interposition vein graft, 64, 65
femoral artery interposition vein graft, 63
sheep models,
carotid artery to jugular vein end-to-side loop graft, 71, 72
carotid interposition vein graft, 72, 73
femoral artery interposition vein graft, 72
Atherosclerosis models,
monkey models, *see* Monkey atherosclerosis models

339